METABOLIC BONE AND MINERAL DISORDERS

CONTEMPORARY ISSUES IN ENDOCRINOLOGY AND METABOLISM
Volume 5

SERIES EDITOR

Jerrold M. Olefsky, M.D.

Professor
Department of Medicine
Head, Division of Endocrinology & Metabolism
University of California, San Diego
School of Medicine
Veterans Administration Medical Center
La Jolla, California

Volumes Already Published

Vol. 1 Diabetes Mellitus: Management and Complications, Jerrold M. Olefsky, M.D., and Robert S. Sherwin, M.D., Editors

Vol. 2 Prolactinomas, Jerrold M. Olefsky, M.D., and Richard J. Robbins, M.D., Editors

Vol. 3 Hypercholesterolemia and Atherosclerosis: Pathogenesis and Prevention, Daniel Steinberg, M.D., Ph.D., and Jerrold M. Olefsky, M.D., Editors

Vol. 4 Growth Abnormalities, Raymond L. Hintz, M.D., and Ron G. Rosenfeld, M.D., Editors

METABOLIC BONE AND MINERAL DISORDERS

Edited by

Stavros C. Manolagas, M.D., Ph.D.

Professor, Department of Medicine
Indiana University School of Medicine
Chief, Endocrinology and Metabolism Section
Veterans Administration Medical Center
Indianapolis, Indiana

Jerrold M. Olefsky, M.D.

Professor, Department of Medicine
Head, Division of Endocrinology & Metabolism
University of California, San Diego
School of Medicine
Veterans Administration Medical Center
San Diego, California

Churchill Livingstone
New York, Edinburgh, London, Melbourne 1988

Library of Congress Cataloging-in-Publication Data

Metabolic bone and mineral disorders.

(Contemporary issues in endocrinology and metabolism; v. 5)
Includes bibliographies and index.
1. Bones—Metabolism—Disorders. 2. Mineral metabolism—Disorders. I. Manolagas, Stavros. II. Olefsky, Jerrold M. III. Series. [DNLM: 1. Bone and Bones—metabolism. 2. Bone Diseases, Metabolic. 3. Minerals—metabolism. W1 C0769MQN v.5/ WE 250 M5867]
RC931.M45M46 1988 616.7′16 88-22864
ISBN 0-443-08586-2

Distributed in the United Kingdom by Churchill Livingstone, Robert Stevenson House, 1–3 Baxter's Place, Leith Walk, Edinburgh EH1 3AF, and by associated companies, branches, and representatives throughout the world.

Accurate indications, adverse reactions, and dosage schedules for drugs are provided in this book, but it is possible that they may change. The reader is urged to review the package information data of the manufacturers of the medications mentioned.

The Publishers have made every effort to trace the copyright holders for borrowed material. If they have inadvertently overlooked any, they will be pleased to make the necessary arrangements at the first opportunity.

Acquisitions Editor: *Kim Loretucci*
Copy Editor: *Ann Ruzycka*
Production Designer: *Melanie Haber*
Production Supervisor: *Jocelyn Eckstein*

Printed in the United States of America

First published in 1988

Contributors

David J. Baylink, M.D.
Distinguished Professor, Department of Medicine
Loma Linda University School of Medicine
Chief, Mineral Metabolism Section
Jerry L. Pettis Veterans Administration Hospital
Loma Linda, California

John P. Bilezikian, M.D.
Professor, Departments of Medicine and Pharmacology
College of Physicians and Surgeons of Columbia University
Attending Physician, Presbyterian Hospital
New York, New York

Bayard D. Catherwood, M.D.
Associate Professor, Department of Medicine
Emory University School of Medicine
Atlanta, Georgia
Chief, Endocrine and Metabolism Section
Veterans Administration Medical Center
Decataur, Georgia

Jack W. Coburn, M.D.
Adjunct Professor, Department of Medicine
University of California, Los Angeles, UCLA School of Medicine
Staff Physician, Nephrology Section
West Los Angeles Veterans Administration Medical Center
Los Angeles, California

Marc K. Drezner, M.D.
Professor, Department of Medicine
Duke University School of Medicine
Durham, North Carolina

Cesar R. Libanati, M.D.
Research Fellow, Department of Medicine
Loma Linda University School of Medicine
Loma Linda, California

Mark W. Lundy, M.D.
Postdoctoral Fellow, Departments of Anatomy and Medicine
Loma Linda University School of Medicine
Loma Linda, California

Robert Marcus, M.D.
Associate Professor, Department of Medicine
Stanford University School of Medicine
Stanford, California
Director, Aging Study Unit
Geriatrics Research, Education, and Clinical Center
Veterans Administration Medical Center
Palo Alto, California

Janet E. Rubin, M.D.
Assistant Professor, Department of Medicine
Emory University School of Medicine
Atlanta, Georgia
Research Associate
Veterans Administration Medical Center
Decataur, Georgia

Isidro B. Salusky, M.D.
Assistant Professor, Department of Pediatrics
Division of Pediatric Nephrology
Director, Pediatric Dialysis Program
University of California, Los Angeles, UCLA School of Medicine
Los Angeles, California

Elizabeth Shane, M.D.
Assistant Professor, Department of Medicine
College of Physicians and Surgeons of Columbia University
New York, New York

Paula H. Stern, Ph.D.
Professor, Department of Pharmacology
Member, Center for Endocrinology and Metabolism
Northwestern University Medical School
Chicago, Illinois

Arch K. Taylor, M.D.
Research Biologist, Mineral Metabolism Section
Jerry L. Pettis Veterans Administration Hospital
Loma Linda, California

Michael P. Whyte, M.D.
Associate Professor, Department of Medicine
Division of Bone and Mineral Diseases
Washington University School of Medicine
Director, Metabolic Research Unit
Shriners Hospital for Children
St. Louis, Missouri

Preface

The understanding of the pathophysiology of bone and mineral disorders and the ability to diagnose and manage these conditions have improved greatly during the last few years. This has been the result of major breakthroughs in basic and clinical research as well as substantial advances in technology. With this book, we intend to provide clinicians with a concise, state-of-the-art update of the area, with particular emphasis on practical aspects of diagnosis and treatment.

The current state of knowledge of bone cell physiology and of the endocrinology of the bone-regulating hormones are discussed in Chapters 1 and 2, respectively. We expect that the reader will find in them important background information for the clinical topics. Chapter 3 is devoted entirely to diagnostic procedures, with emphasis on the usefulness and limitations of the available biochemical, radiologic, and histologic tests. The remaining six chapters cover the major clinical disorders of bone and mineral metabolism. They include the hyper- and hypocalcemias and the primary and secondary abnormalities of the parathyroid gland (Chapter 4); the disorders of Vitamin D metabolism (Chapter 5); and Paget's disease (Chapter 6). The various forms of osteopenia/osteoporosis are dealt with in Chapter 7. In view of the recent explosion of public awareness and interest in this most common disease, we felt that a more extensive coverage of this topic was warranted. Abnormalities of bone associated with renal disease and hyperalimentation are discussed in Chapter 8, and the most common hereditary disorders of skeletal metabolism are presented in Chapter 9.

The contributors, leading authorities in the field, have accepted our challenge to convey pathogenetic, diagnostic, and management concepts in an easy-to-read format with liberal use of illustrations and tables. Editing these chapters and learning from the authors' experiences has been most rewarding to us, and for that we are indebted to them.

Stavros C. Manolagas
Jerrold M. Olefsky

Contents

1 Cellular Physiology of Bone

Paula H. Stern

For a tissue to carry out two functions as essential and diverse as maintenance of calcium homeostasis and support and protection of internal structures of the body, a highly integrated system would be necessary. The derangements that occur in disease states emphasize how well regulated normal bone function is. Recent investigations of bone physiology are revealing the component parts of such a system, including multiple interacting cell types of different stages and a number of newly recognized factors, some locally produced, that could mediate or modulate these interactions. The new knowledge about the characteristics, origin, functions, and hormonal responsiveness of the cells in bone acquired over the last few years has been extensive. This chapter provides an overview of current concepts of the cellular physiology of bone and factors influencing bone cell function. A number of excellent critical reviews addressing different aspects of these questions have been published recently,[1-12] and the reader is referred to them for more extensive treatment of many of these topics.

The complexity of calcium metabolism has led to the use of a variety of models to address the question of how bone functions. In order to focus on a particular question or amplify a particular function, conditions or cells that are distinct from normal bone have often been used. Although caution is indicated in interpreting and applying findings from these artificial models, coincident results from several different model systems can give us confidence that the findings will apply to normal bone tissue.

Several types of bone are present in the body. The limb bones and portions of other bones develop from a cartilaginous template and are termed endochondral. Ossification occurs both within the eroded cartilage, where it forms spongy (trabecular) bone, and beneath the perichondrium, where it develops into more compact bone.[13] The bones of the skull develop from a dense blastemal membrane. Intramembranous ossification begins at different sites in the membrane and results in an expanding meshwork of spicules of trabecular bone. Compact bone is deposited on the inner surface of the periosteum. It is conceivable that these various bone types may differ somewhat in their cellular composition and consequent interactions and hormonal responses. Although this has not been investigated systematically, there are clearly disparities in the in vitro responses of bones from different sites or of different ages.[14-22]

THE CELLS OF BONE: STRUCTURAL AND FUNCTIONAL CHARACTERISTICS, ORIGINS, AND MODELS

The two major functional cell types in bone are osteoblasts and osteoclasts. Osteoblasts are found along the spicules of forming trabecular bone and on the inner surface of the periosteum. They are often cuboidal or low columnar, with nuclei located distal to the bone surface. As would be expected of a cell actively involved in biosynthesis of collagen and other proteins, there is substantial endoplasmic reticulum and a large number of mitochondria. Alkaline phosphatase is characteristically present within the cells and is secreted as an ectoenzyme. Other activities associated with osteoblasts or osteoblastlike cells include the production of osteocalcin, collagenase, and prostaglandins.[23-25] There is evidence that the osteoblasts derive from stromal precursor cells of an undifferentiated type that also have the potential to give rise to adipocytes, chondrocytes, and fibroblasts.[7] Different morphologic stages of the osteoblast have been described, including flatter cells in more mature bone, and osteocytes embedded in the matrix.[6] During remodeling there are changes in the size of the osteoblasts.[9]

Models that have been used extensively to study osteoblast function and hormonal responsiveness include cells isolated from fetal and neonatal calvaria of rodents and to a lesser extent from avian species.[1] Generally these cells have been isolated by enzymatic digestion and the initial cell populations are heterogenous. Investigators have obtained more defined populations by differential dissections, timed digestion, and physical forces applied to the separated cells.[26-28] An alternative approach has been the use of rodent and human cell lines obtained either from osteogenic sarcomas or normal tissues.[29-33] These cell lines display osteoblast characteristics, such as alkaline phosphatase activity. They vary in their ability to synthesize prostaglandins and in their hormonal responsiveness.

Mature osteoclasts are multinucleate cells without mitogenic potential. They are characterized by granular cytoplasm and specific organelles, the ruffled border and clear zone, at the site of apposition to bone. Osteoclasts are characterized by the production of lysosomal enzymes, including a tartrate-resistant acid phosphatase. Carbonic anhydrase activity and the ability to generate hydrogen ions locally in the region of the bone probably play an important role in their activity to resorb bone. The origin of the osteoclast has been extensively investigated. At the present time the evidence is most compelling for a precursor cell of the moncyte cell line being the precursor for the osteoclast as well. The evidence includes fusion studies with examination of characteristics of resulting cells,[34,35] coculture with determination of bone-resorbing activity,[36] and studies with monoclonal antibodies to cell surface antigens.[37-39] Among the models used to study hormonal effects on osteoclast function are mature osteoclasts isolated from avian or mammalian bone by physical removal of cells[40] or enzymatic treatment.[41] Another approach has been to culture marrow cells and evaluate the appearance and activity of multinucleate cells with osteoclastic characteristics.[42,43] Substantial information has been obtained about osteoclast responsiveness by quantitative histomorphometry either in the intact animal or in organ cultures.[43] Although most of the approaches assess the size or number of cells, osteoclast activity and cellular interactions have been evaluated from the ability of osteoclasts to produce excavations on mineralized surfaces.[40]

ENDOGENOUS FACTORS INFLUENCING BONE CELL ACTIVITY

A number of factors may play roles as mediators and modulators of the actions and interactions of the cells within bone. The following sections summarize their effects on bone in general, on bone cell ontogeny, and on cellular metabolic and biochemical processes, including putative second messengers.

Parathyroid Hormone

Parathyroid hormone has several overall effects on bone physiology. The hormone stimulates resorption of mineral and matrix. The effects of parathyroid hormone on bone formation are concentration dependent, with anabolic effects being expressed at low concentrations of the homone and inhibition of collagen synthesis at higher concentrations.[2,3] The exact relationship of these events to the role of parathyroid hormone in the homeostatic regulation of calcium is not clearly established. Receptors for parathyroid hormone have been demonstrated in osteoblasts in intact bone and in cloned osteoblastic osteosarcoma cells.[45,46] It is doubtful that there are receptors for parathyroid hormone on multinucleate osteoclasts. In enriched populations of isolated mature osteoclasts, parathyroid hormone fails to elicit direct effects on osteoclast motility.[47] The evidence supports the concept that the effects of parathyroid hormone to increase osteoclast activity in whole bone are indirectly mediated through a message, either chemical or physical, from osteoblasts.[48,49] Parathyroid hormone treatment elicits shape changes, the responsive cells becoming more stellate.[50] The increase in the number of mature osteoclasts involves fusion of precursor cells and is likely also to involve increased proliferation of a preosteoclastic cell.[10] There is evidence that parathyroid hormone can increase this proliferation, since a delayed component of the effect of parathyroid hormone is decreased by inhibition of DNA synthesis, whereas the more rapid effects of the hormone are resistant to irradiation and hydroxyurea.[51,52]

A universal effect of parathyroid hormone seen in all bone culture systems and osteoblastlike cells is an increase in the production of cyclic AMP, a likely second messenger for parathyroid hormone action.[4,11] Also, cyclic AMP-dependent protein kinase is increased by parathyroid hormone in bone cells and changes in phosphorylation have been observed in bone.[53,54] Increases in intracellular free calcium, another likely second messenger, have been elicited by parathyroid hormone treatment in some, but not all, osteoblastic cells.[55-58] Calcium-dependent phosphorylation in bone is affected by parathyroid hormone.[58a] The substrates for these phosphorylations have not been identified. Enzymatic activities that are altered in bone cells by treatment with parathyroid hormone include alkaline phosphatase in osteoblastic cells and lysosomal enzymes and carbonic anhydrase in osteoclasts.[11] The effects on alkaline phosphatase may be stimulatory or inhibitory depending upon the state of proliferation of the cells. Parathyroid hormone also stimulates secretion of a number of products, including collagenase,[24] prostaglandins,[11,59] and plasminogen activator.[60] These and other locally produced factors could play a role in the communication between cell types in bone.

Vitamin D

1,25-Dihydroxyvitamin D, like parathyroid hormone, has well-established direct effects on bone to stimulate resorption and to depress collagen synthesis. Receptors for 1,25-dihydroxyvitamin D have been demonstrated in osteoblastic cells,[61,62] and, as is the case for parathyroid hormone, direct addition of the vitamin D metabolite to osteoclast-enriched cell isolates has not had effects on motility.[47] Treatment of osteoblastic cells with 1,25-$(OH)_2D_3$ elicits changes in cell shape.[63] Effects of 1,25-dihydroxyvitamin D to inhibit proliferation and enhance differentiation have been demonstrated in a number of cell types,[64] and it has been proposed that an effect of vitamin D to stimulate the differentiation of osteoclast precursors may contribute to the direct effects of vitamin D on bone.[65] 1,25-Dihydroxyvitamin D has been reported to increase or decrease bone alkaline phosphatase, again dependent upon the proliferation state of the cells.[4] Vitamin D metabolites also increase the synthesis of osteocalcin, a calcium-binding protein postulated to have effects on bone mineralization[66] and resorption.[67]

Calcitonin

In intact bone cultures, calcitonin is a general inhibitor of resorption elicited by diverse stimuli. Effects on release of calcium, secretion of lysosomal enzymes, and the morphology of the ruffled border have been described.[12] The inhibitory effects of calcitonin on bone resorption are most likely initiated at the level of the osteoclast. Receptors have been demonstrated on rat osteoclasts,[68] and the hormone added to cultures rich in osteoclasts inhibits their intrinsic or stimulated mobility.[40,47] Calcitonin increases cyclic AMP in bone[12] and this may well be the mediator for the inhibitory effect. Pharmacologic evidence supporting a dual role for cyclic AMP in bone resorption is provided by the biphasic effects of phosphodiesterase inhibitors and forskolin on resorption.[69-72]

Other Systemic Hormones

A number of classic hormones with primary effects on other tissues have distinct actions on bone as well. Estrogens inhibit bone resorption. Although earlier studies provided little support for either receptors or direct effects of estrogens on bone[73-77] recent reports have provided some evidence for both.[78-80] In animal studies, oophorectomy raised and estrogen replacement lowered prostaglandin production by bone.[81] Thyroid hormones stimulate bone turnover in vivo and resorption in bone organ cultures. Receptors for thyroid hormones have been characterized in osteosarcoma cells.[82,83] Effects on alkaline phosphatase and proliferation have been described in cultured bone cells.[83,84] Glucocorticoids have multiple and complex effects on bone, including direct effects to both stimulate and inhibit both bone resorption and bone collagen syntheses.[12] Receptors have been characterized in both normal and osteosarcoma-derived osteoblastic cells.[4] Glucocorticoids also enhance the responses of osteoblasts to parathyroid hormone and 1,25-dihydroxyvitamin D.[4] Other systemic hormones with direct effects on bone include insulin and somatomedin, which stimulate collagen synthesis.[2,3] Two gastrointestinal hormones shown to have direct effects on bone are glucagon, an inhibitor of bone resorption,[85] and vasoactive intestinal peptide, a direct stimulator of resorption.[86]

Prostaglandins

The extensive literature on the effects of prostaglandins on bone and mineral metabolism has been reviewed recently.[87] Certain prostaglandins, notably PGE_1, PGE_2, and PGI_2, like parathyroid hormone and 1,25-dihydroxyvitamin D, stimulate bone resorption and inhibit bone collagen synthesis. However, lower concentrations of prostaglandins stimulate cell replication and collagen synthesis synthesis in fetal rat calvaria.[87] Prostaglandins increase cyclic AMP and cyclic AMP-dependent protein kinase in osteoblastic cells.[4,87] Brief exposures[10-20] to prostaglandins cause osteoblasts from fetal rat calvaria to become more stellate in shape and increased the appearance of intercellular gap junctions.[88] In contrast to parathyroid hormone and 1,25-dihydroxyvitamin D, prostaglandins inhibit motility when applied directly to osteoclast-rich cell isolates.[47] Bone, most likely a subgroup of osteoblasts, has a high capacity for synthesis of prostaglandins.[4,32,87] A number of substances stimulate prostaglandin synthesis in bone and elicit bone resorption through this pathway in responsive culture systems.[15,17,18,20,22]

Growth Factors

A number of growth factors including epidermal growth factor, transforming growth factor, and platelet-derived growth factor have been shown to influence bone resorption and formation.[2,3,12] With the exception of platelet-derived growth factor, which stimulates collagen synthesis, the growth factors that stimulate bone formation are inhibitors of bone collagen synthesis.[3] The characteristics of the bone-resorbing effects of the growth factors are dependent upon the systems used. In calvaria, stimulation of prostaglandin synthesis results in effects on resorption at lower concentrations than in limb bones, where prostaglandin-independent effects are seen.[15,16,20-22] Thrombin, which has mitogenic as well as procoagulant properties, can also increase bone resorption.[17-19] The effects of thrombin can also occur through both prostaglandin-dependent and independent pathways, depending upon the model system. Epidermal growth factor has been shown to stimulate a collagenaselike activity in osteoblastic cells.[89] The potential physiologic importance of some of these growth factors is emphasized by their presence in and production by bone.[90,91]

Immune-Cell-Derived Factors

Interleukins, interferons, and tumor necrosis factors are among the endogenous factors that have been shown to affect resorption. Interleukin 1-β stimulates bone resorption through both prostaglandin-dependent and independent pathways.[92,93] Addition of both parathyroid hormone and interleukin 1-β to bone organ cultures elicited supra-additive effects, suggesting that they may function through different mechanisms.[94] Interleukin 1-β has both stimulatory and inhibitory effects on bone collagen synthesis, dependent upon the treatment protocal.[3] Tumor necrosis factor-α is also an effective stimulator of bone resorption, with biphasic effects on formation.[95-97] Interferons α and γ inhibit bone resorption.[98-100] At lower interferon concentrations, the bone-resorbing effects of interleukin may be more readily antagonized than those of parathyroid hormone.[100] The action of these cytokines on bone constitutes some of the evidence that cells of the immune system are involved in normal bone physiology.[5]

MEDIATORS OF BONE REMODELING

Although pathologic states may result in a clear dominance of bone formation or resorption, normal development and probably normal maintenance of the skeleton undoubtedly require both of these activities acting in a coordinated fashion. A sequence of events has been postulated, which begins with osteoclastic activity and the formation of resorption lacunae.[6,101] Following a reversal phase during which cellular migration takes place, local osteoblastic activity results in the deposition of bone matrix, which becomes mineralized. The actions of many of the agents described above, if tightly regulated, could lead to an integrated pattern of remodeling. Alternatively, a unique factor could be responsible for coordinating the functions of bone. Pursuit of a such a coupling factor, a substance released from resorbing bone that initiates bone formation, has led to the isolation and purification of several mitogenic factors from bone or bone-conditioned medium.[8,102-106] Among the bone-derived factors with stimulatory effects on bone collagen synthesis are transforming growth factor-β, bone-derived growth factor (BDGF), skeletal growth factor, and bone morphogenetic protein. The secretion of a BDGF-like growth factor by a macrophage cell line points up the possibility that other cells resident in bone could play a role in the normal integration of bone remodeling.[107]

CONCLUSION

The research of the past few years has provided considerable new information on the origins of bone cells and the responses of bone and bone cells to a wide range of systemic and local factors. The challenge of the future will be to explain how these interact to produce the highly coordinated picture that constitutes the normal physiology of bone.

REFERENCES

1. Brand JS: Cellular biochemistry of bone formation and resorption. p.423. In Parsons JA (ed): Endocrinology of Calcium Metabolism. Raven Press, New York, 1982
2. Raisz LG, Kream, BE: Regulation of bone formation. N Engl J Med 309:29, 1983
3. Canalis E: The hormonal and local regulation of bone formation. Endocr Rev 4:62, 1983
4. Rodan GA, Rodan SB: Expression of the osteoblastic phenotype. p.244. In Peck WA (ed): Bone and Mineral Research Annual 2. Elsevier, Amsterdam, 1984
5. Baron R, Vignery A, Horowitz M: Lymphocytes, macrophages and the regulation of bone remodeling. p.175. In Peck WA (ed): Bone and Mineral Research Annual 2. Elsevier, Amsterdam, 1984
6. Kahn AJ, Fallon MD, Teitelbaum SL: Structure-function relationships in bone: an examination of events at the cellular level. p.125. In Peck WA (ed): Bone and Mineral Research Annual 2. Elsevier, Amsterdam, 1984
7. Owen M: Lineage of osteogenic cells and their relationship to the stromal system. p.1. In Peck WA (ed): Bone and Mineral Annual 3. Elsevier, Amsterdam, 1985
8. Centrella M, Canalis E: Local regulators of skeletal growth: a perspective. Endocr Rev 6:544, 1985
9. Eriksen EF: Normal and pathological remodeling of human trabecular bone: three

dimensional reconstruction of the remodeling sequence in normals and in metabolic bone disease. Endocr Rev 7:379, 1986
10. Nijweide PJ, Burger EH, Feyen JHM: Cells of bone: proliferation, differentiation, and hormonal regulation. Physiol Rev 66:855, 1986
11. Wong GL: Skeletal effects of PTH. p.103. In Peck WA (ed): Bone and Mineral Research Annual 4. Elsevier, Amsterdam, 1986
12. Mundy GR, Roodman GD: Osteoclast ontogeny and function. p.209. In Peck WA (ed): Bone and Mineral Research Annual 5. Elsevier, Amsterdam, 1987
13. Arey LB: Developmental Anatomy. 6th Ed. WB Saunders, Philadelphia, 1954
14. Krieger NS, Stern PH: Potassium effects on bone: comparison of two model systems. Am J Physiol 245:E303, 1983
15. Tashjian AH Jr, Levine L: Epidermal growth factor stimulates prostaglandin production and bone resorption in cultured mouse calvaria. Biochem Biophys Res Commun 85:966, 1978
16. Raisz LG, Simmons HA, Sandberg AL, Canalis E: Direct stimulation of bone resorption by epidermal growth factor. Endocrinology 107:270, 1980
17. Hoffmann O, Klaushofer K, Koller K, Peterlik M: Prostaglandin-related bone resorption in cultured neonatal mouse calvaria: evaluation of biopotency of nonsteroidal anti-inflammatory drugs. Prostaglandins 30:857, 1985
18. Gustafson GT, Lerner U: Thrombin, a stimulator of bone resorption. Biosci Rep 3:255, 1983
19. Hoffmann O, Klaushofer K, Koller K, et al: Indomethacin inhibits thrombin-, but not thyroxin-stimulated resorption of fetal rat limb bones. Prostaglandins 31:601, 1986
20. Tashjian AH Jr, Voelkel EF, Lazzaro M, et al: Alpha and beta transforming growth factors stimulate prostaglandin production and bone resorption in cultured mouse calvaria. Proc Natl Acad Sci 82:4535, 1985
21. Ibbotson KJ, Harrod J, Gowen M, et al: Human recombinant transforming growth factor (TGF) alpha stimulates bone resorption and inhibits formation in vitro. Proc Natl Acad Sci 83:2228, 1986
22. Stern PH, Krieger NH, Nissenson RA, et al: Human transforming growth factor-alpha stimulates bone resorption in vitro. J Clin Invest 76:2016, 1985
23. Nishimoto SK, Price PA: Secretion of the vitamin K dependent protein of bone by rat osteosarcoma cells. J Biol Chem 255:6579, 1980
24. Sakamoto S, Sakamoto M: Bone collagenase, osteoblasts and cell-mediated bone resorption. p.49. In Peck WA (ed): Bone and Mineral Research Annual 4. Elsevier, Amsterdam, 1986
25. Rodan SB, Rodan GA, Simmons HA, et al: Bone resorption factor produced by osteosarcoma cells with osteoblastic features is PGE_2. Biochem Res Commun 102:1358, 1981
26. Wong GL, Cohn DV: Separation of parathyroid hormone and calcitonin-sensitive cells from non-responsive bone cells. Nature 252:713, 1974
27. Yagiela JA, Woodbury DM: Enzymatic isolation of osteoblasts from fetal rat calvaria. Anat Rec 188:287, 1977
28. Puzas JE, Vignery A, Rasmussen H: Isolation of specific bone cell types by freeflow electrophoresis. Calcif Tissue Int 27:263, 1979
29. Majeska RJ, Rodan SB, Rodan GA: Parathyroid hormone-responsive clonal cell lines from rat osteosarcoma. Endocrinology 107:1494, 1980
30. Forrest SM, Ng KW, Findlay DM, et al: Characterization of an osteoblast-like clonal cell line which responds to both parathyroid hormone and calcitonin. Calcif Tissue Int 37:51, 1985

31. Kodama H, Amagai Y, Sudo H, et al: Establishment of a clonal osteogenic cell line from newborn mouse calvaria. Jpn J Oral Biol 23:899, 1981
32. Shupnik MA, Tashjian AH Jr: Epidermal growth factor and phorbol ester actions on human osteosarcoma cells: characterization of responsive and non-reponsive lines. J Biol Chem 257:12161, 1982
33. Eilon G, Perkins J, Viola MV: Characteristics of a calcitonin-responsive cell line derived from a human osteosarcoma. Cancer Res 43:3763, 1983
34. Kahn AJ, Simmons DJ: Investigation of cell lineage in bone using a chimaera chick and quail embryonic tissue. Nature 258:325, 1975
35. Zambonin Zallone A, Teti A: Autoradiographic demonstration of in vitro fusion of blood monocytes with osteoclasts. Basic Appl Histochem 29:45, 1985
36. Burger EH, van der Meer JWM, van de Gevel J, et al: In vitro formation of osteoclasts from long-term cultures of bone marrow mononuclear phagocytes. J Exp Med 156:1604, 1982
37. Oursler MJ, Bell LV, Clevinger B, Osdoby P: Identification of osteoclast-specific monoclonal antibodies. J Cell Biol 100:1592, 1985
38. Horton MA, Rimmer EF, Lewis D, et al: On the origin of the osteoclast: the cell surface phenotype of rodent osteoclasts. Calcif Tissue Int 37:46, 1985
39. Nijweide PJ, Vrijheid-Lammers T, Mulder RJP, Blok J: Cell surface antigens on osteoclasts and related cells in the quail studied with monoclonal antibodies. Histochemistry 83:315, 1985
40. Chambers TJ: Osteoblasts release osteoclasts from calcitonin-induced quiescence. J Cell Sci 57:247, 1982
41. Hefley TJ, Stern PH: Isolation of osteoclasts from fetal rat long bone. Calcif Tissue Int 34:480, 1982
42. Pharoah MJ, Heersche JNM: 1,25-Dihydroxyvitamin D_3 causes an increase in the number of osteoclast-like cells in cat bone marrow cultures. Calcif Tissue Int 37:276, 1985
43. Roodman GD, Ibbotson KJ, MacDonald BR, et al: 1,25-Dihydroxyvitamin D_3 causes formation of multinucleated cells with several osteoclast characteristics in cultures of primate marrow. Proc Natl Acad Sci 82:8213, 1985
44. Holtrop ME, Raisz LG: Comparison of the effects of 1,25-dihydroxycholecalciferol, prostaglandin E_2, and osteoclast-activating factor with parathyroid hormone on the ultrastructure of osteoclasts in cultured long bones of fetal rats. Calcif Tissue Int 29:201, 1979
45. Silve CM, Hradek GT, Jones AL, Arnaud CD: Parathyroid hormone receptor in intact embryonic chicken bone: characterization and cellular localization. J Cell Biol 94:379, 1982
46. Rizzoli RE, Somerman M, Murray TM, Aurbach GD: Binding of radioiodinated parathyroid hormone to cloned bone cells. Endocrinology 113:1832, 1983
47. Chambers TJ, McSheehy PMJ, Thomson SM, Fuller K: The effect of calcium-regulating hormones and prostaglandins on bone resorption by osteoclasts disaggregated from neonatal rabbit bones. Endocrinology 116:234, 1985
48. Jones SJ, Boyde A: Scanning electron microscopy of bone cells in culture. p.97. In Copp DH, Talmage RV (eds): Endocrinology of Calcium Metabolism. Excerpta Medica, Amsterdam, 1978
49. Rodan GA, Martin TJ: Role of osteoblasts in hormonal control of bone resorption—a hypothesis. Calcif Tissue Int 33:349, 1981
50. Miller SS, Wolf AM, Arnaud CD: Bone cells in culture: morphologic transformation by hormones. Science 192:1340, 1976

51. Feldman RS, Krieger NS, Tashjian AH: Effect of parathyroid hormone and calcitonin on osteoclast formation in vitro. Endocrinology 107:1137, 1980
52. Lorenzo JA, Raisz LG, Hock JM: DNA synthesis is not necessary for osteoclastic responses to parathyroid hormone in cultured fetal rat long bones. J Clin Invest 72:1924, 1983
53. Partridge NC, Kemp BE, Veroni MC, Martin TJ: Activation of adenosine 3′,5′-monophosphate-dependent protein kinase in normal and malignant bone cells by parathyroid hormone, prostaglandin E_2 and prostacyclin. Endocrinology 108:220, 1981
54. Krieger NS, Hefley TJ: Differential effects of parathyroid hormone on protein phosphorylation in two bone cell populations. J Bone Min Res 1(S1):abs 331, 1986
55. Lowik CWGM, van Leeuwen JPTM, van der Meer JM, et al: A two-receptor model for the action of parathyroid hormone on osteoblasts: a role for intracellular free calcium and cAMP. Cell Calcium 6:311, 1985
56. Boland CJ, Fried RM, Tashjian AH Jr: Measurement of cytosolic free Ca^{2+} concentrations in human and rat osteosarcoma cells: actions of bone resorption-stimulating hormones. Endocrinology 118:980, 1986
57. Reid IR, Civitelli R, Halstead LR, et al: Parathyroid hormone acutely elevates intracellular calcium in osteoblastlike cells. Am J Physiol 252:E46, 1987
58. Yamaguchi DT, Hahn TJ, Iida-Klein A, et al: Parathyroid hormone-activated calcium channels in an osteoblast-like clonal osteosarcoma cell line. J Biol Chem 262:7711, 1987
58a. Stewart, PJ, Stern PH: Calcium/phosphatidylserine stimulated protein phosphorylation in bone: effect of parathyroid hormone. J Bone Min Res 2:281, 1987
59. Feyen JHM, van der Wilt G, Moonen P, et al: Stimulation of arachidonic acid metabolism in primary cultures of osteoblast-like cells by hormones and drugs. Prostaglandins 28:769, 1984
60. Hamilton JA, Lingelback SR, Partridge NC, Martin TJ: Stimulation of plasminogen activator in osteoblast-like cells by bone-resorbing hormones. Biochem Biophys Res Comm 122:230, 1984
61. Partridge NC, Frampton RJ, Eisman JA, et al: Receptors for 1,25-$(OH)_2$ vitamin D_3 enriched in cloned osteoblast-like rat osteogenic sarcoma cells. FEBS Lett 115:139, 1980
62. Manolagas SC, Haussler M, Deftos LJ: 1,25-Dihydroxyvitamin D_3 receptor-like macromolecule in rat osteogenic sarcoma cell lines. J Biol Chem 255:4414, 1980
63. Gronowicz G, Egan JJ, Rodan GA: The effect of 1,25-dihydroxyvitamin D_3 on the cytoskeleton of rat calvaria and rat osteosarcoma (ROS 17/2.8) osteoblastic cells. J Bone Min Res 1:441, 1986
64. Suda T, Miyaura C, Abe E, Kuroki T: Modulation of cell differentiation, immune responses and tumor promotion by vitamin D compounds. p.1. In Peck WA (ed): Bone and Mineral Research Annual 4. Elsevier, Amsterdam, 1986
65. Mangelsdorf DJ, Doeffler HP, Donaldson CA, et al: 1,25-Dihydroxyvitamin D_3-induced differentiation in human promyelocytic leukemia cell line (HL-60); receptor-mediated maturation to macarophage-like cells. J Cell Biol 98:391, 1984
66. Price PA, Williamson MK, Haba T, et al: Excessive mineralization with growth plate closure in rats on chronic warfarin treatment. Proc Natl Acad Sci 79:7734, 1982
67. Lian JB, Tassinari M, Glowacki J: Resorption of implanted bone prepared from normal and warfarin-treated rats. J Clin Invest 73:1223, 1984
68. Nicholson GC, Moseley PM, Sexton PM, et al: Abundant calcitonin receptors in isolated rat osteoclasts. J Clin Invest 78:355, 1986

69. Klein DC, Raisz LG: Role of adenosine-3′,5′-monophosphate in the hormonal regulation of bone resorption: studies with cultured fetal bone. Endocrinology 89:818, 1971
70. Lerner U, Fredholm BB, Ransjo M: Transient inhibition on calcium mobilization from cultured mouse calvaria bones by the adenylate cyclase stimulator forskolin. Acta Physiol Scand 120:159, 1984
71. Lorenzo J, Sousa S, Quinton J: Forskolin has both stimulatory and inhibitory effects on bone resorption in fetal rat long bone cultures. J Bone Min Res 1:313, 1986
72. Krieger NS, Stern PH: Effects of forskolin on bone in organ culture. Am J Physiol 252:E44, 1987
73. Stern PH: Inhibition by steroids of parathyroid hormone-induced Ca^{45} release from embryonic bone in vitro. J Pharmacol 168:211, 1969
74. Caputo CB, Meadows D, Raisz LG: Failure of estrogens and androgens to inhibit bone resorption in tissue culture. Endocrinology 98:1065, 1976
75. Canalis E, Raisz LG: Effect of sex steroids on bone collagen synthesis in vitro. Calcif Tissue Res 25:105, 1978
76. Chen TL, Feldman D: Distinction between alpha-fetoprotein and intracellular estrogen receptors: evidence against the presence of estradiol receptors in rat bone. Endocrinology 102:236, 1978
77. Morel G, Boivin G, David L, et al: Immunocytochemical evidence for endogenous calcitonin and parathyroid hormone in osteoblasts from the calvaria of neonatal mice. Absence of endogenous estradiol and estradiol receptors. Cell Tissue Res 240:89, 1985
78. Gray TK, Flynn TC, Gray KM, Nabell LM: 17β-Estradiol acts directly on the clonal osteoblastic cell line UMR106. Proc Natl Acad Sci 84:6276, 1987
79. Komm BS, Sheetz L, Baker M, et al: Bone related cells in culture express putative estrogen receptor mRNA and ^{125}I-17β-estradiol binding. J Bone Min Res 2(S1): abs.237, 1987
80. Erikson EF, Berg NJ, Graham ML, et al: Evidence of estrogen receptors in human bone cells. J Bone Min Res 2(S1):abs.238, 1987
81. Feyen JHM, Raisz LG: Prostaglandin production by calvariae from sham-operated and oophorectomized rats: effect of 17β-estradiol in vivo. Endocrinology 121:819, 1987
82. Rizzoli R, Poser J, Burgi U: Nuclear thyroid hormone receptors in cultured bone cells. Metabolism 35:71, 1986
83. Sato K, Han DC, Fuji Y, et al: Thyroid hormone stimulates alkaline phosphatase activity in cultured rat osteoblastic cells (ROS 17/2.8) through 3,5,3′-triiodo-L-thyronine nuclear receptors. Endocrinology 120:1873, 1987
84. Schmid C, Steiner T, Froesch ER: Triiodothyronine increases responsiveness of cultured rat bone cells to parathyroid hormone. Acta Endocrinol 111:213, 1986
85. Stern PH, Bell NH: Effects of glucagon on serum calcium in the rat and on bone resorption in tissue culture. Endocrinology 87:111, 1970
86. Hohmann EL, Levine L, Tashjian AH Jr: Vasoactive intestinal peptide stimulates bone resorption via a cyclic adenosine 3′,5′-monophosphate-dependent mechanism. Endocrinology 112:1233, 1983
87. Raisz LG, Martin TJ: Prostaglandins in bone and mineral metabolism. p.286. In Peck WA (ed): Bone and Mineral Research Annual 2. Elsevier, Amsterdam, 1984
88. Shen V, Rifas L, Kohler G, Peck WA: Prostaglandins change cell shape and increase intercellular gap junctions in osteoblasts cultured from rat fetal calvaria. J Bone Min Res 1:243, 1986

89. Chikuma T, Kato T, Hiramatsu M, et al: Effect of epidermal growth factor on dipeptidyl-aminopeptidase and collagenase-like peptidase activities in cloned osteoblastic cells. J Biol Chem 95:283, 1984
90. Centrella M, Canalis E: Transforming and nontransforming growth factors are present in medium conditioned by fetal rat calvariae. Proc Natl Acad Sci 82:7335, 1986
91. Centrella M, Canalis E: Isolation of EGF-dependent transforming growth factor (TGFβ-like) activity from culture medium conditioned by fetal rat calvariae. J Bone Min Res 2:29, 1987
92. Gowen M, Wood DD, Ihrie EJ, et al: An interleukin-I-like factor stimulates bone resorption in vitro. Nature 306:378, 1983
93. Heath JK, Saklatvala J, Meikle MC, et al: Pig interleukin-1 (catabolin) is a potent stimulator of bone resorption in vitro. Calcif Tissue Int 37:95, 1985
94. Dewhirst FE, Ago JM, Peros WJ, Stashenko P: Synergism between parathyroid hormone and interleukin 1 in stimulating bone resorption in organ culture. J Bone Min Res 2:127, 1987
95. Bertolini DR, Nedwin T, Bringman T, et al: Stimulation of bone resorption and inhibition of bone formation in vitro by human tumour necrosis factors. Nature 319:516, 1985
96. Tashjian AH Jr, Voelkel EF, Lazzaro M, et al: Tumor necrosis factor-alpha (cachectin) stimulates bone resorption in mouse calvaria via a prostaglandin-mediated mechanism. Endocrinology 120:2029, 1987
97. Canalis E: Effects of tumor necrosis factor on bone formation in vitro. Endocrinology 121:1596, 1987
98. Jilka RL, Hamilton JW: Inhibition of parathormone-stimulated bone resorption by type I interferon. Biochem Biophys Res Commun 120:553, 1984
99. Peterlik M, Hoffman O, Swetly P, et al: Recombinant gamma-interferon inhibits prostaglandin-mediated and parathyroid hormone-induced bone resorption in cultured neonatal mouse calvariae. FEBS Lett 185:287, 1985
100. Gowen M, Nedwin GE, Mundy GR: Preferential inhibition of cytokine-stimulated bone resorption by recombinant interferon gamma. J Bone Min Res 1:469, 1986
101. Frost HM: Tetracycline-based histological analysis of bone remodeling. Calcif Tissue Res 3:211, 1969
102. Farley JR, Tarbaux N, Murphy LA, et al: In vitro evidence that bone formation may be coupled to resorption by release of mitogen(s) from resorbing bone. Metabolism 36:314, 1987
103. Wong GL, Roberts R, Miller E: Production of and response to growth-stimulating activity in isolated bone cells. J Bone Min Res 2:23, 1987
104. Pfeilschifter J, Mundy GR: Modulation of type β transforming growth factor activity in bone cultures by osteotrophic hormones. Proc Natl Acad Sci 84:2024, 1987
105. Farley JR, Baylink DJ: Purification of a skeletal growth factor from human bone. Biochemistry 21:3502, 1982
106. Canalis E, Centrella M, Urist MR: Effect of partially purified bone morphogenetic protein on DNA synthesis and cell replication in calvarial and fibroblast cultures. Clin Orthrop Rel Res 198:289, 1985
107. Cheng S-L, Rifas L, Shen V, et al: J774A macrophage cell line produces PDGF-like and non-PDGF-like growth factors for bone cells. J Bone Min Res 2:467, 1987

2 Endocrine Control of Bone and Mineral Metabolism

Robert Marcus

Calcium is the major extracellular divalent cation. The normal adult man and woman possess about 1300 and 1000 g calcium, respectively. As summarized in Table 2–1, more than 99 percent of whole body calcium is contained in the skeleton, with relatively trivial amounts present in the extracellular fluid.

Among invertebrate phyla, calcium is present mainly as the carbonate salt (e.g., shells). In vertebrates, hydroxyapatite [$Ca_5(OH)(PO_4)_3$], a crystalline complex of calcium and phosphorus, is the primary form. The physiologic roles of calcium are diverse. Intracellular calcium serves as a messenger for transduction of hormone signals, for coupling of neural excitation to muscle contraction, for activating enzyme reactions, and for promoting glandular secretion. As a major component of bone it provides stiffness and support against gravity. As eggshell (here present as carbonate), it protects against dehydration and permits gas exchange. As antler, it is both weapon and ornament.

The biologically important compartments of calcium are those located within cells and in extracellular fluid. Under basal conditions, the ionized calcium level within cells is maintained by energy-dependent calcium pumps at about 0.1 micromolar (10^{-7}M). In response to hormonal, electrical, or mechanical stimuli, a temporary increase in calcium flux raises the ionized calcium toward 10^{-6}M, and permits specific interactions of the cation with calcium-binding proteins to activate numerous intracellular processes. The major cal-

Table 2-1. Distribution of Calcium in the Adult Human Male

	Content (g)	% of Total
Skeleton	1300	99
Soft tissue	7	0.6
Teeth	7	0.6
Plasma	0.35	0.03
Extracellular fluid	0.70	0.07

cium-binding protein in all organisms is calmodulin, a 1700 dalton peptide that binds 4 moles of calcium per mole of protein. Highly conserved throughout evolution, this protein shares substantial homology with other calcium binding proteins, including the vitamin-D-dependent protein described later. For a comprehensive discussion of the roles of intracellular calcium, the reader is referred to the review by Rasmussen.[1]

Of particular importance is the need to maintain extracellular ionized calcium within a fairly narrow concentration range. If calcium is permitted to drop below this level, neural and muscle tissues become increasingly excitable, and muscle twitching, seizures, laryngospasm, and death may occur. Progressively higher levels of calcium may be attended by hyporeflexia, obtundation, renal failure, coma, and death.

In human plasma, calcium circulates at a concentration of about 8.5 to 10.5 mg/dl (2.1 to 2.6 mM). Of this, approximately 50 percent is bound to plasma proteins, primarily albumin, so that the plasma ionized calcium level is about 5 mg/dl (1.25 mM or 2.5 mEq/L). Perhaps 10 percent of total plasma calcium is complexed with anionic buffers, such as bicarbonate and phosphate.

In certain clinical situations, such as malnutrition or liver disease, independent abnormalities in serum albumin levels may change the apparent serum calcium concentration. When this occurs it is useful to correct the calcium value by adding or subtracting 0.8 mg/dl calcium for every 1 g/dl deviation of albumin from 4 g/dl. For example, a patient whose total serum calcium is 8.0 mg/dl with an albumin of 2.5 g/dl would have a corrected calcium level of $(4.0 - 2.5) \times 0.8 + 8.0 = 9.2$ mg/dl, a normal value. A patient whose total calcium is 10.0 mg/dl with an albumin of 2.5 g/dl would have a corrected calcium of $1.5 \times 0.8 + 10.0 = 11.2$ mg/dl, and would be considered hypercalcemic.

The ambient calcium concentration to which saltwater fish are exposed is about 10 mM, and the major challenge for calcium homeostasis is elimination of excessive calcium from the internal milieu. This is accomplished by the concerted action of pituitary and suprarenal hormones on a calcium pump mechanism in the gills. For freshwater fish, amphibians, and land animals, however, calcium is in restricted supply at best. The evolution of a complex series of integrated, hormonally regulated processes permits accommodation to temporary mineral deficiencies and protects against lethal reductions in ionized calcium. The remainder of this chapter will consider these processes and the hormone systems that modulate them.

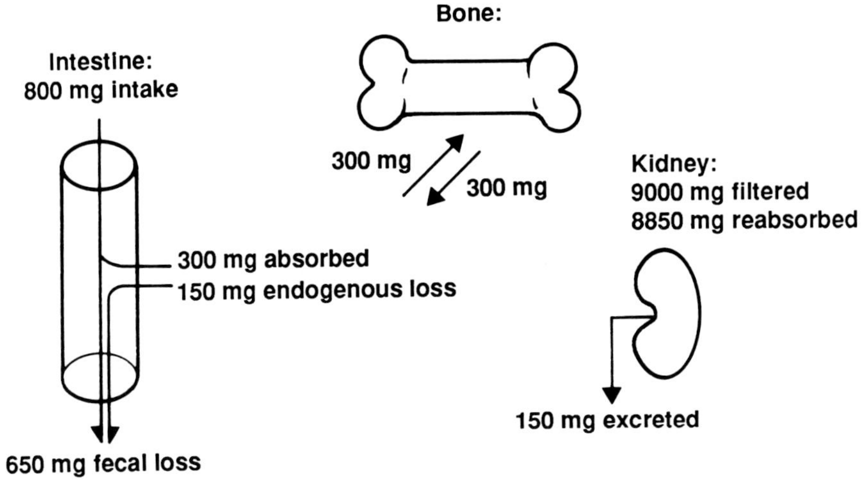

Fig. 2-1 Schematic representation of daily calcium turnover.

COMPONENTS OF THE CALCIUM HOMEOSTASIS SYSTEM

Figure 2–1 illustrates schematically the daily flow of calcium through body compartments. The intestine is the only portal of entry. Intestinal calcium absorption is relatively inefficient, and proceeds by two fundamentally different processes. Facilitated diffusion occurs across the entire small bowel surface, accounting for a substantial portion of net calcium uptake. Active transport occurs in the proximal duodenum, and is highly dependent on vitamin D. Whereas efficiency of calcium absorption declines as calcium intake increases, vitamin D enhances this process at any given mineral intake. A constant loss of calcium into the intestinal lumen amounts to about 150 mg/day, and is contained in secretions and sloughed mucosal cells.

Dietary Considerations

In Western society, calcium is ingested largely (>75 percent) as a component of milk and dairy products (1 quart of milk provides approximately 1100 mg calcium). Calcium is also fairly abundant in some other foods, but its bioavailability may be unpredictable. For example, a high oxalate content may severely constrain calcium absorption from green vegetables. The recommended dietary allowance (RDA) for calcium has been set at 800 mg/day for men and women, with an extra 400 mg recommended during adolescence and pregnancy.[2] This allowance markedly underestimates the needs for women of menopausal age.[3] Although calcium intakes of American men approach RDA values throughout life, major, apparently permanent, deviations of median intakes below this level are seen in girls as early as 12 years of age.[4]

Kidney

Approximately 9000 mg of calcium enter the glomerular filtrate each day. Tubular reabsorption is extremely efficient, with more than 98 percent of the filtered mineral returning to the circulation, predominantly from the proximal nephron. Reabsorption efficiency is highly regulated by parathyroid hormone, but is influenced also by filtered sodium, the presence of nonreabsorbable anions (e.g., SO_4), and diuretic agents. There is no compelling evidence for tubular secretion of calcium in humans. Net urinary calcium excretion is a function of filtered load and reabsorption efficiency. It is influenced to only a modest degree by dietary calcium intake in normal people. When consuming about 400 mg calcium/day, normal men and women should not excrete more than 250 mg/day. With an increase in daily intake of 1000 mg, urinary excretion may be expected to rise by about 50 mg.

Bone

Ionized calcium in the circulation maintains a fairly stable relationship with bone. A labile pool of bone mineral readily exchanges with many constituents of extracellular fluid, including calcium, sodium, and hydrogen ions. A much larger pool, not readily exchangeable, requires active cell-mediated and hormonally regulated resorption for delivery of mineral to the fluid compartment. In young adults, bone resorption and formation are approximately equal, and daily skeletal calcium exchange approaches 300 to 500 mg.

Role of the Skeleton

Mammalian bone serves two basic and occasionally conflicting roles. It provides the structural integrity necessary to withstand the force of gravity, and also serves as the dominant reservoir to support plasma calcium levels. At times when calcium availability is inadequate, blood calcium will be supported at the expense of skeletal mineral.

Bone participates in three fundamental activities. (1) Modeling is the means by which bone achieves and maintains its shape. (2) Repair is a response to fracture. (3) Remodeling is a continuous cycle of breakdown and renewal that occurs throughout life in the bones of humans, primates, and some other mammals. It serves a scavenger function, replacing areas of fatigue damage with new bone. It also constitutes the common pathway through which such diverse stimuli as hormonal or dietary insufficiency affect the rate of bone turnover. The remodeling cycle (Fig. 2–2) leads to gradual accumulation of bone deficits, and in the long run contributes to age-related bone loss. Thus, any agent that increases the degree of remodeling activity will increase the rate of bone loss. For more detailed consideration of remodeling, the reader may consult the review by Marcus.[5]

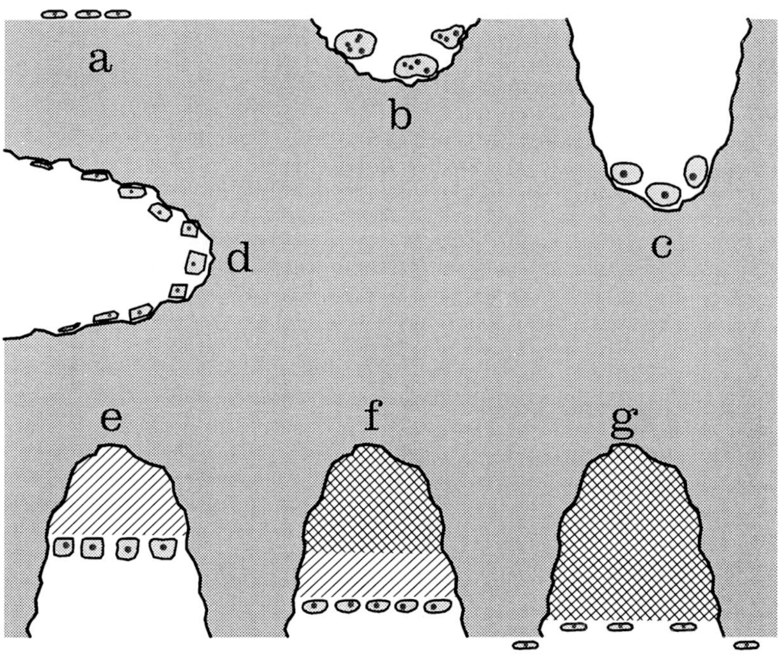

Fig. 2-2 Schematic representation of the bone remodeling cycle. a, About 90 percent of the bone surface is normally at rest. b, Remodeling begins when phagocytic mononuclear cells cluster focally at the bone surface, fuse to become multinucleate osteoclasts, and dig a cavity into the bone. c, When the resorption cavity has reached one-third of final depth, osteoclasts are replaced by mononuclear phagocytes, which continue to remove bone to a depth of about 60 μm. d, Local release of chemical factors attracts osteoblast precursors to the base of the resorption cavity. e, Osteoblasts begin to replace missing bone by secreting new collagen and matrix constituents. f, Mineralization follows matrix production. g, Mineralization is complete. If replacement of resorbed bone were complete, bone would be restored to initial state. However, coupling is not fully efficient, and small bone deficits gradually accrue. These deficits are the basis for age-related bone loss.

THE CALCIUM-REGULATING HORMONES

Parathyroid Hormone

Parathyroid hormone (PTH) is the major peptide hormone involved in calcium homeostasis, its important actions working in concert to elevate blood calcium levels. It is a single peptide chain of 84 amino acids, with biologic activity residing completely within the first amino terminal 34 amino acids. Its secretion is regulated by the calcium concentration of plasma, with even minor reductions leading to a rapid increase in the delivery of hormone to peripheral blood.

Hormone biosynthesis results initially in the formation of a larger, 110 amino acid, biologically inert peptide (pre-pro-PTH) (Fig. 2–3). The amino-terminal "pre" sequence is cleaved upon processing of the nascent peptide in the endoplasmic reticulum. The 90 amino acid pro-PTH is also biologically inactive, and the 6 amino acid "pro" sequence is removed in the Golgi region prior to secretion of intact 1–84 PTH.

The primary physiologic stimulus for PTH secretion is a reduction in the plasma ionized calcium concentration. Such a reduction is reflected in a decrease of intracellular calcium activity within the parathyroid cells, and leads to release of a storage pool of preformed hormone as well as to new hormone synthesis. It is thought that these effects are mediated by a change in cAMP concentration in the parathyroid cell, but the precise details remain unclear. Conversely, elevated plasma calcium levels suppress PTH synthesis and release. Although secretion of some intact PTH persists in the presence of hypercalcemia, most immunoreactive PTH released by the suppressed gland is made up of biologically inert, immunologically reactive cleavage products.

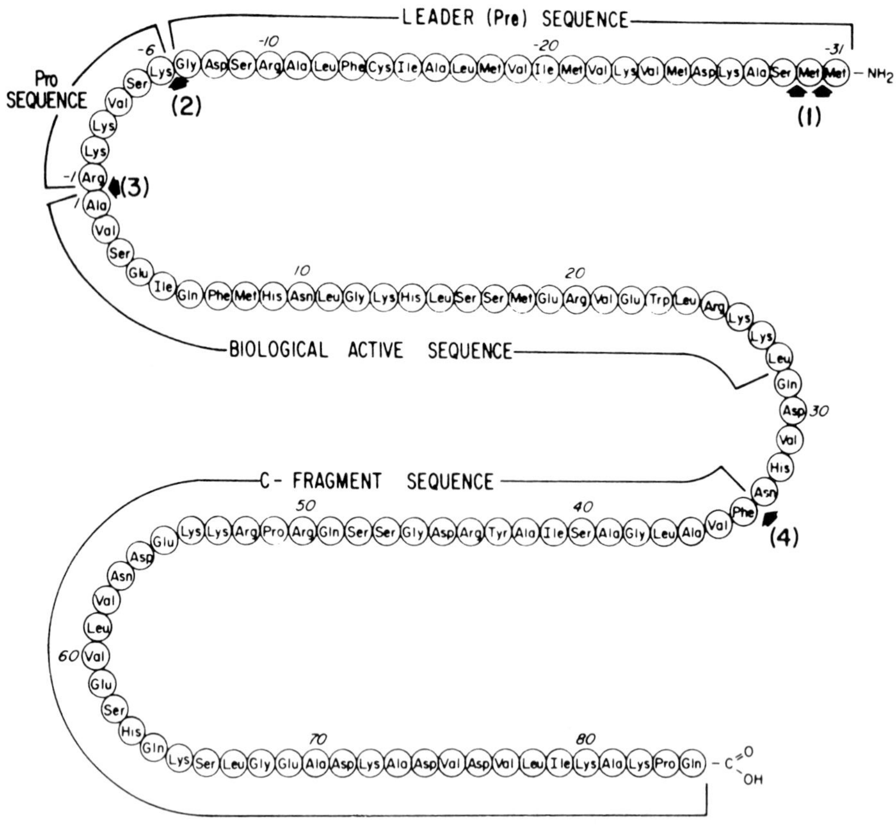

Fig. 2-3 Primary structure of preproparathyroid hormone. (From Habener and Jacobs,[31] with permission.)

Several biologically active agents such as catecholamines and prostaglandins stimulate or inhibit PTH secretion in vitro. Although some evidence exists that these may also modulate hormone secretion in vivo, results have not been consistent, and the magnitude of secretory responses has been far less than those seen with hypocalcemia.

Once in the circulation, PTH is relatively quickly cleaved into an assortment of peptide fragments. The amino terminal 1-34 PTH fragment circulates for a few minutes, and is not generally detectable in plasma. Major carboxyl terminal fragments, such as the 53–84 PTH peptide, circulate for longer periods, and are eliminated by renal excretion. The cleavage pathways have not been fully elucidated, but at least some hormone degradation occurs in the kidney. Evidence has also been presented for an hepatic site of cleavage. With impaired glomerular filtration, plasma levels of carboxyl terminal fragments rise. Since most antisera used in PTH radioimmunoassays recognize portions of the major carboxyl terminal fragments, renal insufficiency may be accompanied by falsely high values for circulating hormone.

Actions

PTH interacts with specific high-affinity receptors located on cell surfaces in its target tissues. This interaction is the proximal step in initiating the primary physiologic actions of the hormone, summarized in Table 2–2.

Kidney

The phosphaturic response to PTH was one of the first actions described for this hormone. A substantial increase in urinary phosphorus is seen within minutes of the injection of exogenous PTH, and chronically low levels of phosphate reabsorption are found in clinical disorders of PTH excess. The calcium-conserving effect of PTH may be masked when hypercalcemia increases the amount filtered by the glomerulus. However, at any given filtered load, there will be less calcium excreted in urine in the presence of PTH than in its absence. Thus, although patients with primary hyperparathyroidism may be hy-

Table 2-2. Major Actions of PTH

Kidney
Promotes phosphate excretion
Promotes calcium conservation
Stimulates formation of calcitriol
Inhibits bicarbonate reabsorption
Bone
Increases resorption (release of both mineral and matrix)
Inhibits osteoblast function
Activates new remodeling units

percalciuric, they do not usually lose as much calcium as do patients with similar degrees of nonparathyroid hypercalcemia. The majority of calcium reabsorption occurs in the proximal tubule. However, it appears that the effect of PTH on calcium handling may reside at more distal sites, particularly the thick ascending segment of the loop of Henle.

Bone

PTH increases the delivery of calcium to the extracellular fluid. This is due to an increase in overall bone resorption, and involves the release of organic matrix components as well as mineral. PTH activates preexisting osteoclasts, and also recruits osteoclast precursor cells into forming new bone remodeling units. Sustained increases in circulating PTH result in characteristic histologic changes in bone. These include an increase in the surface prevalence and number of osteoclasts, and an increase in the proportion of bone surface covered with unmineralized osteoid. Although excessive osteoid surfaces may indicate defective mineralization, they signify in this case a predictable increase in bone-forming surfaces related to an overall increase in remodeling activity.

At the cellular level, changes in both osteoclast and osteoblast function follow PTH treatment. In osteoclasts, PTH leads to the appearance of highly ruffled borders where the cells attach to the bone surface. In addition, PTH stimulates such osteoclast-associated enzyme activities as acid phosphatase and hyaluronic acid synthesis. The nature of these responses has been difficult to unravel, since there are apparently no specific PTH receptors on these cells, nor are the actions of PTH demonstrable in isolated osteoclast preparations. Hormone responsiveness does appear if osteoclasts are cultured in medium exposed to osteoblasts, suggesting a primary role for osteoblasts in mediating the osteoclastic effects of PTH.

Compared to the ambiguities associated with PTH and osteoclast function, the effects of PTH on osteoblasts are relatively straightforward, and generally inhibitory. These include reductions in the formation of type I (bone) collagen, production of alkaline phosphatase, and synthesis of the bone-specific protein, osteocalcin. In addition, PTH stimulates the production of prostaglandin E2 by osteoblasts, and this may be one of several osteoblast-derived agents that ultimately stimulate osteoclasts to initiate resorption. The skeletal effects of PTH have recently been reviewed by Wong.[6]

Intestine

Hypersecretion of PTH leads to increased efficiency of intestinal calcium absorption, but this effect appears to be an indirect consequence of vitamin D activation.

The molecular basis of PTH action is not clear. Binding of the hormone to receptors in kidney and bone stimulates the adenylate cyclase–cyclic AMP system, leading to intracellular accumulation of cyclic AMP and activation of cAMP-dependent protein kinases.[7,8] In kidney, this appears to underlie most, if not all, of the actions of PTH. A unique feature of PTH action on the kidney is an increase in urinary excretion of cAMP. This response to PTH precedes the rise in phosphaturia, and reflects a direct action on the renal tubular cell. Nephrogenous cAMP excretion has found use as a reasonable index of parathyroid status. High levels are observed in patients with hyperparathyroidism, and low levels obtain in hypoparathyroidism. Patients with the genetic disorder pseudohypoparathyroidism show defective generation of nephrogenous cAMP following a PTH challenge.[9] The lesion has not been completely defined, but resides somewhere in the adenylate cyclase enzyme complex.[10,11]

Although cyclic AMP or its analogs can mimic certain aspects of PTH action on bone (e.g., release of enzymes), considerable evidence has accumulated that induction of bone resorption is dissociable from cyclic nucleotide generation. Recent attention has focused on alternative pathways for PTH action. In kidney, the hormone stimulates formation of inositol triphosphate and diacylglycerol, which may activate phospholipid-dependent protein kinases and stimulate cellular calcium uptake.[12] Similar pathways have not been fully elucidated for bone cells, but PTH does rapidly increase intracellular calcium, and it is likely that a calcium-dependent transducing mechanism exists.

Calcitonin

Calcitonin (CT) is a potent hypocalcemic factor whose origins can be traced to early vertebrate evolution. A 32-amino acid single chain peptide, CT is the secretory product of neuroectodermal cells located diffusely throughout the thyroid gland in humans, but contained in separate ultimobranchial bodies in lower vertebrates. Although subtle alterations in the CT molecule permit biologic activity, the only circulating active form of the hormone is the intact molecule. Structure–activity relationships have been conducted with CTs from numerous species. The salmon hormone, which is about 20 times as potent as mammalian calcitonins, has been synthesized and is available for therapeutic use in humans. Recently, synthetic human CT has also been developed for human use.

The major stimulus for CT secretion is hypercalcemia. Secretion of CT increases within minutes of elevating the plasma calcium level in various animals. In humans, most studies of CT secretion have used intravenous calcium or other secretagogues. In pharmacologic doses, pentagastrin is a potent secretagogue, which has led to the suggestion that endogenous gastrin could be an important regulator of CT secretion in vivo. It has been more difficult to demonstrate significant elevations in circulating calcitonin following a calcium-containing meal, although this has been accomplished.[13] Circulating CT has a short half-life, approximately 10 minutes, and depends on renal function for degradation.

The most dramatic response to administered CT is lowering of plasma calcium. The response to a single injection is rapid, and lasts up to 24 hours. The magnitude of the hypocalcemic response is directly proportional to the degree of bone remodeling. Patients with "high-turnover" skeletal disorders, such as Paget's disease or primary hyperparathyroidism, show a more exuberant hypocalcemic response to CT than do normal subjects.

Calcitonin rapidly contracts the characteristic ruffled border of actively resorbing osteoclasts, leading to inhibition of bone resorption, both in vitro and in vivo. It also effectively antagonizes PTH-induced bone turnover, although tachyphylaxis develops following sustained administration.

In kidney, CT acutely stimulates phosphorus excretion, and in this regard is similar to PTH. Calcitonin stimulates natriuresis by a direct effect on the renal tubule. Reported effects on calcium handling are mixed and not of great consequence. Evidence has been presented that CT may independently promote synthesis of 1,25-dihydroxyvitamin D.

Studies of the molecular basis of calcitonin action implicate the adenylate cyclase–cyclic AMP system for both its renal and skeletal effects.[14] However, little attention has been paid to alternative mechanisms, and the question remains open.

Calcitonin probably has a major physiologic role during fish spawning and avian egg laying, and perhaps during mammalian reproduction. Serious questions remain concerning its role in normal humans. Neither the absence of this hormone (as in completely thyroidectomized patients) nor its thousandfold excess (as in patients with thyroid medullary carcinoma) is generally associated with abnormal calcium regulation or skeletal integrity. Moreover, conditions of sustained hypercalcemia are not usually associated with elevated CT blood levels. Nevertheless, the ability of an oral calcium load to provoke an acute rise in circulating hormone is consistent with a role for CT in preventing excessive postprandial calcemic responses.

The most important rationale for measuring CT blood levels is the evaluation of patients suspected of having the neuroectodermal malignancy medullary thyroid carcinoma. This condition, which may be either sporadic or familial, is frequently associated with high circulating CT levels but may sometimes be diagnosed only with provocative testing. In this case, the CT level in blood is measured before and after parenteral administration of calcium or pentagastrin.

Vitamin D

Vitamin D is the fat-soluble substance capable of preventing and curing rickets. In the 70 years since its isolation, major discoveries concerning its metabolic transformations and actions have revolutionized our understanding of mineral homeostasis and metabolic bone disease. The two major forms of vitamin D are vitamin D_2 (ergocalciferol) and vitamin D_3 (cholecalciferol) (Fig.

2–4). Both forms are based on a sterol nucleus in which the B ring has been opened (secosteroid). Ergocalciferol is obtained from the ultraviolet (UV) irradiation of ergosterol in green plants. Cholecalciferol is synthesized in mammalian subcutaneous tissue following sunlight exposure. For practical purposes, vitamins D_2 and D_3 will be referred to simply as vitamin D and considered equivalent.

Although the discovery of vitamin D was based upon the cure of rickets, the action that has been best characterized is its ability to increase the efficiency of intestinal calcium absorption. For many years it was observed that a substantial delay occurred between administration of the vitamin and the first detectable increase in gut calcium transport. This suggested the need for metabolic transformation before the vitamin produces its physiologic effect. The last 20 years have witnessed confirmation of this hypothesis, definition of the regulatory steps, identification of the important metabolites, and characterization of molecular basis of their actions, and represents one of the most exciting chapters in contemporary endocrinology. A comprehensive examination of this

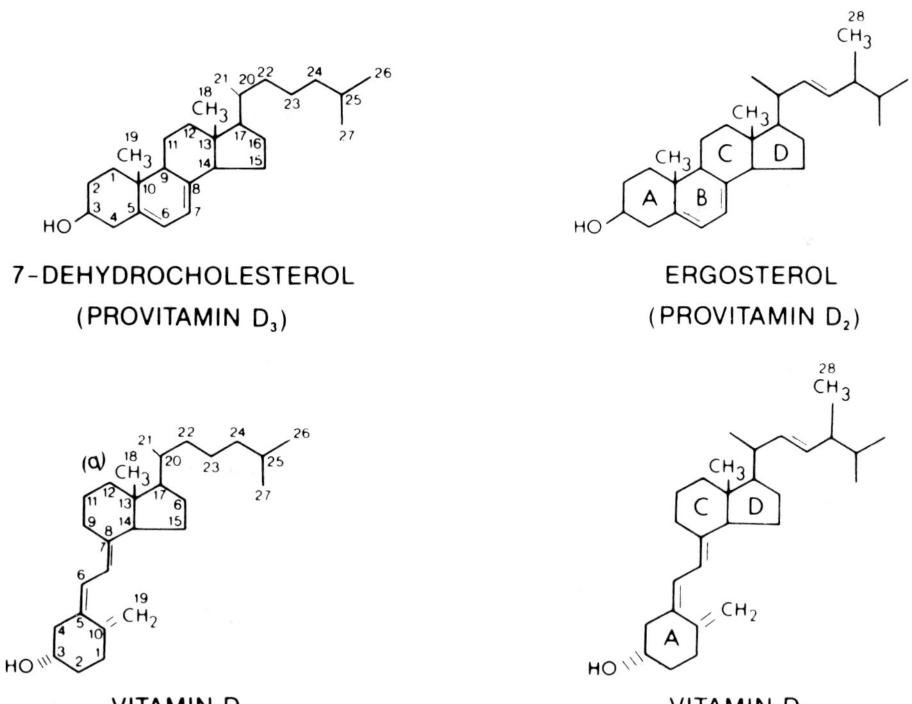

Fig. 2-4 Structures for 7-dehydrocholesterol, ergosterol, vitamin D_3, and vitamin D_2. Numbering system for steroid molecules is shown. During transformation of 7-dehydrocholesterol to vitamin D, the geometric position of ring A is altered, thereby changing the steric orientation of its substituents. However, original designation of the hydroxyl functions on ring A are retained. (From Holick,[32] with permission.)

subject is beyond the scope of this chapter, but the interested reader is referred to several excellent reviews.[15–17]

The steps involved in formation of vitamin D in skin are illustrated in Figure 2–5. A narrow portion of the sunlight spectrum (around 290 nm) splits the B ring in 7-dehydrocholesterol to form a thermolabile compound, previtamin D_3. Over a period of several days, the previtamin undergoes thermal isomerization to vitamin D_3, which, in turn, binds to a specific vitamin-D-binding protein for delivery to the circulation.

Vitamin D itself does not possess biologic activity. The steps that activate it involve two hydroxylations. The first of these, occurring in the liver, is in the carbon 25 position, and results in formation of the biologically active metabolite, 25-hydroxyvitamin D (25 OHD) (Fig. 2–5). This 25 OHD is released into the circulation, where it is the dominant form of vitamin D, with normal plasma concentrations of 20 to 50 ng/ml. Just as with the parent vitamin, 25 OHD is largely bound to vitamin-D-binding protein. Although the 25-hydroxylase is subject to some metabolic control, its activity depends primarily on substrate availability. In cases of vitamin D intoxication, very high levels of 25 OHD are observed.

The 25 OHD is carried in plasma to renal tubular cells, where one of two possible transformations occurs. The most important of these steps is catalyzed by the mitochondrial P-450-dependent enzyme, 1 α hydroxylase, and is the formation of the potent metabolite, 1,25 dihydroxyvitamin D (calcitriol) (Fig. 2–5). The alternative pathway results in synthesis of 24,25 dihydroxy vitamin D, a compound of considerably reduced potency. Which of these two pathways predominates is the result of exquisite regulatory control. The major factors that promote calcitriol formation are PTH, hypophosphatemia or phosphorus depletion, and hypocalcemia. Factors favoring 24 hydroxylation are hyperphosphatemia or phosphorus loading, hypercalcemia, and hypoparathyroidism. In an interesting example of short-loop feedback, calcitriol itself induces the activity of the 24 hydroxylase.

Calcitriol formation is enhanced at times of calcium need. This occurs by a direct effect of hypocalcemia on the 1 α hydroxylase, as well as indirectly through the action of PTH. For example, a low calcium intake leads to transient reductions in plasma ionized calcium and compensatory hypersecretion of PTH. PTH directly stimulates renal 1 α hydroxylase, an effect that is augmented by its action to increase phosphorus excretion and deplete tissue phosphorus levels. Elevated calcitriol production then increases calcium absorption efficiency, with restoration of the ionized calcium concentration. In the absence of PTH the calcitriol response to induced hypocalcemia is severely reduced, so PTH appears to be the most important modulator of 1 α hydroxylase activity. Calcitriol in plasma is largely bound to the vitamin-D-binding protein. Circulating levels are only 1/1000th those of 25 OHD (25 to 75 pg/ml), but calcitriol is also about 1000 times more potent than 25 OHD.

In addition to the primary regulators of 1 α hydroxylase, other physiologic and hormonal factors modulate calcitriol production. Estrogen markedly increases calcitriol formation in birds, and appears to have a similar action in

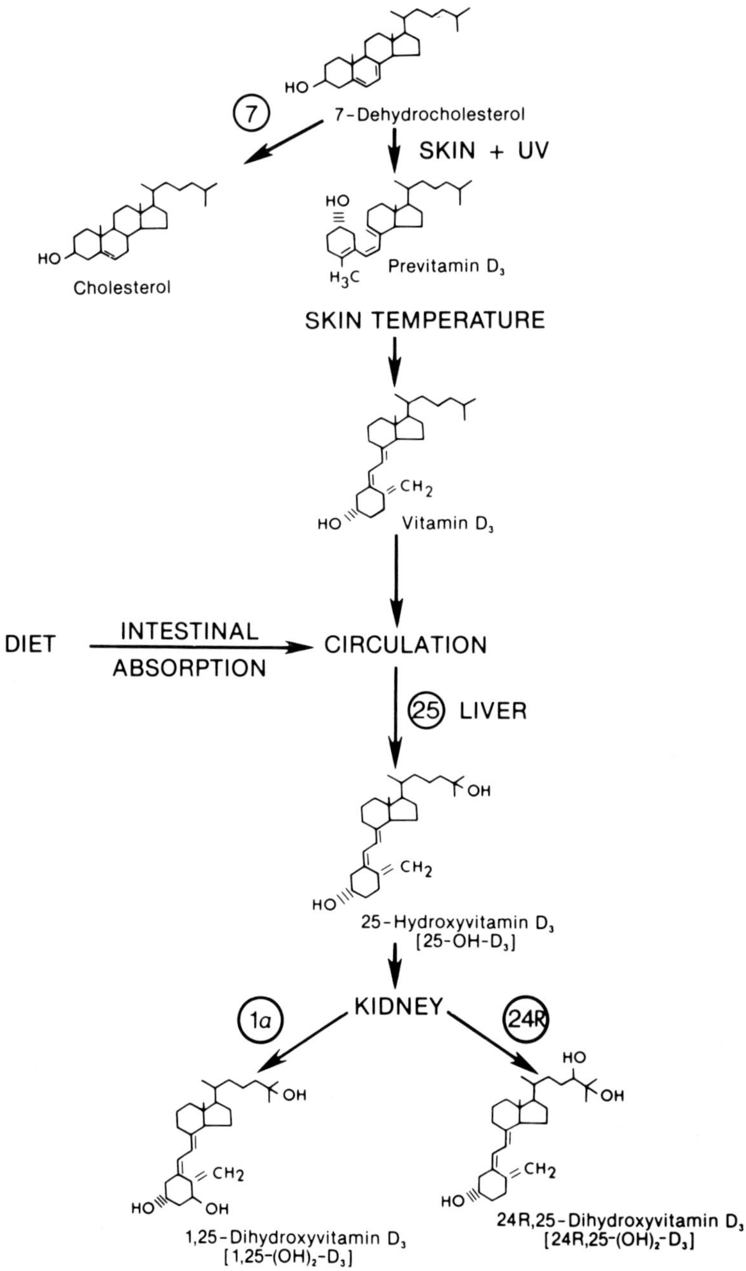

Fig. 2-5 Photobiogenesis and metabolic pathways for vitamin D production and metabolism. Circled letters and numbers denote specific enzymes: 7, 7-dehydrocholesterol reductase; 25, vitamin D-25 hydroxylase; 1 *a*, 25 OHD-1 α hydroxylase; 24R, 25 OHD-24R hydroxylase. (From Holick,[32] with permission.)

mammals and humans. Circulating calcitriol levels are clearly higher in pregnant and estrogen-treated women, but the degree to which this represents increased availability of active calcitriol, rather than an apparent rise due to increased vitamin D binding protein, has not been completely resolved.

Excess thyroid hormone reduces calcitriol levels, and this may reflect the action of thyroxine on bone to increase plasma ionized calcium and suppress PTH secretion. The suggestion has been made that the anabolic hormones growth hormone and prolactin modulate calcitriol production, but information in this regard is still incomplete.

Alternative sources of calcitriol exist under certain circumstances. Placental synthesis has been demonstrated, as well as local synthesis in bone cells. However, the kidney remains the primary source of circulating calcitriol, and levels remain extremely low in anephric humans or in patients with renal failure. Recent evidence suggests that macrophages and lymphocytes possess 1 α hydroxylase activity, and may produce very high calcitriol levels that underlie hypercalcemia in patients with various granulomatous disorders, such as sarcoidosis, tuberculosis, and lymphomas.

Vitamin D Action

The molecular basis of vitamin D action is similar to that of other steroid hormones. Thus, following passive entry into a target cell calcitriol binds specifically to high-affinity receptors associated with nuclear chromatin. In turn, the hormone-receptor complex alters DNA transcription leading to increases or decreases of specific proteins that mediate the effects of this molecule.

In the intestine, calcitriol rapidly increases calcium transport, a process largely occurring in the duodenum. The precise mechanisms underlying this action are complex and remain unresolved. Calcitriol increases the synthesis of a calcium-binding protein (CaBP), but since this occurs after the transport response, its relationship to calcium transport is unclear. Activities of calcium-dependent ATPase and alkaline phosphatase are induced by calcitriol, and may partly underlie the changes in calcium transport. Calcitriol also stimulates net jejunal phosphorus absorption, but little information about the specific basis for this action exists.

Calcitriol action in kidney is relatively obscure. The vitamin appears not to regulate renal phosphorus handling. An interation with PTH on tubular calcium reabsorption is likely, but has been incompletely studied. Its most consistent action appears to be the induction of 24 hydroxylation and suppression of further 1 hydroxylation.

Bone

Skeletal effects of vitamin D deficiency have been recognized for more than 100 years. The consequence of inadequate mineral deposition is identified as rickets in growing skeletons, whereas its occurrence in mature bone is called osteomalacia. Characteristic abnormalities of osteomalacic bone consist of a decrease in the prevalence of osteons actively forming bone, a decrease in the skeletal mineral apposition rate, and an increased surface prevalence and mean thickness of osteoid seams.[5] The degree to which these abnormalities reflect the absence of vitamin D itself rather than the poor supply of calcium and phosphorus accompanying vitamin D deficiency continues to be a matter of conjecture. Adequate concentrations of calcium and phosphorus are clearly necessary for mineralization, and vitamin D deficiency is associated with poor intestinal absoprtion of both. However, specific high-affinity receptors for calcitriol are found in osteoblasts; calcitriol modifies collagen production in bone cells; and calcitriol directly stimulates production of the gamma carboxyglutamic acid-containing peptide, osteocalcin, in osteoblasts. Thus, it appears that vitamin D also plays a direct role in normal bone cell physiology.

Calcitriol directly stimulates resorption in cultured embryonic bone. Because this process is primarily osteoclast-mediated, there has been some concern that specific calcitriol receptors have not been located in osteoclasts. However, it now appears that osteoclastic bone resorption in response to several agents, including PTH and calcitriol, could be mediated indirectly via interactions with osteblasts.

Miscellaneous Functions

Analysis of the distribution of calcitriol receptors in mammalian tissues strongly implies that physiologic roles for vitamin D may extend beyond those already discussed. With respect to calcium metabolism, two are of particular interest. Presence of specific high-affinity binding of calcitriol in parathyroid cells suggests that vitamin D may directly regulate PTH secretion. Recent data that skin keratinocytes may be a target tissue for calcitriol suggest that calcitriol may exert feedback control over vitamin D synthesis.

A variety of other tissues have been shown to respond to vitamin D. Vitamin D therapy rapidly increases muscle strength in rachitic children. Whether this reflects the mineral environment or is directly due to the vitamin is not clear. Pancreatic islets have receptors for calcitriol, and insulin secretion is modulated by vitamin D status. It is possible, therefore, that other calcium-dependent secretory processes may be directly influenced by vitamin D.

One of the most exciting new areas concerning vitamin D relates to cellular differentiation. This will not be discussed further in this chapter, since it does not relate directly to calcium homeostasis. The interested reader should consult the review by Suda et al.[18]

Human Vitamin D Adequacy

In Western society, sunlight exposure provides about 90 percent of total vitamin D, the remainder coming largely from fortified dairy products. The serum level of 25 OHD gives the best overall index of vitamin D nutritional status, but it is difficult to reach a consensus on "normal" levels because of the wide variation in UV exposure from one geographic region to the next. Most of the published literature originates from northern Europe or from the northeastern United States. In these areas, adverse climate prevents many people from being out of doors for substantial portions of the year. In addition, even if people in northern regions venture outside during winter, the UV spectrum of available sunlight may not support endogenous vitamin D synthesis.

The level of 25 OHD that defines vitamin D "adequacy" has not been determined. Traditional concerns have focused on levels below which osteomalacia is found,(6 to 8 ng/ml), but recent evidence suggests that different criteria may be appropriate. Calcitriol production may be impaired in elderly people. Although this may be related in part to a primary abnormality in kidney function, it may also represent a degree of substrate insufficiency. By this formulation marginal vitamin D from nutritional sources cannot support normal calcium absorption and leads to compensatory hypersecretion of PTH. The latter maintains plasma calcium levels in the normal range by activating the 1 α hydroxylase, increasing calcitriol production to whatever extent is possible, and also by increasing bone remodeling activity. Thus, plasma calcium is maintained at the cost of PTH-dependent bone loss. According to this model, vitamin D adequacy could be defined as that level of 25 OHD at which PTH secretion is minimized. Current evidence supports that this level is about 15 to 20 ng/ml.[19]

Age-Related Changes in Calciotropic Hormones

Circulating immunoreactive PTH levels increase with age in normal men and women.[20,21] The basis for this change is not entirely clear. The earliest demonstrations used radioimmunoassays responsive to carboxyl-terminal hormone fragments. Since glomerular filtration rate declines with age, these studies could not distinguish fragment retention from increased hormone secretion. However, recent use of assays sensitive only to intact PTH or its aminoterminal fragment confirms that the steady-state concentration of biologically active hormone rises with age.[22] The stimulus for increased hormone production is not certain, but may be a compensation for inadequate vitamin D status and/or impaired intestinal calcium absorption.

Most studies in humans suggest that circulating levels of 25 OHD decrease with age and undergo significant seasonal fluctuation, being higher in months of increased sunlight exposure. However, the majority of this literature originates from northern Europe and northernmost United States. Studies originating from more temperate environments do not consistently confirm significant age-related decreases in vitamin D status in healthy populations, and impressive seasonal variation may be restricted primarily to young people who experience intense solar irradiation during summer months. However, given the propensity for many older individuals to avoid sunlight and to minimize consumption of dairy products, it is likely that marginal vitamin D deficiency is extremely common among elderly North Americans.

CT levels are lower in women than in men,[23] and are reported to decrease with age.[24] Relative calcitonin deficiency has been suggested to contribute to increased bone loss in elderly women.[23] However, studies with newer, more accurate radioimmunoassays for this hormone have failed to confirm the presence of age- or estrogen-related changes in circulating CT,[25] so a major role for calcitonin deficiency in age-related bone loss or in the pathogenesis of osteoporosis remains in doubt.

Effect of Pregnancy

Since the average fetus acquires 30 g calcium during gestation, pregnancy has been considered traditionally to constitute a challenge to the maternal skeleton. It is now clear that robust adaptations to pregnancy more than compensate for fetal mineral needs. These adaptations reflect both the high estogen environment and increased weight-bearing of pregnant women. Elevations in circulating free and bound calcitriol accompany increased estrogen production, and are mirrored in improved calcium absorption and balance. The extent to which elevated calcitriol production may reflect placental 1 α hydroxylase activity is unknown. Calcitonin levels rise during pregnancy and may play a role in protecting the maternal skeleton.[26,27] A recent demonstration that serum levels of the osteoblast-derived peptide, osteocalcin, decrease during pregnancy supports the conclusion that bone remodeling is suppressed starting in the second trimester.[28] Changes in circulating PTH during pregnancy are not well-defined, and reported increases during the second trimester have not been confirmed consistently.

Regulation of Plasma Calcium

By tradition, PTH action on bone has been considered the primary means by which adjustments are made in minute-to-minute alterations in plasma calcium levels. Nordin and Peacock[29] have summarized weaknesses in this model, and proposed that the kidney is probably more important for maintaining plasma calcium under relatively normal conditions, with increased contributions from bone when hypocalcemic stresses are particularly intense or prolonged. They calculated that if a subject is in skeletal balance, that is, if he or she is neither gaining nor losing bone, if intestinal calcium absorption is constant, and if the glomerular filtration rate remains at 100 ml/min, 98 percent reabsorption of filtered calcium would produce a serum calcium concentration of 6 mg/dl. Were reabsorption efficiency to increase to 99 percent, the serum calcium level would rise to about 12 mg/dl. Thus, minor alterations in the efficiency of renal calcium handling may elicit major changes in plasma calcium level. Additional work in rats supports a critical role for the kidney in maintaining plasma calcium, with a relatively important skeletal contribution in young, rapidly growing animals, and in animals exposed to sustained dietary calcium deficiency.[30]

The relative importance of bone and kidney to calcium homeostasis in humans remain incompletely defined, but a primary role for the kidney under usual daily conditions of feeding and fasting remains attractive. Accordingly, the following model for calcium homeostasis can be proposed tentatively. Reduction in plasma calcium levels are quickly registered by the parathyroid glands, which increase PTH secretion. PTH promotes tubular reabsorption of calcium in the kidney, which generally suffices to restore plasma calcium to normal. Under prolonged exposure to high levels of PTH, renal production of calcitriol levels rises. This effect is magnified by phosphorus depletion, achieved through the classic phosphaturic effect of PTH, and leads over a period of days to weeks to increased intestinal calcium absorption. Finally, when the calcemic stress is particularly severe or persistent, PTH-dependent activation of remodeling results in mobilization of calcium from the skeleton.

When plasma calcium levels rise, PTH secretion is suppressed, and tubular calcium reabsorption decreases. The decrease in circulating PTH increases renal phosphorus conservation, and both of these reduce calcitriol production, thereby decreasing intestinal calcium absorption. Finally, bone remodeling is suppressed.

Thus, one may construct a coherent model for calcium homeostasis in humans based on the participation of two hormones, PTH and calcitriol, and involving the hierarchic contributions of kidney, intestine, and bone. The importance of other hormones in humans, such as calcitonin, to this scheme remains unsettled, but it is likely that these modulate the parathyroid–vitamin D axis rather than serving as primary regulators.

ACKNOWLEDGMENTS

This work was supported in part by NIH Grant No. AGO4458-03A3 and by the Research Service, Veterans Administration. The manuscript was expertly prepared by Ms. Susan Singh.

REFERENCES

1. Rasmussen, H: The calcium messenger system. N Engl J Med 314:1164, 1986
2. Committee on Dietary Allowances, Food and Nutrition Board, National Research Council: Recommended Dietary Allowances, National Academy of Sciences, Washington, DC, 1980, p. 125
3. Heaney, RP, Recker, RR, Saville PD: Calcium balance and calcium requirements in middle-aged women. Am J Clin Nutr 30:1603, 1977
4. Carroll MD, Abraham S. Dresser CM: Dietary Intake Source Data 1976–1980. DHHS Publication No. (PHS) 83-1681. US Government Printing Office, Washington, DC, 1983
5. Marcus R: Normal and abnormal bone remodeling in man. Annu Rev Med 38:129, 1987

6. Wong GL: Skeletal effects of parathyroid hormone. p. 103. In Peck WA (ed): Bone and Mineral Research Annual. Vol. 4. Elsevier Biomedical, Amsterdam, 1986
7. Chase LR, Aurbach GD: Parathyroid function and the renal excretion of 3′-5′ adenylic acid. Proc Natl Acad Sci USA 58:518, 1967
8. Chase LR, Aurbach GD: Renal adenyl cyclase: anatomically separate site for parathyroid hormone and vasopressin. Science 159:545, 1968
9. Chase LR, Melson GL, Aurbach GD: Pseudohypoparathyroidism: defective excretion of 3′,5′-AMP in response to parathyroid hormone. J Clin Invest 48:1832, 1969
10. Farfel Z, Brickman AS, Kaslow HR, et al: Defect of receptor-cyclase coupling protein in pseudohypoparathyroidism. N Engl J Med 303:237, 1980
11. Downs, RW, Jr., Levine MA, Drezner MK, et al: Deficient adenylate cyclase regulatory protein in renal membranes from a patient with pseudohypoparathyroidism. J Clin Invest 71:231, 1983
12. Hruska KA, Moskowitz D, Esbrit P, et al: Stimulation of inositol triphosphate and diacylglycerol production in renal tubular cells by parathyroid hormone J Clin Invest 79:230, 1987
13. Austin LA, Heath H III, Go VLW: Reulation of calcitonin secretion in normal man by changes of serum calcium within the physiologic range. J Clin Invest 64:1721, 1979
14. Heersche JNM, Marcus R, Aurbach GD: Calcitonin and the formation of 3′-5′-AMP in bone and kidney. Endocrinology 94:241, 1974
15. Haussler MR, McCain TA: Vitamin D metabolism and action (2 parts). N Engl J Med 297:974, 1977
16. Norman AW, Henry HL: Vitamin D to 1,25-dihydroxycholecalciferol: evolution to a steroid hormone. Trends Biochem Sci 4:14, 1979
17. DeLuca HF: Metabolism and mechanism of action of vitamin D-1982, p. 7. In Peck WA (ed): Bone and Mineral Research Annual. Vol. 1. Excerpta Medica, Amsterdam, 1983
18. Suda T, Miyaura C, Abe E, Kuroki T: Modulation of cell differentiation, immune responses and tumor promotion by vitamin D compounds. p. 1. In Peck WA (ed): Bone and Mineral Research Annual. Vol. 4. Elsevier Biomedical, Amsterdam, 1986
19. Bouillon RA, Auwerx JH, Lissens WD, Pelemans WK: Vitamin D status in the elderly: seasonal substrate deficiency causes 1,25-dihydroxycholecalciferol deficiency. Am J Clin Nutr 45:755, 1987
20. Wiske PS, Epstein S, Bell NH, et al: Increases in immunoreactive parathyroid hormone with age. N Engl J Med 300:1419, 1979
21. Marcus, R, Madvig P, Young G: Age-related changes in parathyroid hormone and parathyroid hormone action in normal humans. J. Clin Endocrinol Metab 58:223, 1984
22. Young G, Marcus R, Minkoff JR, et al: Age-related rise in parathyroid hormone in man: the use of "intact" and "mid-molecule" antisera to distinguish hormone secretion from retention. J Bone Min Res 2:367, 1987
23. Hillyard CJ, Stevenson JC, MacIntyre I: Relative deficiency of plasma-calcitonin in normal women. Lancet 1:961, 1978
24. Shamonki IM, Frumar AM, Tataryn IV, et al: Age-related changes of calcitonin secretion in females. J Clin Endocrinol Metab 50:437, 1980
25. Body JJ, Heath H III: Estimates of circulating monomeric calcitonin: physiological studies in normal and thyroidectomized man. J Clin Endocrinol Metab 57:897, 1983
26. Samaan NA, Anderson GD, Adam-Mayne ME: Immunoreactive calcitonin in the mother, neonate, child and adult. Am J Obstet Gynecol 121:622, 1975

27. Stevenson JC, Hillyard C, MacIntyre I, et al: A physiological role for calcitonin: protection of the maternal skeleton. Lancet 2:769, 1979
28. Cole DE, Gundberg, CM, Stirk LJ, et al: Changing osteocalcin concentrations during pregnancy and lactation: implications for maternal mineral metabolism. J Clin Endocrinol Metab 65:290, 1987
29. Nordin BEC, Peacock M: The role of the kidney in serum calcium homeostasis. p. 472. In Taylor S, Foster G (eds): Calcitonin. Heineman, London 1969
30. Kalu DN, Hadji-Georgopoulos A, Foster GV: Effect of calcium deprivation on parathyroid hormone-mediated bone and kidney contributions to the maintenance of plasma calcium in rats. J Endocrinol 64:299, 1975
31. Habener JF, Jacobs JW: Biosynthesis and control of secretion of the calcium-regulating peptides. p. 145. In Parsons JA(ed): Endocrinology of Calcium Metabolism. Raven Press, New York, 1982
32. Holick MF: Vitamin D: Relevance for Clinical Medicine. Nichols Institute, Los Angeles, 1981

3 Diagnostic Tests for Metabolic Bone and Mineral Disorders

Arch K. Taylor
Mark W. Lundy
Cesar R. Libanati
David J. Baylink

In the past a major difficulty in the diagnosis and management of metabolic bone diseases has been the lack of convenient and accurate means by which the metabolic state of the bone could be monitored. Remarkable advances have been made in diagnostic methods, particularly in the realm of densitometric methods, so that accurate diagnosis of metabolic bone diseases can now be made. These densitometric methods, along with other methods such as biochemical assays and bone biopsy analysis, are discussed in this chapter. The focus is on the strengths and weaknesses of each method and the indications for each.

RADIOLOGIC AND DENSITOMETRIC MEASUREMENTS

A variety of methods, described under the general classification of radiologic and densitometric measurements, are available for the diagnosis and monitoring of metabolic bone diseases. Chief among these are radiographs, single and dual photon absorptiometry, quantitative computer tomography, and bone scans. This section discusses the advantages and disadvantages of each of these methods and their use in the diagnosis and monitoring of metabolic bone diseases, with a special emphasis on the diagnosis of osteoporosis.

Radiographs

The visualization of skeletal tissue on radiographs is the oldest of the noninvasive methods of diagnosing metabolic bone disorders and remains one of the best tools for evaluating the severity of osteoporosis. These tests are quick, site-specific, noninvasive, allow for multiple measurements at the same site, available in most communities, and compared to the other techniques discussed in this section, relatively inexpensive. The major disadvantage of this method is its insensitivity. At least 30 percent of the bone mineral must be lost before changes can be detected on radiographs of the spine.[1] This deficiency makes this technique of little use for monitoring the effect of treatment on bone density in diseases such as osteoporosis or for identifying persons at risk for this disease. Certain characteristics attributed to the presence of osteoporosis can, however, be identified using spinal radiography. These include a diffuse radiolucency of the vertebrae accompanied by "pencil thin" cortices and accentuated vertical trabeculii, wedging of the vertebrae with the anterior height more than 15 percent less than the posterior height, collapsed vertebra, and biconcavity, which is especially seen in the lumbar vertebra in association with an expansion of the intervertebral discs.[2] Although atraumatic anterior wedging of the thoracic vertebrae is pathognomonic of osteoporosis, the presence of posterior wedging or the collapse of a single vertebra with no apparent involvement of any other vertebra is most likely due to trauma or a local lesion such as can be seen with a metastatic malignancy,[1,2] and is less likely due to osteoporosis. Although it is the most common cause of deformed vertebra, it must be remembered that osteoporosis is not the only bone disease that can cause these deformities and that other diseases can occur along with typical osteoporosis.

Another radiographic technique involves the measurement of cortical bone thickness of the metacarpals.[3] The inner and outer diameters of the cortical bone cylinder are measured using calipers and, if we assume that the bone is a true cylinder, the values obtained can be used to determine indices such as cortical thickness and cross-sectional cortical area.[4] These indices can then be used to differentiate normal from severely osteoporotic women. The technique is inexpensive and reproducible and can be used to detect both endosteal and periosteal changes. It does, however, have a significant drawback. In early osteoporosis, the cortical bone of the appendicular skeleton is less involved in bone loss than the trabecular bone of the axial skeleton. Because of this, changes in the cortical thickness of the metacarpals can only be detected in the advanced stages of the disease, when vertebral fractures are already present. Thus, significant loss of bone from the spine can occur in the presence of normal cortical bone indices. It, therefore, cannot be used for the early detection of osteoporosis or for screening to identify the population at risk for the disease. Additionally, the introduction of more automated and precise photon densitometric measurements has led to a decrease in the use of this technique for the diagnosis and monitoring of bone diseases.

Single Photon Absorptiometry

Single photon absorptiometry (SPA) was one of the earliest quantitative techniques of bone analysis developed.[5] Like radiographs of the metacarpal bones, SPA can only assess the appendicular bones of the skeleton. This is because the highly collimated single energy beam requires a constant thickness of soft tissue around the bone to obtain valid results. SPA does not differentiate trabecular and cortical components of the bone; the entire cross section of the bone, classically the distal radius, is assayed. SPA measures both the bone mineral content (BMC) and the bone width (BW). The bone mineral density (BMD) per unit area can then be estimated by dividing the BMC by the BW at the site examined. This is the easiest, least expensive, and most reproducible of the bone densitometric methods. It does, however, suffer from the same drawback as the measurement of the metacarpal cortical thickness described above. The radius, like the metacarpals, is primarily cortical bone. Because of this, there is a good correlation between the BMC of the radius and the BMC of the other long bones and with the total skeletal mass,[6,7] which consists of 80 percent cortical bone. However, the correlation with the bone density of the spine, which is made up of about 65 percent trabecular bone,[8] is weak. Although a low radial BMC is almost invariably indicative of a low spinal density, a normal radial BMC does not exclude the existence of osteoporosis. Although these problems exist, SPA of the radius has been used in research studies to evaluate the effectiveness of therapy on osteoporosis. Estrogen treatment of perimenopausal women has been shown to prevent loss of bone density of the radius as measured with SPA.[9] On the other hand, response to fluoride treatment, which has been shown to increase bone volume in the axial skeleton, could not be detected using this method.[10] This demonstrates the need for the appropriate choice of technique to monitor each skeletal site when evaluating the effectiveness of various treatments for osteoporosis.

Dual Photon Absorptiometry

The major advantage of bone density assessment by dual photon absorptiometry (DPA), as opposed to that by SPA, is that DPA measurements are done at two distinct energy levels instead of one.[11] This overcomes the requirement by SPA for a constant thickness of soft tissue around the bone and enables it to be used for the measurement of any skeletal site. This method is particularly useful for measuring the hip and the spine, areas that are inaccessible for measurements by SPA and are at high risk for fractures in patients with osteoporosis. A second advantage of the dual energy method is that mineral content measurements are less influenced by variations in marrow fat content of the bone. Marrow fat content of the spine increases in the elderly and, unless corrected for, tends to cause misleading results in determinations of spinal densities.

With today's technology DPA is the best method for measuring the BMC of the hip, a site of major clinical interest in osteoporosis. When care is taken to ensure proper positioning of the femur, these measurements are reproducible and can be used to identify patients at risk for hip fractures and for monitoring changes occurring with time.

On the other hand, DPA measurements of the spine are subject to several methodologic problems. First, DPA measures the density of the entire vertebral body including the spinous processes and not just the trabecular bone, the most important determinant of vertebral strength.[12] A second problem, especially among the elderly, is the presence of compression fractures. A compression of the vertebral body, which reduces the vertebral volume and thereby increases its density, will give the appearance of a normal, or possibly above normal, bone density for the vertebra in question. Since DPA measurements are done on a number of vertebrae, the existence of fractures in any one or more of these will produce a falsely elevated BMC unless caution is taken to exclude compressed vertebrae from the measurements, which is not always easy. Similar falsely elevated densities can occur as a result of degenerative joint disease, osteophytes, or aortic calcifications, all of which are common in the elderly.[4] In spite of these difficulties, DPA, with its relatively low exposure to radiation, low cost, and widespread availability, may be the method of choice for screening younger adults (i.e., less than 50 years of age) for spinal bone densities. Before this can be advocated, however, a strong relationship between bone mineral content, as measured by DPA, and spinal fractures, must be documented.

Quantitative Computed Tomography

Another densitometric method is quantitative computed tomography (QCT). Similar to the photon absorptiometry methods, QCT exists in both single and dual energy modes and can be used to examine the bones of both the axial and appendicular skeleton. The major advantage of QCT over DPA is its ability to differentiate the trabecular bone densities of the vertebrae from the cortical bone densities, which allows a direct measurement of the most reactive part of the vertebra. This is of great importance since the trabecular component of the vertebrae has been shown, both in vitro and in vivo, to be the most important determinant of vertebral strength.[12] This ability, along with its ability to isolate and analyze precisely a region of interest within a three-dimensional slice, allows accurate measurements that are unaffected by degenerative joint disease, osteophytes, or aortic calcifications, all of which affect the accuracy of DPA.[13]

The initial problem of standardizing density values, especially between different machines, has been addressed through the use of special calibration phantoms containing solutions of various concentrations of K_2HPO_4, which have radiologic attenuation properties similar to those of hydroxyapatite. The measured density of the region of interest of the vertebra, usually the trabecular region, is compared to the known densities of the phantom and is calculated[13] in equivalents of K_2HPO_4. Using this method, Genant and co-workers report a 3 to 4 percent coefficient of variation between scanners, indicating that results obtained on a scanner at one site can be compared to those obtained using different scanners at different sites.[14]

Although single energy QCT provides a reliable method for determining trabecular spinal densities, it does have some disadvantages. The measurements require at least 20 minutes to perform and patients, particularly the elderly osteoporotic, complain about the uncomfortable position and the hard scanning table. Additionally, it is costly and does not adjust for increasing marrow fat in the elderly. Although the influence of marrow fat in density measurements can be overcome by the use of dual energy QCT, this occurs with a loss of precision and an increase in radiation dose. Because of this, dual energy QCT is currently used only in clinical research studies. Despite these disadvantages, the ability of single energy QCT to assess accurately the spinal trabecular bone density allows it to be more quantitative and more definitive than DPA for the diagnosis of osteoporosis, and, in particular, for the identification of the population at risk for fractures before these occur.

The major problem of using spinal bone density measurements, as assessed by either DPA or QCT, as a means of diagnosis resides in the difficulty in establishing a working definition for osteoporosis. Attempts to establish normal ranges of spinal densities that would distinguish normals from osteoporotics (i.e., those more than two standard deviations below the mean value of the normal range) have proven unsuccessful, except in young adults between the ages of 20 and 40. This is because bone densities, unlike some other body parameters, normally decrease with age as a continuous variable.[15] As a result, the normal range gradually merges with the osteoporotic, making it difficult to distinguish between the two. Because of this investigators have taken a new approach to addressing this problem,[13,16] and have sought to define an absolute density level, rather than an age-adjusted one, to predict fracture risk. An operational definition of this *fracture threshold* is the absolute theoretical vertebral trabecular bone density level that can be used to classify patients into two groups: those with a high risk for nontraumatic spinal fractures and those with a low risk. In a study of 100 female patients referred to our clinic for evaluation of osteoporosis, we were able to show a strong negative correlation between the number of vertebral fractures per patient as well as the presence of vertebral fractures versus the trabecular vertebral body density as determined by QCT.[17] Based on these data we have assigned an operational fracture threshold for women at 100 mg/cm^3 and quantitatively define osteoporosis as occurring in persons having a trabecular vertebral body density of 100 mg/cm^3 or less. The value for men was somewhat higher (around 130 mg/cm^3); however, the number of men in the study was small and this value is just an estimate. It should be pointed out here that fracture threshold is being used to identify those with an increased risk of nontraumatic fractures and not as an absolute value to say who will or will not suffer from fractures. In this study all women had at least one fracture when their density was below 70 mg/cm^3, while no women with densities above 103 mg/cm^3 had spinal fractures (Fig. 3-1). Between these two values there was a continuum of increasing fracture risk with decreasing density, with a 50 percent risk at 85 mg/cm^3. Our vertebral fracture threshold value is similar to that reported by other investigators. The major clinical value of such a threshold is that it can be used to identify patients at imminent risk for fracture before irreversible spinal deformity occurs. For example, an early menopause patient with a spinal bone density of 110 would predictably have a density of 100 in about 3 years due to the documented rate of bone loss of 3 to 5 percent per year during the early menopause. Thus, although this patient's level is above the fracture threshold and would probably have no symptoms of osteoporosis, it would be possible to predict that she would develop the disease within 3 to 5 years. This would indicate the vital need to inititate prophylactic therapy at this time and the importance of monitoring the effectiveness of the treatment indicated. In addition, any female patient whose level falls below 100 mg/cm^3 requires a form of therapy to increase vertebral bone density above the fracture threshold. For such patients we routinely use fluoride therapy,[18] which increases density at a rate of 12 mg/cm^3/year.

Unfortunately, because of the expense involved and the presently limited number of instruments available to doing these determinations, mass screening by QCT is not yet a feasible technique.

Bone Scans

The use of bone scans or total skeletal scintigrams is a radiologic method that takes advantage of the increased skeletal uptake of technetium 99 labeled diphosphonates in sites of bone formation. These sites will then appear as "hot spots" on skeletal scintigrams.

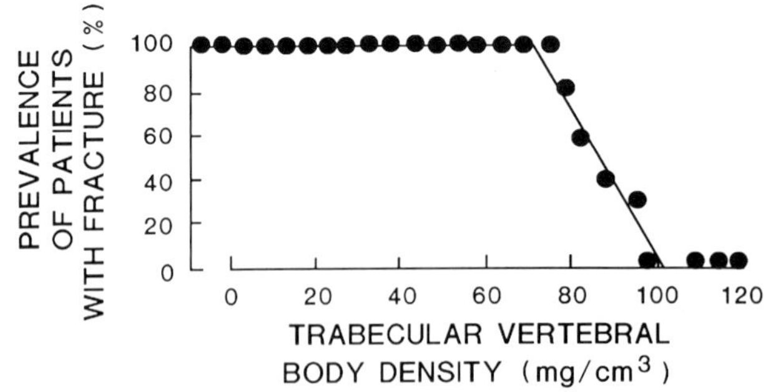

Fig. 3-1 Relationship between percentage of patients with fractures and trabecular vertebral body density (TVBD). Prevalence of patients with vertebral body fractures in 100 female patients as a function of TVBD. Each point represents the mean of four patients.

Bone scans, although not usually required in the diagnosis and evaluation of osteoporosis, can be utilized to detect stress fractures that may not yet be apparent on radiographs. The early detection of these fractures and their proper treatment, particularly at the hip, can reduce the need for surgery. On the other hand, bone scans have proved to be valuable in the identification of local bone lesions such as can be seen in Paget's disease and metastatic bone disease, since these lesions will also appear as "hot spots" on bone scans. Finally, bone scans can also be used to delineate sites of degenerative joint disease.

In summary, the diagnosis and monitoring of spinal-density-related bone disease can best be accomplished by QCT, with the greatest disadvantages being the expense of the measurements and the discomfort to the patient. On the other hand, DPA is an excellent method for monitoring hip densities. Radiographs of the thoracic and lumbar spine remain a valuable method for detecting fractures and can be useful for the diagnosis of osteoporosis when other more sensitive methods are not available.

BONE-SPECIFIC BIOCHEMICAL MARKERS AND HORMONES

A second group of methods for diagnosing metabolic bone disorders involves the use of urine and serum assays for various bone-specific biochemical markers or hormones. The major advantage of these assays is that they can be used to monitor short-term changes in the physiologic state of the patient. They are not, however, site-specific and thus can only be used as a means of monitoring general overall skeletal trends. Although the use of single assays can be beneficial in the diagnosis of some diseases such as Paget's disease and hyperparathyroidism, it is often necessary to use a battery of different assays to characterize properly some disorders. For example, some bone metabolic diseases, such as postmenopausal osteoporosis, result in normal or near-normal levels of the various bone markers, making the diagnosis of these diseases, based on individual biochemical assays alone, difficult if not impossible. However, since bone mass is maintained through a coupling of bone formation with bone resorption, a patient with elevated but normal resorption, and depressed but normal formation would be experiencing a negative bone balance and be at risk for osteoporosis. On the other hand, a reversal of this relationship between bone formation and bone resorption as a result of therapy would indicate an increase in bone mass. Although present biochemical assays are not sensitive enough to be used in this manner, new assays, some of which are discussed in this section, are being developed, and their use in the assessment of bone balance in metabolic bone diseases is being studied. All biochemical abnormalities must be interpreted only after taking into consideration the entire clinical situation, including radiologic and densitometric results and, occasionally, bone biopsy results.

Bone Formation Markers

The formation of new bone by osteoblasts (bone-forming cells) can be monitored by the measurement of serum levels of various markers of bone formation such as alkaline phosphatase, osteocalcin (bone gla protein), and possibly the terminal extensions of procollagen.

Alkaline Phosphatase

The most commonly used marker for bone formation is serum alkaline phosphatase (AlP). Since the relationship between increases in serum AlP and increases in osteoblastic activity was first reported,[19] substantial amounts of evidence have been amassed linking AlP and bone formation.[20,21] However, AlP has been isolated from several different tissues, including bone, liver, kidney, intestine, and placenta.[22] Of these, except during pregnancy, only the bone and the liver contribute significant amounts to the serum levels of AlP in normal adults. Skeletal AlP is primarily located in the membrane of osteoblasts[23]; however, the mechanism of its release into the extracellular fluid and its actual role in bone formation remain unknown. Nonetheless, serum levels of AlP have been shown to correlate with bone formation in patients who demonstrate a high rate of bone turnover, such as those with Paget's disease.[24] During these times, the skeletal isozyme constitutes the majority of the serum AlP. For conditions associated with normal or below normal rates of bone formation, the skeletal isozyme usually contributes around 50 percent of the total AlP activity. In order to demonstrate a good correlation with bone formation in these cases, it is necessary to identify the contribution that the skeletal isozyme makes to the total serum level.

Several methods to separate the skeletal isozyme from the hepatic isozyme have been described. These include heat denaturation, chemical inhibition of kinetic activity, electrophoretic separation, and immunologic specificites.[25–28] None of these existing methods has proven entirely adequate. Since the skeletal isozyme is more sensitive to heat denaturation than the hepatic isozyme,[29] some investigators have attempted to quantitate the isozyme levels by comparing the total activity before and after heating the serum samples[29]; however, this method has proven to be subject to interference and to give only a rough estimate of the skeletal isozyme.[22,30] A method combining heat denaturation and chemical inhibition is very tedious, requires careful controls for even moderate reproducibility, and does not lend itself to the examination of a large number of samples.[29] The electrophoretic separation methods of determining the skeletal isozyme are also not convenient for examining large numbers of samples, and overlapping of the skeletal and the hepatic isozymes can make the quantitation of these enzymes by densitometry difficult.[22] Immunologic assays using polyclonal antibodies have been developed[31]; however, because the hepatic, renal, and skeletal isozymes are the product of a single gene,[32] existing assays have not been able to differentiate between them. With the introduction of monoclonal antibody techniques, the development of immunoassays that are able to differentiate between these isozymes may occur in the near future. Recently, a new assay, based on the ability of wheat germ lectin specifically to absorb the skeletal isozyme from the serum due to differences in the post-translational modifications of the carbohydrate side chains of the molecule, has been introduced.[33] Although this assay is thought to differentiate the skeletal AlP from other serum AlPs, more testing is needed to confirm the usefulness of this procedure.

Because of these difficulties in measuring the specific isozymes of AlP, clinical examinations usually include determinations only of the total AlP activity. Total serum AlP activity, consisting of a summation of the activities of the isozymes derived from a number of various organs including bone, liver, and intestine, should be considered to be a useful but rather insensitive marker for the rate of bone formation. Except in cases of large increases in bone formation, as is seen in Paget's disease, total AlP can not be used as a specific index of osteoblast function.

The normal levels of serum AlP are determined by age, sex, and hormonal status. There is an increase in total AlP, which can be attributed to the skeletal isozyme, during childhood and periods of adolescent growth.[34] During adulthood, total AlP levels remain relatively constant, with men having slightly higher levels of both total and skeletal AlP than women.[34,35]

Elevated total AlP levels are seen in a number of metabolic bone diseases including Paget's disease, renal osteodystrophy, vitamin D deficiency, primary and secondary hyperparathyroidism, osteomalacia, primary and metastatic cancers of the bone, acromegaly, and fractures.[36,37] On the other hand, low levels of serum AlP are usually seen only in hypophosphatasia, a rare disorder of mineralization, and sometimes in hypoparathyroidism. Besides bone disorders, elevated serum levels of AlP can also result from diseases of the liver and gastrointestinal tract, from hyperthyroidism, and from the ectopic production of the enzyme by tumors.[36]

For monitoring the response of various diseases to treatment, serial measurements of total AlP levels are more useful than single measurements. For example, serial measurements of total AlP in osteoporotic patients being treated with fluoride show an increase in AlP that is fluoride-dependent and that can be associated with a response to the treatment.[10,38] A single determination of AlP may fail to indicate such an increase, since the time between the start of therapy and the initial increase in activity varies and the increase is not always sustained. Further evidence of the usefulness of serial measurements of total AlP can be seen in the treatment of Paget's disease. Treatment with calcitonin or diphosphonates will bring about a decrease in the serum levels of AlP while an exacerbation of the disease is accompanied by an increase in AlP.[39–41]

Although total AlP can be a useful index of the rate of bone formation, because it reflects an accumulation of isozymes from a number of organs (especially bone and liver), a variety of diseases must be considered in the interpretation of elevated levels of AlP, particularly when only a single determination is made. With the development of better assays for the measurement of the various isozymes, quantitation of the skeletal AlP should prove to be of greater use in the diagnosis and treatment of metabolic bone diseases.

Osteocalcin

A second biochemical index of bone formation is osteocalcin (OC). Osteocalcin, also called bone gla protein or BGP, is a vitamin-K-dependent calcium-binding protein found in bone.[42,43] It is a 49-amino-acid protein with a molecular weight of 5800, which is synthesized by osteoblasts and constitutes up to 20 percent of the noncollagenous proteins found in bovine bone.[43] One of the unusual properties of this protein is the presence of gamma-carboxyglutamic acid residues, which confers a high affinity for hydroxyapatite.[44,45] Although OC is found primarily in the bone, small amounts can be detected in the serum. Evidence indicates that this circulating OC is an index of bone formation and not bone resorption.[46,47]

Serum OC is usually measured using radioimmunoassays developed against bovine OC.[37,48–50] Although the use of these assays in clinical studies is still experimental, data accumulated indicate that measurements of circulating OC can be indicators of bone turnover. This is true even in situations of concurrent liver disease resulting in high serum AlP caused by increases in the circulating level of liver AlP. In general, serum levels of OC are raised in diseases characterized by increases in bone turnover such as primary and secondary hyperparathyroidism, Paget's disease, bone metastasis, fractures, and renal osteodystrophy.[37,51] In contrast, low levels of OC have been reported in patients with low bone turnover, such as those with hypoparathyroidism.[37,51] Two exceptions to the correlation of OC levels with bone formation are in patients treated with high doses of 1,25 dihydroxyvitamin D (1,25-D), and in patients with renal failure. 1,25-D is a regulatior of OC synthesis and high doses can increase OC levels without a corresponding increase in bone formation.[52] Serum OC is normally rapidly cleared by glomerular filtration.[46] Impaired renal function causes an accumulation of immunoreactive fragments that will be detected in the immunoassays, giving rise to high serum levels of OC.[53]

Care must be taken when interpreting serum OC results. In addition to the possibility of high serum levels caused by impaired renal function or treatment with high doses of 1,25-D, OC has also been shown to undergo a large diurnal variation, peaking during the late night and early morning and dropping during the late morning and early afternoon.[54] Because of this, it is important that samples be taken at the same time each day, especially when serial measurements are being done to monitor progress during treatment.

Although the accumulated research is promising, further studies are required to determine the value of OC measurements in the diagnosis and management of patients with metabolic bone disease.

Procollagen Peptide

Like OC measurements, assays for procollagen peptides have been limited to clinical research and have not yet found their way into routine clinical testing.

Collagen is the most abundant protein in bone, accounting for 90 to 95 percent of the total.[55] The basic structure of type I collagen, the type found in bone, consists of two α_1-(I) and one α_2-chain coiled around each other, forming a "right-handed" triple helix.[56] These molecules are produced as precursor molecules called procollagen, which have substantial extensions at both the aminoterminal and carboxyterminal ends compared to the final collagen molecule.[57] The procollagen is secreted as an intact molecule with a molecular weight of approximately 450,000 daltons.[58] Prior to insertion into the existing extracellular matrix, the terminal ends are proteolytically removed.[59] Radioimmunoassays for the carboxyterminal peptide have been developed that allow circulating levels of the peptide to be measured.[60]

To date, the studies done using these assays have been sparse but promising, with most of them centering on investigations of Paget's disease.[61,62] As would be expected, serum from patients with Paget's disease contain high levels of type I procollagen peptides compared to serum of normal individuals.[61] In addition, a decrease in the level of the peptide was observed following treatment of the disease with calcitonin or diphosphonates.[61] On the other hand, osteogenesis imperfecta, a disease characterized by defective collagen production, has been shown to have low levels of circulating procollagen peptides.[63]

Although these data are few, this assay may prove to be a valuable test for diagnosing metabolic bone diseases since, unlike A1P and OC, whose biological functions during bone formation are unknown, a direct relationship between procollagen peptide synthesis and new bone-specific collagen formation can be shown.

Bone Resorption Assays

Changes in bone resorption are clinically more difficult to detect. There are no good, simple assays for markers of bone resorption. Those that are available include assays for urinary hydroxyproline and serum tartrate-resistant acid phosphatase.

Hydroxyproline

The most commonly used marker for bone resorption is urinary hydroxyproline. Hydroxyproline is an amino acid produced as a result of a posttranslational modification of proline during collagen synthesis, and is found almost exclusively in collagen.[55,64] During collagen turnover, it is released into the serum and cleared from the body in the urine. There are, however, some difficulties in using hydroxyproline as a marker of bone resorption. First, hydroxyproline is found in all collagens and not just type I.[55] Therefore, it cannot be considered as a marker entirely specific for bone. Second, a large portion of the hydroxyproline is degraded in the liver into materials that cannot be detected by assays for hydroxyproline.[65,66] Because of this, hydroxyproline cannot be used as an absolutely quantitative method for the analysis of collagen breakdown. Finally, it has been suggested that about 10 percent of the urinary hydroxyproline is indicative of formation, and not resorption, being released during the proteolytic processing of procollagen.[67] Even with these drawbacks, the measurement of urinary levels of hydroxyproline remains the most widely used marker for monitoring rates of bone resorption.

Normal values for hydroxyproline excretion are dependent on several factors including age, sex, body size, and dietary intake of collagenous material.[35,67,68] Similar to the markers of bone formation, urinary hydroxyproline levels are elevated during childhood and adolescent growth, which are times of increased skeletal turnover.[35,67] In adults, higher 24-hour levels are reported for men than for women.[69] This is generally due to the larger size of men and their greater collagen mass. When body size is corrected for by reporting hydroxyproline/creatinine ratios, this difference disappears.[69] Finally, dietary hydroxyproline is rapidly absorbed in the intestine and excreted into the urine.[69] To prevent this from contributing significantly to the urinary levels of hydroxyproline, patients are usually placed on a diet free of collagen-containing foods for the day before and the day of the urine collection.

The greatest clinical application for monitoring urinary hydroxyproline is as an index of bone-resorptive activity in Paget's disease and as a method of monitoring treatment. Effective treatment of the disease with calcitonin or diphosphonates will bring about a decrease in the 24-hour excretion of hydroxyproline. In addition, elevated levels of hydroxyproline are also found in patients with hyperparathyroidism, osteomalacia, hyperthyroidism, and acromegaly.[67,68]

Tartrate-Resistant Acid Phosphatase

A second, less commonly used marker for bone resorption is the serum tartrate-resident acid phosphatase (TR-AcP). Osteoclasts, the cells responsible for bone resorption, can be differentiated from other bone cells in histologic sections by the presence of TR-AcP,[69] an enzyme similar to the TR-AcP found in serum.[69,70] Currently, TR-AcP can be measured in one of two ways: either with an enzyme immunoassay using antibodies produced against the AcP isolated from the spleen of a patient with hairy cell leukemia[71], or with a colorimetric assay in the presence of sodium tartrate.[72,73] Although both of these methods of determining TR-AcP have been published, the assays have not yet been established as routine clinical assays and are limited to use in clinical research.

The normal values for TR-AcP vary with age, sex, and hormonal status in a manner similar to that of the other markers of bone turnover. High levels, found during childhood and adolescence, decline after puberty and remain relatively constant throughout adulthood.[35] There are not many reports on the use of measurements of TR-AcP in the diagnosis or monitoring of metabolic bone disease. However, the available data indicate that measurements of serum levels of TR-AcP may be of value in evaluating osteoclastic activity in bone turnover. In a recent report, it was shown that both Paget's disease patients, who have increased bone turnover, and immobilized patients, who have an imbalance in bone turnover in favor of resorption, have increased serum levels of TR-AcP.[73] In contrast to these patients, those with low turnover compared to normal, such as patients with hypoparathyroidism, have lower than normal levels of serum TR-AcP.[73]

Even though the actual cellular source of the serum TR-AcP has not yet been established, available evidence indicates that serum levels of the enzyme may come to be an excellent marker for monitoring the rate of bone resorption.

Hormonal Assays

In addition to the measurement of the indices of bone formation and bone resorption, additional diagnostic information about bone and calcium metabolism can be obtained through assays of calcium-regulating hormones. The two most important hormones involved with calcium homeostasis are parathyroid hormone and the metabolites of vitamin D, especially 1,25 dihydroxyvitamin D.

Parathyroid Hormone

Parathyroid hormone (PTH) is produced by the parathyroid glands and released into the circulation at a basal level and also in proportion to a decrease in serum levels of calcium. Thus, hypocalcemia stimulates the release of PTH, which, in turn, works to increase the circulating levels of calcium through a direct effect of the hormone on the bone and kidney, and an indirect action on the intestine mediated by the effect of PTH to increase serum levels of 1,25 dihydroxyvitamin D (1,25-D). PTH directly increases bone resorption by stimulating the action of osteoclasts, the cells responsible for bone resorption.[74] Calcium, released from the skeletal reservoir during resorption, enters the circulation and increases the serum level of calcium making it available for use by the body. PTH acts on the kidneys to bring about an increase in the renal reabsorption of calcium by the kidney tubules, which reduces loss of calcium in the urine.[75] Finally, PTH stimulates renal production of 1,25-D, the active metabolite of vitamin D, which, in turn, increases the intestinal absorption of dietary calcium.[76,77]

PTH is initially synthesized as a 115-amino-acid precursor and is processed into the 84-amino-acid active polypeptide before secretion.[78–81] When secretion of the intact peptide is inhibited by high levels of serum calcium, the intracellular PTH is further metabolized and secreted as biologically inactive fragments.[82–85] Intact circulating PTH is rapidly cleared from the serum by metabolic cleavage in the kidney and liver,[86] forming biologically inactive midmolecule and carboxyterminal fragments, and biologically active aminoterminal fragments.[87] Because the clearance rate of the C-terminal fragments is much lower than that of either the intact molecule or the N-terminal fragment,[88] C-terminal fragments are the predominant peptides found in normal serum.

Radioimmunoassays for determining serum levels of PTH have been developed using bovine PTH, human PTH, and synthetic fragments of human PTH.[84,89,90] Interpretation of the results from these assays is dependent upon the specificity of the antisera used. Antisera that recognize the biologically inactive midmolecule and C-terminal fragments have proven to be of greater use in the diagnosis of primary hyperparathyroidism than antisera specific for the more rapidly cleared N-terminal fragments. On the other hand, levels of the midmolecule and C-terminal fragments, which are normally cleared by the kidneys, can be very high in patients with renal failure and, consequently, antisera that recognize the biologically active N-terminal fragments or the intact molecule may be more useful in the monitoring of parathyroid function in these patients.

Although the most important use for PTH assays is to differentiate between primary hyperparathyroidism and other causes of hypercalcemia such as hypercalcemia of malignancy, they can also be used to examine calcium homeostasis in elderly osteoporotic persons. For example, a patient with hypercalciuria accompanied by low serum PTH levels probably has either increased bone resorption due to a non-PTH mechanism or hyperabsorption of calcium in the intestine. On the other hand, hypercalciuria with elevated PTH levels is indicative of a renal leak of calcium. These distinctions are important because the cause of the elevated urinary calcium dictates the appropriate therapy. On the other hand, elevated serum PTH levels with normo- or hypocalcemia in the absence of hypercalciuria indicates the presence of a secondary hyperparathyroidism resulting from a vitamin D deficiency or calcium malabsorption. An increase in dietary calcium or treatment with vitamin D in these patients will usually result in a decrease in the serum levels of PTH.

Although PTH assays are useful in the diagnosis and monitoring of various metabolic bone diseases, due to the existence of circulating fragments with varying biological activities and metabolic clearance rates, it is important to know the specificity of the antisera before making any final interpretation of the results.

Vitamin D

Vitamin D, a steroid hormone, comes primarily from two sources. Vitamin D_3 (cholecalciferol) is produced as a result of ultraviolet irradiation of the skin, while vitamin D_2 (ergocalciferol) is obtained primarily in the diet in fortified dairy products. Whatever the original source of it, vitamin D is essentially biologically inactive and requires enzymatic transformation to become metabolically active. This two-step process starts in the liver, where the hormone undergoes an initial hydroxylation forming 25-hydroxyvitamin D (25-D).[91] This metabolite is further hydroxylated in the kidney, as a response to elevated

PTH, forming 1,25-D, the biologically active form of the hormone.[92] The 1,25-D then acts on the cells of the intestine to increase dietary calcium absorption. Other metabolites of vitamin D, such as 24,25 dihydroxyvitamin D and 1,24,25 trihydroxyvitamin D, have been identified but their biologic significance has not been established.

Vitamin D and its metabolites can be measured from extracted serum using either radioimmunoassays or receptor binding assays.[93] Except in cases of extreme hepatic dysfunction, the conversion of vitamin D to 25-D depends on the serum level of vitamin D. Because of this, low 25-D levels are generally seen only in cases of vitamin D deficiency resulting from poor nutrition, the inability to get adequate exposure to the sun, such as in the chronically ill bedridden patient, or vitamin D malabsorption. Elevated 25-D levels are seen only in those who are exposed to large amounts of sun, such as lifeguards, and in subjects receiving large doses of vitamin D. Disorders associated with either elevated or depressed levels of 1,25-D are also known to exist. In chronic renal failure, there is an impairment of the renal enzyme responsible for the hydroxylation of 25-D into 1,25-D, resulting in a low serum level of 1,25-D.[94] In addition, normal to low levels of 1,25-D are found in hyperthyroidism, immobilization, type I vitamin-D-dependent rickets, and vitamin-D-resistant rickets. In contrast to these diseases, elevated 1,25-D levels can be found in some patients with primary hyperparathyroidism, as a result of renal stimulation by the elevated PTH levels, type II vitamin-D-resistant rickets, and idiopathic hypercalciuria.[95]

In summary, biochemical assays can be of considerable use in the diagnosis of metabolic bone diseases; however, interpretation of the results should take into account the clinical history of the patient. The changes in the biochemical markers and hormones discussed in this chapter associated with various metabolic bone diseases are shown in Table 3-1.

Table 3-1. Bone-Specific Biochemical Markers and Hormones

	Bone Formation Marker			Bone Resorption Marker		Hormonal Effectors	
	Serum Skeletal Alkaline Phosphatase	Serum Osteocalcin	Serum Procollagen	Serum Tartrate-Resisant Acid Phosphatase	Urinary Hydroxypudine	Serum Parathyroid Hormone	Serum 1,25D
Osteoporosis	→,(↑)	→,(↑)	?	?	→	↑,→,↓	→
Osteomalacia	↑,↑↑	?	?	?	↑	→,↑	→,↓
Primary hyperparathyroidism	→,↑	↑	?	↑	↑	↑	→,↑
Secondary (renal) hyperparathyroidism	↑	↑	?	↑	NA	↑	↓
Hypoparathyroidism	→	?	?	↓	→,↓	↓	↓
Immobilization	→	?	?	↑	↑	→,↓	→,↓
Bone metastasis	↑	↑	?	↑	↑	→,↓	→,↓
Paget's disease	↑↑	↑,(↑)	↑	↑	↑↑	→	→

→, Normal; ↑, increased; ↓, decreased; (↑), slightly increased; ?, unknown; NA, not appropriate.

HISTOLOGIC ANALYSIS OF BONE BIOPSIES

A third method for diagnosis of metabolic bone diseases is the histologic analysis of bone biopsies. Biopsies are no longer used for the routine diagnosis of osteoporosis or other metabolic bone diseases because of their invasive, painful nature, and because of recent advances in densitometric and biochemical methods that provide information similar to that obtained from bone biopsy analysis. Occasionally, however, biopsies, which allow the direct examination of bone tissue, are necessary to confirm a diagnosis. Histologic examination of bone is most useful for evaluation of skeletal disorders such as Paget's disease, renal osteodystrophy, osteomalacia, and metastatic bone disease.

Bone biopsies remain an essential tool when conducting clinical research on the pathogenesis and treatment of skeletal disorders, since parameters of bone metabolism can be directly assessed and quantitative measurements can provide information on the rates of bone formation and bone resorption. The histomorphometric (or quantitative) analysis of mineralized bone specimens has contributed greatly to our current understanding of the mechanisms underlying normal bone physiology and the pathogenesis of many skeletal diseases. Many excellent reviews are available on quantitative histologic analysis of metabolic bone disease.[99–101] We will describe briefly the preparation of bone specimens for analysis, the parameters that are measured, and their biologic significance. We will also discuss the advantages and disadvantages of using bone biopsies to identify skeletal disorders. Analysis of bone biopsies is also useful for the diagnosis of metastatic bone diseases and other pathologic bone marrow conditions; however, a discussion of these disorders, of which there are many good reviews,[96–98] is outside the scope of this chapter.

Biopsy Procedure and Specimen Preparation

Bone biopsies can be obtained for qualitative analysis from nearly any skeletal site.[102,103] To obtain the larger core samples needed for quantitative histomorphometry,[104] a manual or electric drill with an internal diameter of 4 to 8 mm is used.[105] The ilium or the iliac crest is generally used as a sampling site for quantitative histologic specimens because it is easily accessible, offers the opportunity for repeated biopsies, and allows observations on both cortical and trabecular bone. Few complications have been reported with the use of these biopsy techniques.[106]

Bone specimens are fixed in neutral-buffered formalin overnight, dehydrated in graded alcohols, and embedded in a methacrylate mixture described in detail by Gruber et al.[107] Mineralized specimens embedded in plastic are used rather than demineralized specimens in paraffin because the latter introduces artifactual shrinkage of the tissue, removes intravital bone markers such as tetracyclines, and prevents clear identification of the unmineralized bone matrix (osteoid). Because of this, mineralized bone specimens are preferred for qualitative analysis, and are required for quantitative analysis of bone biopsies.

Sections of mineralized bone (5 to 7 μm), which allow identification of cell and tissue parameters, are obtained with a special microtome, such as a Reichart-Jung Autocut Model 1140, designed for cutting hard-tissue specimens. Sections are then stained with Goldner's stain[108] for clear identification of the mineralized and unmineralized bone and the bone marrow cells. Information on the amount of bone and the extent of bone formation can be obtained from these sections. Additional sections are stained histochemically for acid phosphatase to identify osteoclasts[109] in order to obtain an index of bone resorption.

Although qualitative examination of Goldner's- and acid-phosphatase-stained sections provides most of the information needed to confirm a diagnosis, in some cases the question is whether the bone is mineralizing properly. Administration of an intravital bone label, usually tetracycline, prior to obtaining the biopsy, identifies sites of active bone formation and mineralization. Thus, a distinct label indicates normal mineralization, while a wide label suggests impaired mineralization.

The use of tetracyclines is essential in quantitative histomorphometry. When two courses of tetracycline are administered, the rate of bone formation at the cell and tissue levels can be determined.[110] The protocol for tetracycline administration is tetracycline HCl (250 mg three times/day) for 3 days, followed by declomycin (250 mg three times/day) 10 to 21 days later for 3 days. The biopsy should be obtained 5 to 7 days after the last label is given. Following processing of the biopsy, unstained sections (10 to 20 μm) are viewed by fluorescent microscopy (Fig. 3-2). The two types of tetracycline are used be-

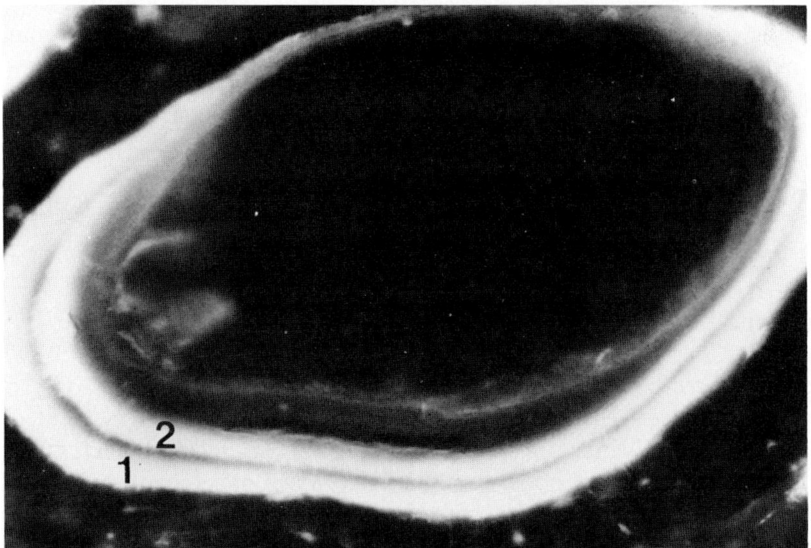

Fig. 3-2 Doubly labeled tetracycline surface in a 10 μm thick section of iliac crest bone biopsy examined by fluorescent microscopy. The time between administration of the first, inner label (1) and the second, outer tetracycline label (2) was 14 days.

cause they fluoresce at different colors (although Fig. 3-2 is black and white, the labels when viewed are yellow or orange), allowing for the identification of each type of label.

A number of methods have been described for the quantitative analysis of bone biopsies. The method requiring the least equipment, but which is time-consuming, is the point count method using a grid system.[111] Semiautomatic techniques are available that require more equipment but allow more rapid, less tedious measurements, and the data are automatically collected and initial calculations are performed.[104,112] For the semiautomatic methods a microscopic image is obtained by using a camera lucida, by projecting the image using a series of mirrors, or by using a video camera to produce a television display of the image. In each case, an operator traces the microscopic image onto a digitizing tablet that interfaces with a computer. The various parameters can then be calculated by the computer on the data stored in memory.

Measurement Parameters

The parameters examined in bone biopsies will be similar whether they are viewed qualitatively (i.e., estimation of the parameter by visual inspection) or measured for quantitative analysis. These parameters are designed to provide information on the amount and structure of bone, the rate at which bone is formed and removed, and the types of cells contained in the bone marrow. The following parameters can be examined qualitatively or measured for quantitative analysis: mineralized bone area, osteoid area, osteoid length, osteoid width, resorbed (scalloped) bone surface, and the number of acid-phosphatase-positive osteoclasts. When possible, the length of tetracycline-labeled bone surface, and the distance between two successive tetracycline labels, is also determined.

Bone Area

The structure of bone provides information on the amount of bone and on the remodeling process. The bone area normally occupies 20 percent of the tissue area.[113] Trabeculae appear as continuous, branching spicules of bone connected to the cortical bone. In a disease of low bone density such as osteogenesis imperfecta or various types of osteoporosis, the cortices are thin and porous, and the trabeculae are few and far between and may appear as isolated pieces of bone within the marrow spaces.[114,115] In contrast, in osteopetrosis, a disease characterized by excess bone, the tissue area becomes completely filled with bone.[116]

Bone-Forming Surface

Bone formation is assessed from measurements made on the Goldner's stained sections, or on unstained tetracycline-labeled sections. The length of bone-forming surface is indicated by either the length of osteoblast-covered bone surface, the length of osteoid surface (normally 20 percent of the bone surface), or the length of tetracycline-labeled bone surface (10 to 15 percent of the bone surface).[113] The osteoid-covered bone surface may increase to greater than 30 percent in patients with Paget's disease[117] or hyperparathyroidism.[118] Levels of bone-forming surface can also be high in certain stages of renal osteodystrophy,[119] usually associated with a secondary hyperparathyroidism.[120]

A low osteoid length is occasionally associated with osteoporosis; however, osteoid length is usually within the normal range in this disorder.[99] Because of the heterogeneity in all the parameters of bone turnover in osteoporosis, including the length of osteoid, bone biopsies are rarely helpful for determining the cause of bone loss. Biopsies can, however, indicate the efficacy of agents used for the treatment of osteoporosis. The most successful agent for treatment of spinal osteoporosis is fluoride,[121,122] which increases osteoid length linearly with each year of fluoride therapy.[123] This increase in osteoid length appears to be due to a direct stimulation of osteoblast proliferation.[124]

Osteoid Width

Another index of bone formation and mineralization is provided by the osteoid width. The width of osteoid seams is dependent on the rate at which osteoblasts form bone matrix (termed the matrix apposition rate or the linear rate of bone formation, which represents the width of new bone matrix added per unit time), and the delay (lag time) prior to the initiation of the mineralization of newly deposited matrix. The mean width of the osteoid seams is approximately 10 μm. When the linear rate of matrix formation increases, and the lag time remains relatively constant, osteoid width will increase. This is what is seen in Paget's disease, hyperparathyroidism, and other cases with high bone formation rates.

Another cause of wide osteoid seams is osteomalacia.[125] If mineralization is impaired, the lag time increases, causing the osteoid seams to become wider. Although the osteoid width in mild osteomalacia may appear similar to that caused by rapid bone formation, osteoid width increases dramatically in severe osteomalacia. Subsequently, osteoid volume may increase from the normal 5 percent to greater than 20 percent of the bone area (Fig. 3-3). The definitive identification of osteomalacia is provided by tetracycline labels. These labels allow measurement of the mineralization lag time, which is increased in osteomalacia. In addition, when wide osteoid seams are the result of an increase

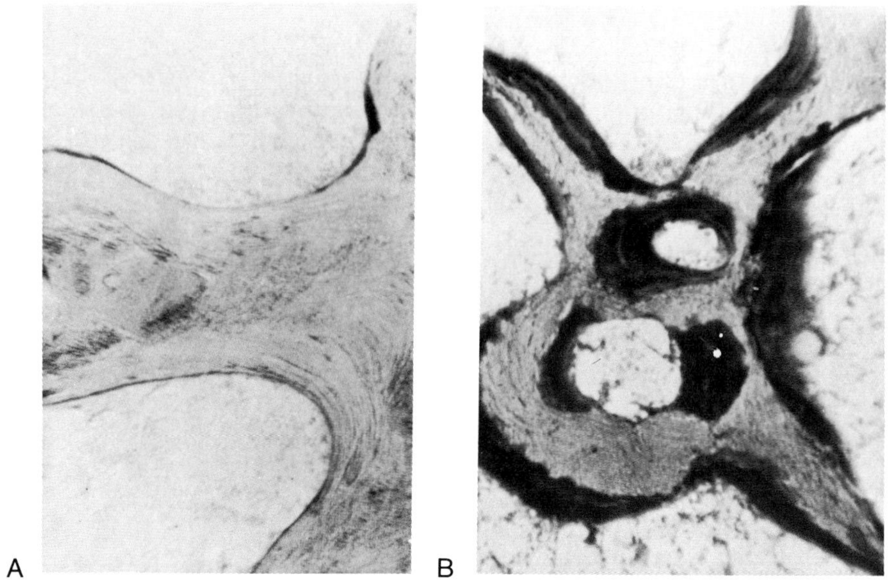

Fig. 3-3 These Goldner's-stained sections illustrate the difference between normal (**A**) and osteomalacic bone (**B**). The mineralized bone stains lighter than the unmineralized osteoid matrix (black). In osteomalacia, an increase in both the length and width of the osteoid contributes to the increased osteoid volume.

in the linear rate of bone formation, as in Paget's disease, the labels remain clear and distinct. On the other hand, in osteomalacia, tetracycline labels will be wide and indistinct or may even be absent. The most common cause of osteomalacia is vitamin D deficiency. In severe cases of vitamin D deficiency osteoid matrix is slowly deposited at a given formation site along the bone surface; however, the onset of mineralization may be delayed for years (or until the patient is treated with vitamin D). In this situation tetracycline labels will not be apparent beneath wide osteoid seams and the osteoid will meet the corresponding cement lines.[125,126]

Determination of Bone Formation Rates

Although bone biopsies are no longer routinely used for the diagnosis of metabolic bone diseases, histomorphometry is very useful for assessing therapeutic regimens using experimental agents. When using bone biopsies to monitor drug therapies, it is essential to analyze the biopsies quantitatively. This requires the use of tetracycline labels to measure the rate of bone formation.[129] Bone formation rates can be determined once the length of bone surface involved in formation and the matrix apposition rate are known. The length of bone-forming surface is indicated by the tetracycline-labeled bone surface.[130]

Tetracycline is incorporated into bone only when bone contains 20 percent or less of the maximum mineral content, and continued mineral deposition locks tetracycline in the bone.[131] The matrix apposition rate, which can be calculated after the administration of two courses of tetracycline, is determined by dividing the distance between the labels by the number of days between tetracycline administrations. Thus, the bone formation rate (mm^2 bone matrix/mm^2 tissue area/day) can be calculated as:

$$\text{matrix apposition rate (mm/day)} \times \frac{\text{tetracycline length (mm)}}{\text{tissue area (mm}^2\text{)}}$$

This equation is often calculated with a volume referent (mm^3), which requires a correction factor,[111] but this complicated derivation actually changes the values only slightly.

Bone Resorption

Although it is not possible to measure directly the rate of bone resorption, the length of resorbed (scalloped) bone surface and the number and size of osteoclasts can provide an index of the amount of bone resorption. For example, in Paget's disease the number and size of osteoclasts are increased in localized areas of rapid bone resorption.[117] The number of nuclei per cell also increases, reaching as many as 100 per cell. In hyperparathyroidism a generalized increase in the number of osteoclasts occurs throughout the skeleton.[119] The high osteoclastic activity may produce excavating lesions within the bone, resulting in thin, distorted trabeculae. In contrast to these diseases, very few osteoclasts are apparent in osteopetrosis[116]; normal bone formation and low bone resorption thus produce large amounts of bone.

As stated previously, bone biopsies are rarely used for the diagnosis of osteoporosis. One reason for obtaining biopsies is to identify subjects with a high bone resorption rate, because agents such as calcitonin and diphosphonates are available to decrease resorption effectively.[132] An increase in osteoclast number can confirm the presence of increased bone resorption suggested by increases in serum acid phosphatase and urinary hydroxyproline (see the section on Biochemical Markers).

Woven Bone

Other parameters observed in bone biopsies can also be used to characterized disease processes. Normal bone consists of layers of collagen fibers oriented in alternating directions, which appear as light–dark layers using polarized light microscopy. In contrast, during rapid bone formation such as in Paget's disease, the collagen fibers of the bone matrix are not aligned in any direction. When this bone is examined by polarized light microscopy, the birefringent collagen fibers appear in a criss-cross woven pattern.

Marrow Fibrosis

Another characteristic of rapid bone formation is fibrous tissue in the marrow at the bone surface. Bands of fibrous tissue are apparent at osteoid surfaces in hyperparathyroidism,[120,133] while fibrous tissue may completely fill the bone marrow in Paget's disease[117] and fibrous dysplasia.[134]

Cement Lines

The pattern of bone remodeling is apparent from the pattern of cement lines within the trabecular spicules. Cement lines are formed at sites where resorption stops and formation begins. These lines can be detected because the material produced to hold the old and the new bone together has a different staining characteristic than the rest of the bone matrix. The result is the formation of crescent-shaped lines that are usually parallel to the long axis of the trabeculae. In Paget's disease, this pattern of cement lines is drastically altered. The cement lines form a mosaic pattern, not seen in other bone diseases, which is indicative of short alternative bone formation and bone resorption cycles distributed in a haphazard fashion throughout the affected bone tissue (Fig. 3-4).

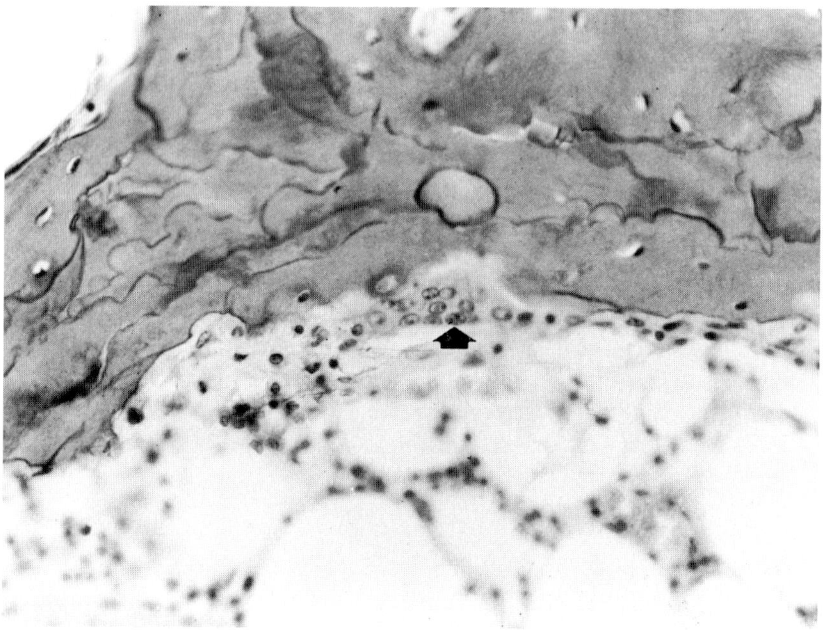

Fig. 3-4 The moasic of dark cement lines in this demineralized section stained with hematoxylin and eosin is typical of trabecular bone in Paget's disease. The large, multinucleate osteoclast within a Howship's lacunae (arrow) is also typical of the many osteoclasts found in Paget's disease of bone.

SUMMARY

The diagnosis of metabolic bone disease, including osteoporosis, and the monitoring of the effects of therapy, can now be accomplished earlier and more accurately due to the development of new techniques that can assess skeletal metabolism and bone density. These techniques include densitometric assessment of bone, assays of biochemical markers of bone metabolism, and histomorphometric determination of bone turnover.

The densitometric techniques have the advantages of being noninvasive, site-specific, and, especially true of QCT, able to differentiate cortical from trabecular bone mass. In many instances these densitometric techniques are sufficient for clinical diagnosis of certain metabolic bone diseases. Disadvantages of these techniques include their current expense and limited availability. In addition, when monitoring drug responses, months to years of therapy may be required before changes in bone density can be detected.

Biochemical markers of bone metabolism can be used to examine the pathogenesis of metabolic bone diseases. They are minimally invasive and can indicate response to therapy within days to weeks of starting a new regimen. Disadvantages of these assays are that they describe total skeletal changes, and they do not differentiate between cortical and trabecular metabolism. Skeletal abnormalities or responses to treatment that are site-specific may be masked if they are small compared to the total skeletal influence. Although the number of currently available biochemical markers that have been definitively validated is limited, the future holds promise for the development of new, sensitive assays that can be of great use in the diagnosis and monitoring of metabolic bone diseases.

The major advantage provided by histomorphometric analysis of bone biopsies is that it enables the direct identification of the mechanisms of the disease process. Since it allows a direct determination of both the cell number and the cell activity, it provides a more detailed examination of the pathogenesis of metabolic bone diseases than assays of biochemical markers. In addition, histomorphometry is the most definitive means to assess osteomalacia and Paget's disease, although in the latter it is rarely necessary. It can potentially provide an early indication of the skeletal response to therapeutic agents, though the use of biochemical markers is often more appropriate for this purpose. The major disadvantage of histomorphometric analysis of bone biopsies is the invasive nature of the technique, which limits the number of repeat biopsies and prevents mass surveys. Another disadvantage is the poor precision of the various parameters measured. Finally, few laboratories provide histomorphometric analysis of bone biopsy specimens because the processing and measurement procedure is very time-consuming and requires special equipment.

REFERENCES

1. Jennings J, Baylink D: Osteoporosis. p.466. In Calkins E, Davis PJ, Ford AB (eds): The Practice of Geriatrics. WB Saunders, Philadelphia, 1986
2. Gruber HE, Baylink DJ: The diagnosis of osteoporosis. J Am Geriatr Soc 29:490, 1981
3. Horsman A, Simpson M: The measurement of sequential changes in cortical bone geometry. Br J Radiol 48:470, 1975
4. Wahner HW, Dunn WL, Riggs BL: Assessment of bone mineral. Part 1. J Nucl Med 25:1134, 1984
5. Cameron JR, Soreson J: Measurement of bone mineral in vivo: an improved method. Science 142:230, 1963
6. Mazess RB: Estimation of bone and skeletal weight by direct photon absorptiometry. Invest Radiol 6:52, 1971
7. Manzke E, Chesnut CH, Wergedal JE, et al: Relationship between local and total bone mass in osteoporosis. Metabolism 24:605, 1975
8. Mazess RB: Noninvasive methods for quantitating trabecular bone. p.85. In Avioli LV (ed): The Osteoporotic Syndrome. Grune & Stratton, Orlando, 1983
9. Christiansen C: Prophylactic treatment for age-related bone loss in women. p.587. In Christiansen C, Arnaud CD, Nordin BEC, et al (eds): Osteoporosis. Aalborg Stiftsbogtrykkeri, Copenhagen, Denmark, 1984
10. Farley SMG, Wergedal JE, Smith LC, et al: Fluoride therapy for osteoporosis: characterization of the skeletal response by serial measurements of serum alkaline phosphatase activity. Metabolism 36:211, 1987
11. Mazess RB: Advances in single- and dual-photon absorptiometry. p.57. In Christiansen C, Arnaud CD, Nordin BEC, et al (eds): Osteoporosis. Aalborg Stiftsbogtrykkeri, Copenhagen, Denmark, 1984
12. Brassow F, Crone-Muenzebrock W, Weh L, et al: Correlations between breaking load and CT absorption values of vertebral bodies. Eur J Radiol 2:99, 1982
13. Richardson ML, Genant HK, Cann CE, et al: Assessment of metabolic bone diseases by quantitative computed tomography. Clin Orthop Rel Res 195:224, 1985
14. Genant HK, Cann CE, Ettinger B, et al: Quantitative computed tomography for spinal mineral assessment: current status. J Comput Assist Tomogr 9:602, 1985
15. Riggs BL, Wahner HW, Dunn WL, et al: Differential changes in bone mineral density of the appendicular and axial skeleton with aging. J Clin Invest 67:328, 1981
16. Wahner HW, Dunn WL, Riggs BL: Assessment of bone mineral. Part 2. J Nucl Med 25:1241, 1984
17. Odvina CV, Wergedal JE, Libanati CR, et al: Relationship between trabecular vertebral body density and fractures. A quantitative definition of osteoporosis. Metabolism 37:221, 1988
18. Farley SM, Libanati CR, Schulz EE, Baylink DJ: Fluoride therapy for osteoporosis: progressive increase in spinal bone density and effective management of side effects. Thirty-third Annual Meeting, Orthopaedic Res Soc 12:260, 1987
19. Robison R: The possible significance of hexose phosporic esters in ossification. Biochem J 17:286, 1923
20. Marie PJ, Travers R: Continuous infusion of 1,25-dihydroxyvitamin D_3 stimulates bone turnover in the normal mouse. Calcif Tissue Int 35:418, 1983
21. Canalis E: Effect of hormones and growth factors on alkaline phosphatase activity and collagen synthesis in cultured rat calvariae. Metabolism 32:14, 1983

22. Moss DW: Alkaline phosphatase isoenzymes (review). Clin Chem 28:2007, 1982
23. Gothlin G, Ericsson JLE: Fine structural localization of alkaline phosphomonoesterase in the fracture callus of the rat. Isr J Med Sci 7:488, 1971
24. Nagent de Deuxchaisnes C, Krane SM: Paget's disease of bone: clinical and metabolic observations. Medicine 43:233, 1964
25. Green S, Antiss CL, Fishman WH: Automated differential isoenzyme analysis. II. The fractionation of serum alkaline phosphatase into liver, intestinal, and other components. Enzymologia 41:9, 1971
26. Gorman L, Statland BE: Clinical usefulness of alkaline phosphatase isoenzyme determinations. Clin Biochem 10:171, 1977
27. Lum G, Catrou P, Liuzza G, Kokatnur M: Clinical assessment of the electrophoretic separation of alkaline phosphatase isoenzymes. Am J Clin Pathol 80:682, 1983
28. Alpers DH, Goodwin CL, Young GP: Quantitation of human intestinal and liver/bone alkaline phophatase in serum by rocket electroimmunoassay. Anal Biochem 140:129, 1984
29. Farley JR, Chestnut CH III, Baylink DJ: Improved method for quantitative determination in serum of alkaline phosphatase of skeletal origin. Clin Chem 27:2002, 1981
30. Fishman WH: Perspectives on alkaline phosphatase isoenzymes. Am J Med 56:617, 1984
31. Lehmann FG: Intestinal alkaline phosphatase: an immunoprecipitation method for the determination of feces. Biochem Biophys Acta 616:41, 1980
32. McKenna MJ, Hamilton TA, Sussman HH: Comparison of human alkaline phosphatase isoenzymes. Biochem J 181:67, 1979
33. Behr W, Barnert J: Quantification of bone alkaline phosphatase in serum by precipitation with wheat-germ lectin: a simplified method and its clinical plausibility. Clin Chem 32:1960, 1986
34. Krabbe S, Christiansen C: Longitudinal study of calcium metabolism in male puberty. Acta Paediatr Scand 73:745, 1984
35. Stepan JJ, Tesarova A, Havranek T, et al: Age and sex dependency of the biochemical indices of bone remodeling. Clin Chem Acta 151:273, 1985
36. Wolf PL: Clinical significance of increased or decreased serum alkaline phosphatase isoenzymes. Clin Lab Med 6:525, 1986
37. Price PA, Parthemore JG, Deftos LT: New biochemical marker for bone metabolism. J Clin Invest 66:878, 1980
38. Mariano-Menez MR, Farley SM, Tudtud LA, et al: Fluoride therapy in osteoporosis: skeletal response and management of side-effects. Clin Res 35:155A, 1987
39. Delmas PD, Chapuy MC, Vignon E, et al: Long-term effects of dichloromethylene diphosphonate in Paget's disease of the bone. J Clin Endocrinol Metab 54:837, 1982
40. Altman RD: Long-term follow-up of therapy with intermittant etidronate disodium in Paget's disease of bone. Am J Med 79:583, 1985
41. Smith ML, Fogelman I, Ralston S, et al: Correlation of skeletal uptake of 99mTc-diphosphonate and alkaline phosphatase before and after oral diphosphonate therapy in Paget's disease. Metab Bone Dis Rel Res 5:167, 1984
42. Hauschka PV, Lian JB, Gallop PM: Direct identification of the calcium-binding amino acid, gamma-carboxyglutamate, in mineralized tissue. Proc Natl Acad Sci USA 72:3925, 1975

43. Price PA, Otsuka AS, Posen JW, et al: Characterization of a gamma-carboxyglutamic acid-containing protein from bone. Proc Natl Acad Sci USA 73:1447, 1976
44. Poser JW, Esch FS, Ling NC, Price PA: Isolation and sequence of the vitamin K-dependent protein from human bone. J Biol Chem 255:8685, 1980
45. Hauschka PV, Carr SA: Calcium-dependent alpha-helical structure in osteocalcin. Biochemistry 21:2538, 1982
46. Price PA, Williamson MK, Lothringer JW: Origin of the vitamin K-dependent bone protein found in plasma and its clearance by kidney and bone. J Biol Chem 256:12760, 1981
47. Brown JP, Delmas PD, Malaval L, et al: Serum bone Gla-protein: a specific marker for bone formation in postmenopausal osteoporosis. Lancet 1:1091, 1984
48. Gundberg CM, Lian JB, Gallop PM: Measurements of gamma-carboxyglutamate and circulating osteocalcin in normal children and adults. Clin Chem Acta 128:1, 1983
49. Price PA, Nishimoto SK: Radioimmunoassay for the vitamin K-dependent protein of bone and its discovery in plasma. Proc Natl Acad Sci USA 77:2234, 1980
50. Gundberg CM, Wilson PS, Gallop PM, Parfitt AM: Determinant of osteocalcin in human serum: results with two kits compared with those by a well-characterized assay. Clin Chem 31:1720, 1985
51. Lukert BP, Higgins JC, Stodkopf MM: Serum osteocalcin is increased in patients with hyperthyroidism and decreased in patients receiving glucocorticoids. J Clin Endocrinol Metab 62:1056, 1986
52. Price PA, Baukol SA: 1,25-dihydroxyvitamin D_3 increases synthesis of the vitamin K-dependent bone protein by osteosarcoma cells. J Biol Chem 255:11660, 1980
53. Gundberg CM, Weinstein RS: Multiple immunoreactive forms of osteocalcin in uremic serum. J Clin Invest 77:1762, 1986
54. Gundberg CM, Markowitz ME, Mizruchi M, Rosen JF: Osteocalcin in human serum: a circadian rhythm. J Clin Endocrinol 60:736, 1985
55. Prockop DJ, Kivirikko KI, Tuderman L, Guzman NA: The biosynthesis of collagen and its disorders. N Engl J Med 301:12, 1979
56. Martin GR, Byers PH, Piez KA: Procollagen. Adv Enzymol 42:167, 1975
57. Merry AH, Harwood R, Wooley DE, et al: Identification and partial characterization of the non-collagenous amino- and carboxy-terminal extension peptides of cartilage procollagen. Biochem Biophys Res Commun 71:83, 1976
58. Timpl R, Glanville RW: The aminopropeptide of collagen. Clin Orthop 158:224, 1981
59. Fessler LI, Morris NP, Fessler JH: Procollagen: biological scission of amino and carboxyl extension peptides. Proc Natl Acad Sci USA 72:4905, 1975
60. Taubman MB, Goldberg B, Sherr CJ: Radioimmunoassay for human procollagen. Science 186:1115, 1974
61. Simon LS, Krane SM, Wortman PD, et al: Serum levels of type I and III procollagen fragments in Paget's disease of bone. J Clin Endocrinol Metab 58:110, 1984
62. Russel GG, Beard DJ, Cameron EC, et al: Biochemical markers of bone turnover in Paget's disease. Metab Bone Dis Rel Res 3:255, 1981
63. Prockop DJ, Kivirikko KI: Heritable diseases of collagen. N Engl J Med 311:376, 1984
64. Harwood R, Grant ME, Jackson DS: Collagen biosynthesis: characterization of subcellular fractions from embryonic chick fibroblasts and the intracellular localization of protocollagen prolyl and protocollagen lysyl hydroxylases. Biochem J 144:123, 1974
65. Lowry M, Hall DE, Brosnan JT: Hydroxyproline metabolism by the rat kidney:

distribution of renal enzymes of hydroxyproline catabolism and renal conversion of hydroxyproline to glycine and serine. Metabolism 34:955, 1985
66. Woessner JF Jr: Catabolism of collagen and noncollagen protein in the rat uterus during post-partum involution. Biochem J 83:304, 1962
67. Smith R: Collagen and disorders of bone. Clin Sci 59:215, 1980
68. Orwoll ES, Belsey RE: The laboratory evaluation of osteopenia. Clin Lab Med 4:763, 1984
69. Hodgkinson A, Thompson T: Measurement of the fasting urinary hydroxyproline: creatinine ratio in normal adults and its variation with age and sex. J Clin Pathol 35:807, 1982
70. Minkin C: Bone acid phosphatase: tartrate-resistant acid phosphatase as a marker of osteoclast function. Calcif Tissue Int 34:285, 1982
71. Lam KW, Lee PF, Li CY, Yam LT: Immunological and biochemical evidence for identity of tartrate-resistant isoenzymes of acid phosphatases from human serum and tissue. Clin Chem 26:420, 1980
72. Lam KW, Siemens M, Sun T, et al: Enzyme immunoassay for tartrate-resistant acid phosphatase. Clin Chem 28:467, 1982
73. Lau WKW, Onishi T, Wergedal JE, et al: Characterization of, and assay for, human serum tartrate-resistant acid phosphatase activity: A potential assay to assess bone resorption. Clin Chem 33:458, 1987
74. Thompson ER, Baylink DJ, Wergedal JE: Increases in number and size of osteoclasts in response to calcium or phosphorus deficiency in the rat. Endocrinology 97:283, 1975
75. Armitage EK: Parathyrin (parathyroid hormone): metabolism and methods of assay. Clin Chem 32:418, 1986
76. Garabedian M, Holick MF, DeLuca HF, Boyle IT: Control of 25-hydroxy-cholecalciferol metabolism by parathyroid glands. Proc Natl Acad Sci USA 69:1673, 1972
77. Schachter D, Rosen SM: Active transport of Ca^{45} by the small intestine and dependence on vitamin D. Am J Physiol 196:357, 1959
78. Habener JF, Potts JT: Biosynthesis of parathyroid hormone. Part 1. N Engl J Med 299:580, 1978
79. Habener JF, Potts JT: Biosynthesis of parathyroid hormone. Part 2. N Engl J Med 299:635, 1978
80. Habener JF, Rosenblatt M, Dee PC, Potts JT: Cellular processing of preproparathyroid hormone involves rapid hydrolysis of the leader sequence. J Biol Chem 254:10596, 1979
81. Habener JF, Kemper BW, Potts JT, Rich A: Calcium-independent intracellular conversion of proparathyroid hormone to parathyroid hormone. Endocrin Res Commun 1:239, 1974
82. Habener JF, Kemper B, Potts JT: Calcium-dependent intracellular degradation of parathyroid hormone: a possible mechanism for the regulation of hormone stores. Endocrinology 97:431, 1975
83. Flueck JA, DiBella FP, Edis AJ, et al: Immunoheterogeneity of parathyroid hormone in venous effluent serum from hyperfunctioning parathyroid glands. J Clin Invest 60:1367, 1977
84. Marx SJ, Sharp ME, Krudy A, et al: RIA for the middle region of human PTH—studies with a radioiodinated synthetic peptide. J Clin Endocrinol Metab 53:76, 1981
85. Roos BA, Lindall AW, Aron DC, et al: Detection and characterization of small midregion parathyroid hormone fragments in normal and hyperparathyroid glands

and sera by immunoextraction and region-specific radioimmunoassays. J Clin Endocrinol Metab 53:709, 1981
86. Corvilain J, Manderlier T, Struyven J, et al: Metabolism of human PTH by the kidney and the liver. Horm Metab Res 9:239, 1977
87. Canterbury JM, Bricker LA, Levey GS, et al: Metabolism of bovine parathyroid hormone. Immunological and biological characteristics of fragments generated by liver perfusion. J Clin Invest 55:1245, 1975
88. Berson SA, Yallow RS: Immunochemical heterogeneity of parathyroid hormone in plasma. J Clin Endocrinol Metab 28:1037, 1968
89. DiBella FP, Gilkinson JB, Flueck J, Arnaud CD: Carboxy-terminal fragments of human parathyroid hormone in parathyroid tumors. J Clin Endocrinol Metab 46:604, 1978
90. Papapoulos SE, Manning RM, Hendy GN, et al: Studies of circulating parathyroid hormone in man using a homologous amino-terminal specific immunoradiometric assay. Clin Endocrinol 13:57, 1980
91. Blunt JW, Tanaka Y, DeLuca HF: The biological activity of 25-hydroxycholecalciferol, a metabolite of vitamin D_3. Proc Natl Acad Sci USA 61:1503, 1968
92. Fraser DR, Kodicek E: Unique biosynthesis by kidney of a biochemically active vitamin D metabolite. Nature 228:764, 1970
93. Bickle DD (ed): Assay of Calcium-Regulating Hormones. Springer-Verlag, New York, 1983
94. DeLuca HF: Vitamin D: Metabolism and Function. Springer-Verlag, New York, 1979
95. Shen FH, Baylink DJ, Nielsen RL, et al: Increased serum 1,25-dihydroxyvitamin D in idiopathic hypercalciuria. J Lab Clin Med 90:955, 1977
96. Burkhardt R, Frisch B, Bartl R: Bone biopsy in haematological disorders. J Clin Pathol 35:257, 1982
97. Krause JR: Bone Marrow Biopsy. Churchill Livingstone, Edinburgh, 1981
98. Frisch B, Lewis SM, Burkhardt R, Bartl R: Biopsy Pathology of Bone and Bone Marrow. CRC Press, Boca Raton, FL, 1985
99. Parfitt AM: The coupling of bone formation to bone resorption: a critical analysis of the concept and its relevance to the pathogenesis of osteoporosis. Metab Bone Dis Rel Res 4:1, 1986
100. Jaworski ZFG: Histomorphometric characteristics of metabolic bone disease. p.241. In Recker RR (ed): Bone Histomorphometry: Techniques and Interpretation. CRC Press, Boca Raton, FL, 1983
101. Melsen F, Moselkilde L, Kragstrup J: Metabolic bone disease as evaluated by bone histomorphometry. p.265. In Recker RR (ed): Bone Histomorphometry: Techniques and Interpretation. CRC Press, Boca Raton, FL, 1983
102. Ellis LD, Jensen WN: Needle biopsy of bone and marrow. An experience with 1,445 biopsies. Arch Intern Med 114:213, 1964
103. DeSantos LA, Lukeman JM, Wallace S, et al: Percutaneous needle biopsy of bone in the cancer patient. AJR 130:641, 1978
104. Sherrard DJ, Baylink DJ, Wergedal JE, et al: Quantitative histologic studies on the pathogenesis of uremic bone disease. J Clin Endocrinol Metab 39:119, 1974
105. Bordier P, Matrajt H, Miracet L, Hioco D: Mésure histologique de la masse et de la resorption des travées osseuses. Pathol Microbiol 12:1238, 1964
106. Duncan H, Sudhaker DR, Parfitt AM: Complications of bone biopsy. Metab Bone Dis Rel Res 2S:483, 1980

107. Gruber HE, Stauffer ME, Thompson ER, Baylink DJ: Diagnosis of bone disease by core biopsies. Semin Hematol 18:258, 1981
108. Goldner JA: A modification of the Masson trichrome technique for routine laboratory purposes. Am J Pathol 14:237, 1938
109. Evans RA, Dunstan CR, Baylink DJ, et al: Histochemical identification of osteoclasts in undecalcified sections of human bone. Min Electrolyte Metab 2:179, 1979
110. Frost HM: Bone histomorphometry: Choice of marking agent and labeling schedule. p.37. In Recker RR (ed): Bone Histomorphometry: Techniques and Interpretation. CRC Press, Boca Raton, FL, 1983
111. Parfitt AM: Sterologic basis of bone histomorphometry: theory of quantitative microscopy and reconstruction of the third dimension. p.53. In Recker RR (ed): Bone Histomorphometry: Techniques and Interpretation. CRC Press, Boca Raton, FL, 1983
112. Smith JM, Jee WSS: Automated skeletal histomorphometry. p.285. In Recker RR (ed): Bone Histomorphometry: Techniques and Interpretation. CRC Press, Boca Raton, FL, 1983
113. Malluche HM, Meyer W, Sherman D, Massry SG: Quantitative bone histology in 84 normal American subjects. Calcif Tissue Int 34:449, 1982
114. Shapiro JR, Triche T, Rowe DW, et al: Osteogenesis imperfecta and Paget's disease of bone. Biochemical and morphologic studies. Arch Intern Med 143:2250, 1983
115. Pope FM, Cheah KSE, Nicholls AC, et al: Lethal osteogenesis imperfecta congenita and a 300 base pair gene deletion for an l(I)-like collagen. Br Med J 288:431, 1984
116. Shapiro F, Glimcher MJ, Holtrop ME, et al: Human osteopetrosis. A histological, ultrastructural and biochemical study. J Bone J Surg 62A:384, 1980
117. Meunier PJ, Coindre JM, Edouard CM, Arlot ME: Bone histomorphometry in Paget's disease. Arthritis Rheum 23:1095, 1980
118. Moselkilde L, Melsen F: A tetracycline based histomorphometric evaluation of bone resorption and bone turnover in hyperthyroidism and hyperparathyroidism. Acta Med Scand 204:97, 1978
119. Wilde CD, Jaworski ZFG, Hitt O, et al: Cellular-level bone resorption in chronic renal failure and primary hyperparathyroidism. Calcif Tissue Res 12:137, 1973
120. Garner A, Ball J: Quantitative observations on mineralized and unmineralized bones in chronic renal azotaemia and intestinal malabsorption syndrome. J Pathol Bacteriol 91:545, 1966
121. Riggs BL: Treatment of osteoporosis with sodium fluoride: an appraisal. p.35. In: Bone and Mineral Research Annual. Vol. 2. Elsevier, Amsterdam, 1983
122. Kanis JA, Meunier PJ: Should we use fluoride to treat osteoporosis?: a review. Q J Med 210:145, 1984
123. Lundy MW, Baylink, DJ, Hodgsen SF, Riggs BL: A double blind placebo controlled study of fluoride therapy in osteoporosis: preliminary histological results. J Bone Min Res 2(Suppl1):379, 1987
124. Farley JR, Wergedal JE, Baylink DJ: Fluoride directly stimulates proliferation and alkaline phosphatase activity of bone-forming cells. Science 222:330, 1982
125. Frame B, Parfitt AM: Osteomalacia: current concepts. Ann Intern Med 89:966, 1978
126. Aviol LV, Raisz LG: Metabolic bone disease. Clin Endocrinol Metab 9:177, 1980
127. Ward MK, Feest TG, Ellis HA, et al: Osteomalacic dialysis osteodystrophy: evidence for a waterborne aetiologic agent, probably aluminum. Lancet 1:841, 1978

128. Andress DL, Maloney NA, Endres DB, Sherrard DJ: Aluminum-associated bone disease in chronic renal failure: High prevalence in a long-term dialysis population. J Bone Min Res 1:391, 1986
129. Frost HM, Villaneuva AR, Roth H, et al: Tetracycline bone labelling. J New Drugs 1:206, 1961
130. Melsen F, Mosekilde L: Interpretation of single labels after in vivo double labeling. Metab Bone Dis Rel Res 2S:171, 1980
131. Frost HM: Tetracycline-based histological analysis of bone remodeling. Calcif Tissue Res 3:211, 1969
132. Krane SM: Etidronate disodium in treatment of Paget's disease of bone. Am Intern Med 96:619, 1982
133. Melsen F, Mosekilde L, Christesen MS: Interrelationship between bone histomorphometry, s-iPTH and calcium-phosphorus metabolism in primary hyperparathyroidism. Calcif Tissue Res 24S:16, 1977
134. Ehrig V, Wilson DR: Fibrous dysplasia of bone and primary hyperparathyroidism. Ann Intern Med 77:234, 1972

4 Disorders of Calcium and the Parathyroid Glands

John P. Bilezikian

In this chapter, the major disorders associated with hypercalcemia and hypocalcemia are discussed with particular emphasis on those diseases seen most commonly in clinical medicine. Their presentation, diagnosis, and management are considered in the context of our current understanding of the mechanism and pathophysiology of these disorders. Information relative to basic aspects of bone physiology (Chapter 1) and endocrine control of bone and mineral metabolism (Chapter 2) provides relevant background to this chapter.

HYPERCALCEMIC DISORDERS

The differential diagnosis of hypercalcemia includes many potential causes but few likely ones (Table 4-1). In hospitalized patients or those evaluated in the outpatient setting, the major distinction to be made is between hypercalcemia due to primary hyperparathyroidism and hypercalcemia due to malignancy. The long list of other causes of hypercalcemia enters the differential diagnosis only after these two common causes have been excluded. Fewer than 10 percent of hypercalcemic patients have disorders other than primary hyperparathyroidism or malignancy.

Table 4-1. Causes of Hypercalcemia

Most common
Primary hyperparathyroidism
Malignant disease
Multiple myeloma
Carcinoma (lung, breast, esophageal, head and neck, renal, ovarian, bladder)
Lymphoproliferative (T cell, B cell, acute leukemia, HIV-associated)
Uncommon
Hyperthyroidism
Vitamin D intoxication
Sarcoidosis
Lithium administration
Immobilization
Recovery phase of acute renal failure
Drug-induced
Thiazide diuretics
Lithium
Estrogens
Androgens; in treatment of breast cancer
Tamoxifen
Theophylline toxicity
Rare
Adrenal insufficiency
Tuberculosis, histoplasmosis, leprosy, coccidioidomycosis and other granulomatous diseases
Vitamin A intoxication
Hypophosphatasia
Familial hypocalciuric hypercalcemia
Milk-alkali syndrome

Primary Hyperparathyroidism

Primary hyperparathyroidism is the most common cause of hypercalcemia in the outpatient setting and constitutes a major etiology in all hypercalcemic patients. A rare disease in the first half of the twentieth century, primary hyperparathyroidism is now relatively common, occurring[1] with an incidence of 1 : 500 to 1 : 1000. Undoubtedly, the increased incidence of primary hyperparathyroidism is due to the widespread clinical use of the multichannel autoanalyzer.[2] The condition is frequently discovered incidentally in individuals whose serum calcium is measured in the course of an evaluation for some other reason. Women are affected more commonly than men by a ratio of 3 : 2. Primary hyperparathyroidism occurs in patients at all ages but its peak incidence is in the sixth decade.

Over 80 percent of patients with primary hyperparathyroidism harbor a single adenoma. Double adenomas are distinctly unusual. The typical parathyroid adenoma is less than 1 g but may uncommonly be as large as 10 g. Histologic examination shows a collection of chief cells crowding out a rim of normal parathyroid tissue. Cystic elements within the adenomatous gland suggests the possibility of a newly recognized, rare familial form of primary hyperparathyroidism: familial cystic parathyroid adenomatosis.[3] In a minority of patients with primary hyperparathyroidism (15 to 20 percent), the pathologic process affects all glands as a multiglandular hyperplasia. Although four-gland parathyroid hyperplasia may occur sporadically, it is more commonly seen in association with multiple endocrine neoplasia, type I or II. Rarely, in fewer than 1 percent of patients, primary hyperparathyroidism is due to parathyroid carcinoma. The presence of malignancy is established by several histologic features (mitoses, vascular invasion, fibrous trabeculae), and/or by the presence of metastases to contiguous (thyroid, neck muscles, esophagus) or distant (cervical lymph nodes, lung, liver, bone) tissues.[4]

The pathophysiology of primary hyperparathyroidism involves a change in the relationship between extracellular calcium and its control of parathyroid hormone secretion. The concurrent elevation in the serum calcium and the parathyroid hormone level implies that the "set point" at which a given concentration of calcium normally controls the secretion of parathyroid hormone is altered. Alternatively, it is possible that the increased secretory rate of parathyroid hormone in primary hyperparathyroidism is due to increased tissue mass without a change in the set point for calcium. Evidence exists for both mechanisms in adenomatous disease, whereas in multiglandular parathyroid hyperplasia the set point appears to be normal.[5]

The underlying cause in the majority of patients with primary hyperparathyroidism is unknown. With molecular approaches, it is apparent that the disease is best described as clonal[6] and not multicellular, as proposed several years ago.[7] Rarely, there is a history of radiation to the neck during childhood among patients who appear with the disease as adults.[8] The familial forms of primary hyperparathyroidism, which in the aggregate affect a small minority of patients overall, are best described as autosomal dominant disorders. The two forms of multiple endocrine neoplasia (types I and II) include multiglandular parathyroid disease as prominent components. Familial primary hyperparathyroidism, in which only parathyroid disease appears to be transmitted in a genetic pattern, is most uncommon.

Signs and Symptoms

The signs and symptoms of primary hyperparathyroidism should be differentiated from those due to hypercalcemia per se from any cause. Involvement of the skeleton, a classic feature of primary hyperparathyroidism, is not widely appreciated any more because of the relatively mild nature of hyperparathyroidism at the time of presentation. Nevertheless, in those populations without ready access to medical care, osteitis fibrosa cystica is still seen. The earliest sign of osteitis fibrosa cystica is subperiosteal resorption of the distal phalanges. In more advanced skeletal disease, the skull, clavicle, long bones, and pelvis may be involved by the same pathologic process. Examples of overt bone involvement, as noted in conventional radiographs, are shown in Figure 4-1. This kind of apparent bone disease is seen in less than 10 percent of patients with primary hyperparathyroidism, consistent with the clinical impression that the disorder is infrequently associated with overt skeletal disease.

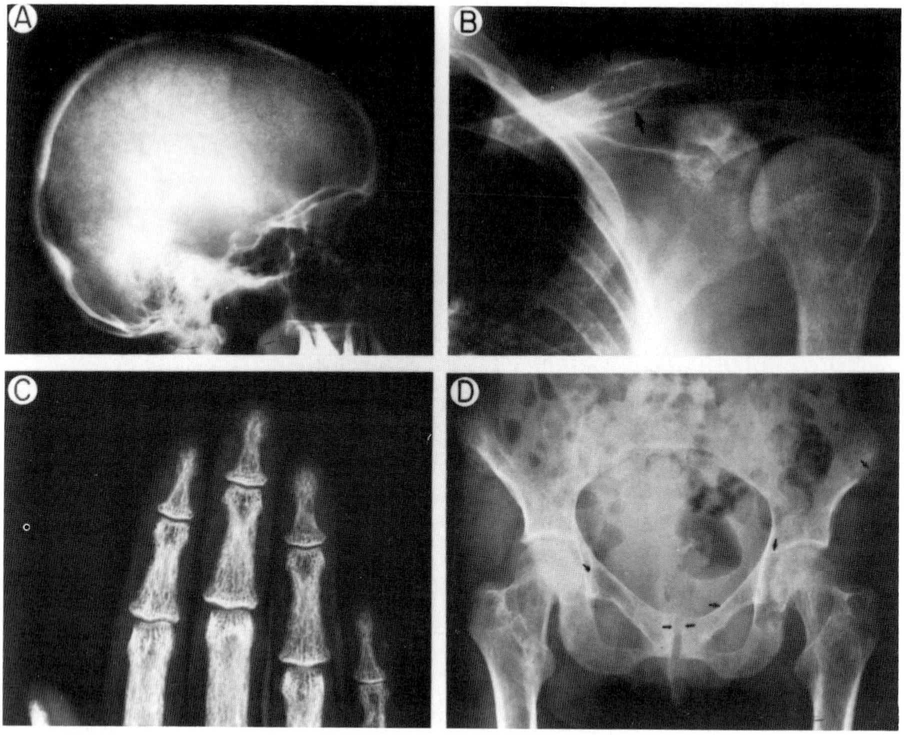

Fig. 4-1 Radiographic representations of osteitis fibrosa cystica in primary hyperparathyroidism. **(A)** Salt and pepper erosions of the skull. **(B)** Clavicle; arrow shows healed fracture. **(C)** Subperiosteal bone resorption of the digits. **(D)** Cortical erosions; arrows at pubis show oseolytic resorption, and arrows elsewhere represent brown tumors. (Courtesy of Dr. John Doppman, NIH.)

On the other hand, it is possible that parathyroid bone disease exists in a greater percentage of patients with primary hyperparathyroidism but that our detection methods are not yet sophisticated enough to detect it. As a new generation of methodologies is applied to this issue, the prevalence of bone disease in patients without clear-cut radiologic signs may become greater. Photon absorptiometry and computed tomography are newer, noninvasive technologies that hold great promise. Recent use of single and dual photon absorptiometry, in fact, is detecting reduced cortical bone density among patients without overt bone disease.[9,10] Recognition among hyperparathyroid subjects of diminished cortical bone mineral density with relative preservation of trabecular bone is consistent, moveover, with the physiologic actions of parathyroid hormone. A scanning electron micrograph of a bone biopsy specimen obtained from a patient with primary hyperparathyroidism illustrates that cortical bone is affected preferentially over trabecular bone by the hyperparathyroid process (Fig. 4-2).

Bone disease in primary hyperparathyroidism can be detected with even

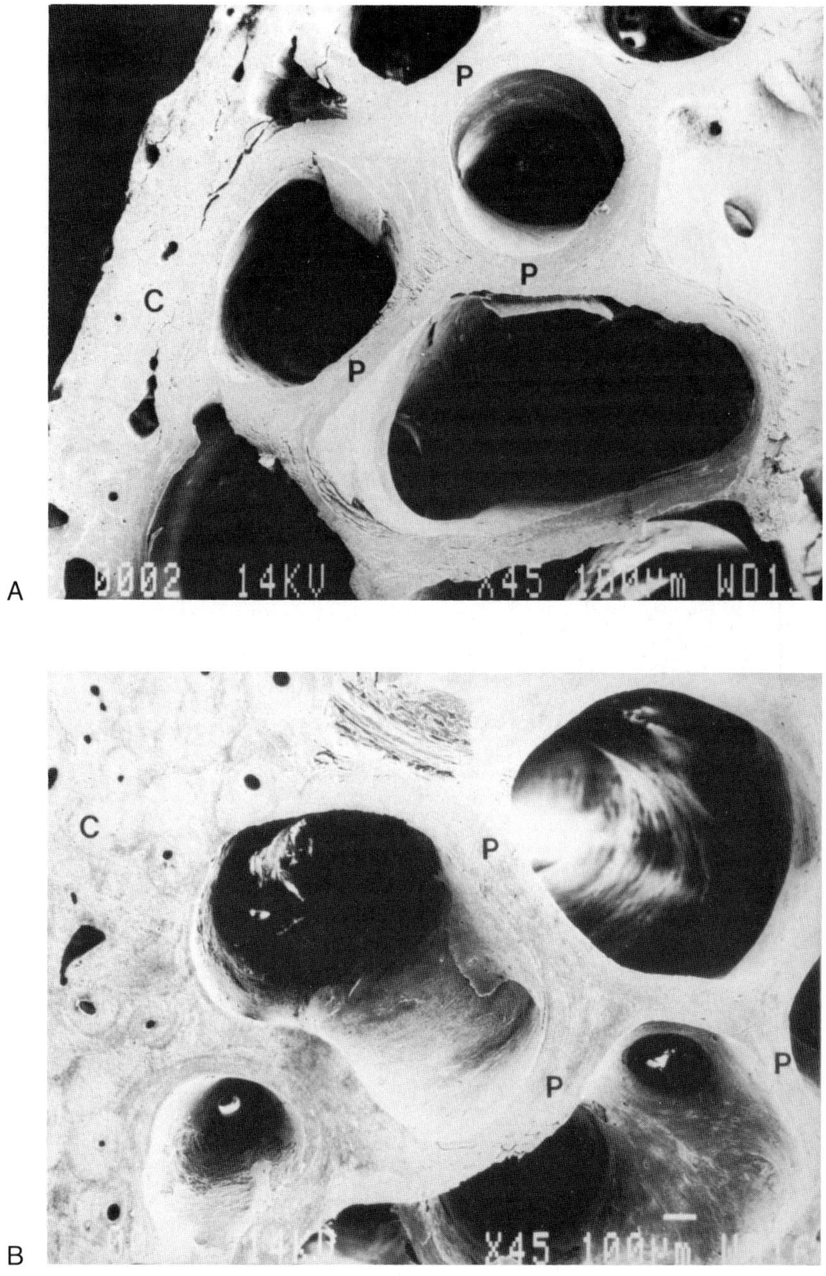

Fig. 4-2 Primary hyperparathyroidism seen by scanning electron microscopy. Findings in a 45-year old man with primary hyperparathyroidism **(A)** are compared to the presentation of normal bone from an age- and sex-matched normal subject **(B)**. Note that the trabecular plates (P) are conserved in hyperparathyroidism, but that the cortex (C) is considerably thinner. The loss of cortical bone along with preservation of the trabecular plates contrasts with the presentation by SEM of osteoporosis (Chapter 5). The field width is 2.4 mm in each case and the magnification is the same for normal and hyperparathyroid bone. (Courtesy of Dr. David Dempster, Helen Hayes Hospital.)

A

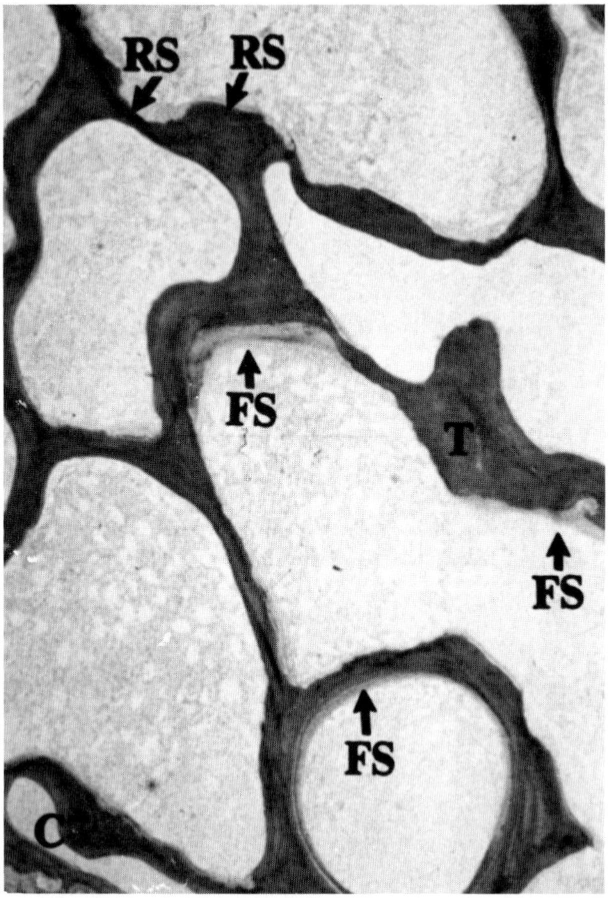

Fig. 4-3 Histologic features of bone in primary hyperparathyroidism: **(A)** Marked elevations of bone resorption and bone formation surfaces are 13 percent and 36 percent of total trabecular surface, respectively. C, cortical bone; T, trabecular bone; RS, resorption surface; FS, formation surface. (*Figure continues.*)

greater sensitivity by histomorphometric analysis of the percutaneous bone biopsy specimen. Although the bone biopsy is being performed with increasing frequency in the field of metabolic bone disease, its application in primary hyperparathyroidism is still as a research tool. Early studies have indicated that evidence for hyperparathyroid bone disease is being seen even among patients who appear to be asymptomatic.[11] Cortical width, formation, and resorption surfaces, as well as the bone formation rate are most likely to be affected in primary hyperparathyroidism. Consistent with the information obtained by densitometry, trabecular bone volume appears to be normal in patients with primary hyperparathyroidism. Examples of histomorphometric features of primary hyperparathyroidism are shown in Figures 4-3 and 4-4.

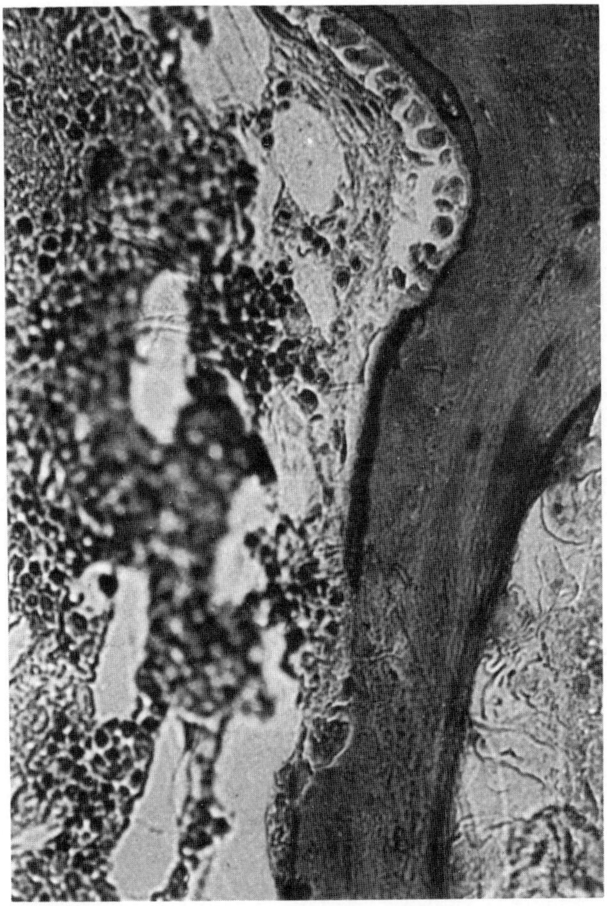

B

Fig. 4-3 (*Continued*). **(B)** A higher power view of the same biopsy. Note the active osteoclasts in scalloped resorption lacunae adjacent to team of osteoblasts busily depositing new, unmineralized osteoid over mineralized bone. In all cases, cortical bone is thin and porous. (Courtesy of Dr. David Dempster, Helen Hayes Hospital.)

It remains to be established whether these more sensitive methodologies by which bone involvement can be appreciated in primary hyperparathyroidism will be useful in predicting those who are at greater risk for complications of the disease. It also remains to be established whether more readily available markers of primary hyperparathyroidism, such as circulating parathyroid hormone, bone GLA protein, and others, are predictive of the information that can be obtained by analysis of bone biopsy specimens.

The kidney is the other major organ classically involved in primary hyperparathyroidism. Nephrolithiasis and nephrocalcinosis are the most common manifestations. Whereas 30 percent of the hyperparathyroid population used to present with kidney stones, the incidence today is approximately 10 percent.

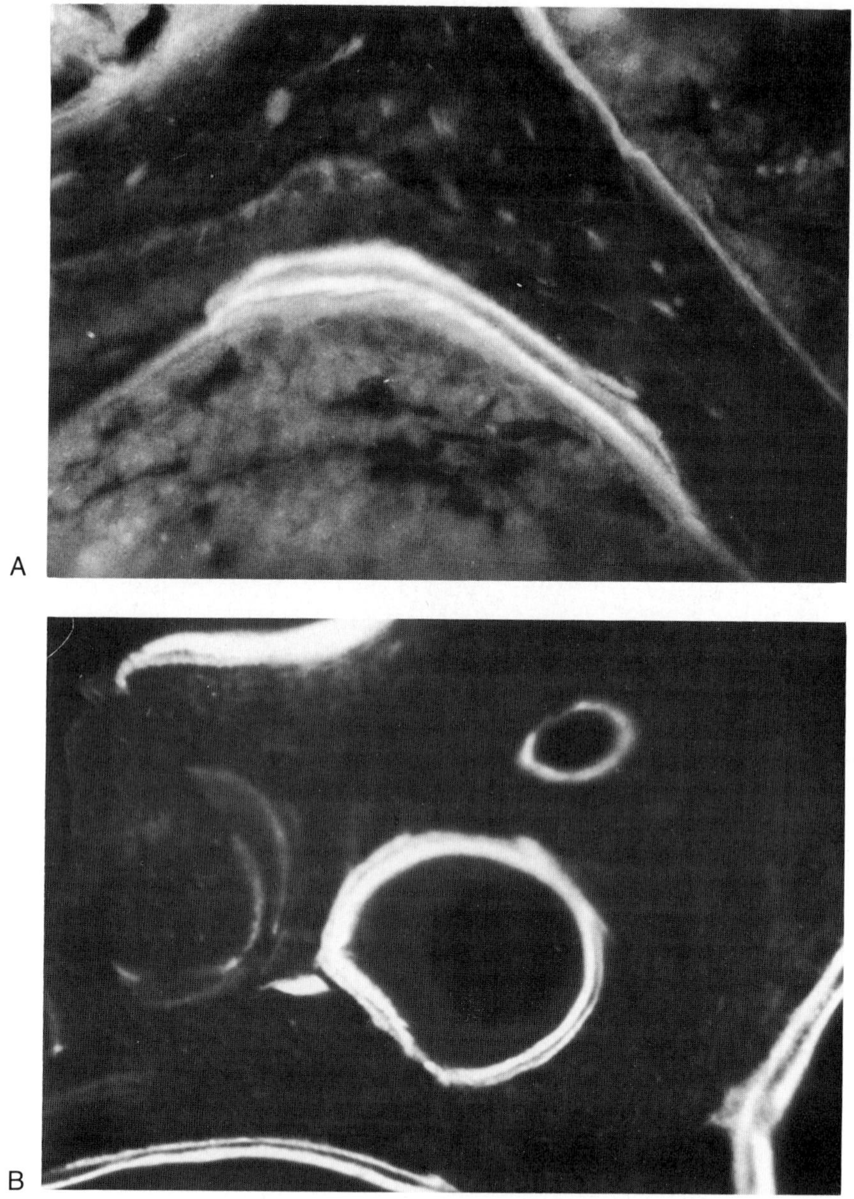

Fig. 4-4 Tetracycline uptake in bone in primary hyperparathyroidism. A normal pattern of tetracycline fluorescence **(A)** is shown in comparison to the pattern in a patient with primary hyperparathyroidism **(B)**. Note the extensive deposition of tetracycline labels along virtually the entire trabecular surface, indicating enhanced bone formation rate in primary hyperparathyroidism. The hyperparathyroid specimen is the same as shown in Figure 4-3. (Courtesy of Dr. David Dempster, Helen Hayes Hospital.)

As with overt hyperparathyroid bone disease, the reduced incidence of nephrolithiasis is a likely consequence of earlier detection of the disease. Hypercalciuria is appreciated perhaps more commonly than renal stones. Urinary calcium excretion greater than 250 mg daily may be seen in as many as 20 percent of patients. The most subtle renal manifestation of primary hyperparathyroidism is a reduced creatinine clearance rate in the absence of any other definable cause for impaired renal function.

There are a number of other potential complications of the hyperparathyroid state. Prominent among these is involvement of the neuromuscular system, which may well be responsible for the proximal muscle weakness and easy fatigability seen in some patients with primary hyperparathyroidism.[12] The gastrointestinal tract may be involved with peptic ulcer disease or pancreatitis. It is not clear, however, whether these potential gastrointestinal complications are pathophysiologically related to the hyperparathyroid state or whether the association with peptic ulcer and/or pancreatitis is based upon their common appearance in the population at large. Similarly, the increased incidence of hypertension among hyperparathyroid subjects may not be evidence of a causal relationship.[13] The list of systems potentially affected in primary hyperparathyroidism also includes the joints (gout and pseudogout[14]), the blood (anemia[15]), and the mind (depression[16]).

Clinical Forms

Primary hyperparathyroidism has different presentations due to its modern clinical profile, its potential for complications, and its different genetic forms (Table 4-2). The most common form of primary hyperparathyroidism is an asymptomatic disease characterized by mild, chronic hypercalcemia. The serum calcium level is usually within 1 mg/dl above the upper limit of normal. There are no other laboratory abnormalities and the patient has no specific or general complaints. Asymptomatic primary hyperparathyroidism constitutes by far the most common presentation of the disease today. In marked contrast, a very small number of patients with primary hyperparathyroidism have life-threatening hypercalcemia, a condition termed acute primary hyperparathy-

Table 4-2. Clinical Presentations of Primary Hyperparathyroidism

Asymptomatic hypercalcemia
Bone or stone disease
Other recognized complications (neuromuscular, gastrointestinal, articular, hematologic, central nervous system)
"Normocalcemic" hyperparathyroidism
Acute primary hyperparathyroidism
Parathyroid carcinoma
Multiple endocrine neoplasia, type I or II
Familial primary hyperparathyroidism
Familial cystic parathyroid adenomatosis
Neonatal hyperparathyroidism

roidism or parathyroid crisis.[17] One-fourth of patients with acute primary hyperparathyroidism have a previous history of mild, asymptomatic hypercalcemia, but at presentation their calcium level is greater than 15 mg/dl and symptoms of hypercalcemia are invariably present. The serum parathyroid hormone concentration is remarkably elevated, as much as 20 times normal. Bone and stone disease are often present together. Another unusual form of primary hyperparathyroidism, parathyroid carcinoma, is impossible to differentiate from acute primary hyperparathyroidism on clinical grounds but the markedly elevated parathyroid hormone levels in these two conditions do differentiate them from severe hypercalcemia of malignancy, in which parathyroid hormone levels are not elevated. It is important to consider the diagnosis of acute primary hyperparathyroidism or parathyroid carcinoma in life-threatening hypercalcemia because they are both theoretically curable disorders.

Occasionally, primary hyperparathyroidism will be diagnosed in the patient who presents with a kidney stone. Although unusual, the diagnosis should therefore be considered in any patient who has renal stone disease. In these patients, the serum calcium level is elevated, as is the case in virtually all forms of primary hyperparathyroidism. On a single determination, however, the serum calcium level may be normal. A form of primary hyperparathyroidism in which the serum calcium is frequently normal has been called *normocalcemic primary hyperparathyroidism.* It is more accurately described as *intermittent normocalcemic primary hyperparathyroidism* because patients with this condition do demonstrate hypercalcemia when they are monitored regularly.

Other clinical presentations of primary hyperparathyroidism occur in association with the familial syndromes. Of great interest is familial hypocalciuric hypercalcemia (FHH), a disorder not believed to be primarily a parathyroid disease, seen in kindreds of children with neonatal hyperparathyroidism, a life-threatening disorder of the parathyroid glands.[18] Finally, the recent description of familial cystic parathyroid adenomatosis calls attention to a disorder of the parathyroids characterized by recurrent disease as multiple glands become sequentially involved over a period of years. Most perplexing is the description of kindreds that appear to contain all three disorders: FHH, neonatal hyperparathyroidism, and familial cystic parathyroid adenomatosis.[3]

Diagnosis and Evaluation

Hypercalcemia is a virtually constant finding in primary hyperparathyroidism. It is difficult to make the diagnosis without hypercalcemia. Less common, but present in approximately one-third of patients, is hypophosphatemia. In most patients, the serum phosphorus level is in the lower range of normal, between 2.5 and 3.0 mg/dl. Even more uncommon is an increased serum level of alkaline phosphatase, reflecting the presence of bone disease. If the serum alkaline phosphatase is elevated, however, the urinary hydroxyproline excretion, which is a more direct index of bone turnover, will also be elevated. Mild hyperchloremia may be present, reflecting the action of parathyroid hormone to influence acid-base handling by the kidney. Hypercalciuria is present in only a minority of patients. The absence of excessive urinary calcium excretion among most patients with primary hyperparathyroidism is due to the effect of parathyroid hormone in facilitating renal conservation of calcium.

The most useful diagnostic test for primary hyperparathyroidism is the parathyroid hormone level per se. With rare exceptions, an elevation in the parathyroid hormone level along with hypercalcemia indicates the presence of hyperparathyroidism. The diagnostic utility of the radioimmunoassay for parathyroid hormone is due to three factors. First, the assays have been improved in recent years to the point where assays for parathyroid hormone that detect the midregion or C-terminal fragments of the molecule will be elevated in over 90 percent of the patients with documented primary hyperparathyroidism.[19] The second reason for the improved diagnostic utility of the radioimmunoassay for parathyroid hormone is recognition that malignancy, the most common other cause of hypercalcemia, is rarely associated with elevated levels of the hormone. Finally, the other causes of hypercalcemia (Table 4-1) are not associated with elevated levels of parathyroid hormone. Two exceptions worthy of note, namely lithium-associated and thiazide-associated hypercalcemia, are readily determined by history and further evaluation (see below). An example of the diagnostic usefulness of the several different commercially available radioimmunoassays for parathyroid hormone, especially as they distinguish primary hyperparathyroidism from hypercalcemia of malignancy and normal subjects, is illustrated in Figure 4-5.

The 1,25 dihydroxyvitamin D level is elevated in a substantial number of patients with primary hyperparathyroidism, but the importance of this finding relates more to possible pathophysiologic subgroups of patients than to diagnosis of the disease. Other disorders associated with hypercalcemia, particularly granulomatous disease, lymphomas, and vitamin D toxicity, may be associated with elevations in 1,25 dihydroxyvitamin D. With respect to primary hyperparathyroidism, one group of investigators has presented data to suggest that elevated levels of 1,25 dihydroxyvitamin D occur among patients who absorb abnormally large amounts of calcium from the gastrointestinal tract.[20] It is suggested that these patients may be at greater risk of kidney stones. On the other hand, a more recent report suggests that patients with primary hyperparathyroidism do not regulate the amount of 1,25 dihydroxyvitamin converted from its precursor, 25 hydroxyvitamin D,[21] suggesting that subgrouping of patients on the basis of 1,25 dihydroxyvitamin D levels may relate more to the amount of precursor substrate, 25-hydroxyvitamin D, than to any other pathophysiologic feature.

Treatment

The definitive therapy for primary hyperparathyroidism is surgical removal of the abnormal gland(s). In the hands of an experienced surgeon, the operation is successful over 90 percent of the time.[22] It is important to empha-

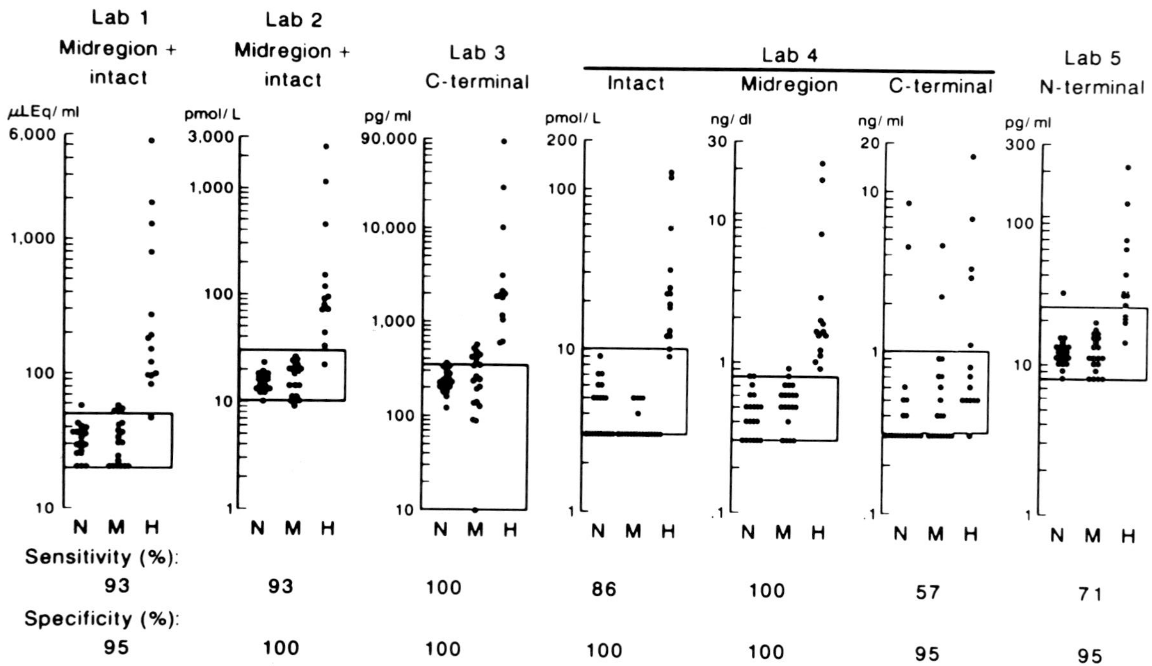

Fig. 4-5 Serum parathyroid hormone levels in 20 normal persons (N), 20 patients with humoral hypercalcemia of malignancy (M), and 14 patients with hyperparathyroidism (H), as assayed by 5 different laboratories. The open boxes in each scale represent the normal range. Laboratory assays 1,3,4, and 5 are available commercially. (From Lufkin et al.,[19] with permission.)

size that parathyroid surgery requires a surgeon with experience in the nuances and potential technical problems that may be encountered during the procedure. The operation can be prolonged and difficult because parathyroid glands are not always found in their classic locations, *para* to the thyroid gland. In particular, the inferior parathyroid glands may be found within the substance of the thyroid gland, in retroesophageal locations, and in the mediastinum. Moreover, the parathyroid adenoma does not always appear as a distinctive, oval-shaped, brownish-red gland. After the adenoma is located and confirmed as such by frozen section diagnosis, the surgeon attempts to identify the other gland on the same side of the neck. If the gland is normal, some surgeons will not seek to identify parathyroid tissue on the other side of the neck because the presence of two adenomas is most unusual. On the other hand, if hyperplastic tissue is discovered, the accepted operative procedure is to identify all glands and to remove the majority of tissue, leaving the patient with enough parathyroid substance to maintain a normal serum calcium level. This approach calls for the removal of approximately 3.5 glands in most cases. Some surgeons will remove all parathyroid tissue and transplant a small remnant in the patient's forearm.

Postoperatively, the patient may experience a period of mild, transient hypocalcemia until the normal, suppressed parathyroid tissue becomes active once again. During this time, there may be mild symptoms of neuromuscular irritability such as paresthesias of the extremities. In patients with evidence of overt bone disease, the postoperative course can be stormy as the skeleton seeks calcium with great avidity and causes prolonged, profound hypocalcemia (hungry bone syndrome). The calcium level, however, eventually returns to normal.

A more permanent complication of parathyroid surgery is hypoparathyroidism. Hypoparathyroidism does not always occur in the weeks to months following surgery but rather may develop years later. In this situation, it is believed that the functioning parathyroid tissue, left with a marginal blood supply at the time of surgery, is rendered hypofunctional with further compromise of vascular integrity over the years. Recurrent laryngeal nerve damage at the time of surgery can lead to chronic hoarseness, another permanent complication of the operation.

Localization of Abnormal Parathyroid Tissue

Noninvasive attempts to localize parathyroid tissue are not reliable enough yet to recommend the procedure for all patients who are to undergo parathyroid surgery. A noninvasive approach would be desirable in view of the fact that the greatest difficulty of parathyroid surgery is finding the abnormal gland. At the present time, localization procedures are indicated most strongly for patients with a previous history of neck surgery in whom anatomic landmarks are likely to have been distorted. Moreover, for those who have had unsuccessful surgery for primary hyperparathyroidism, it is more likely for the adenoma to be found ultimately in an aberrant site in the neck than in the mediastinum, which is another potential location.

The current interest in noninvasive methods for localizing parathyroid tissue has centered on sonography, computed tomography, and scintigraphy.[23] With no method, however, has the resolving power been refined yet to the point where adenomas can be repeatedly and reliably identified. Nevertheless, these approaches are under active investigation and it is likely that in the future noninvasive methods for locating parathyroid tissue will be more useful than at the present time. Examples of scintigraphy, sonography, and computed tomography are shown in Figures 4-6 and 4-7.

Other localization procedures used to identify parathyroid tissue preoperatively are arteriography and selective venous catheterization, which are more invasive procedures.[24] These two methods, especially when used together, may provide anatomic and functional identification of the adenoma. The success of

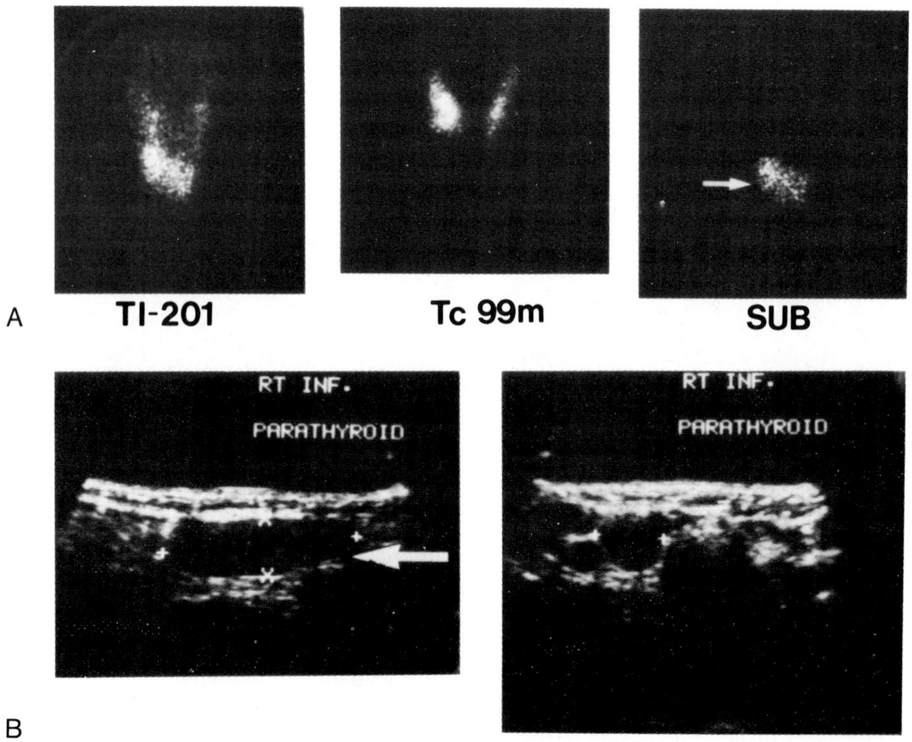

Fig. 4-6 Localization of parathyroid tissue by scintigraphy and ultrasound. **(A)** Thallium 201 (Tl 201) technetium 99m (Tc 99m) parathyroid scans in an elderly patient with hypercalcemia and elevated serum parathyroid hormone levels. Scintigram shows increased thallium uptake in tne inferior aspect of the right lobe of the thyroid, which is confirmed by subtraction (sub) image (arrow). **(B)** High-resolution parathyroid sonogram in same patient in sagittal (left) and transverse (right) planes confirm presence of enlarged parathyroid gland. At surgery, a 1200 mg right inferior (RT INF) parathyroid adenoma was removed. (From Winzelberg,[23] with permission.)

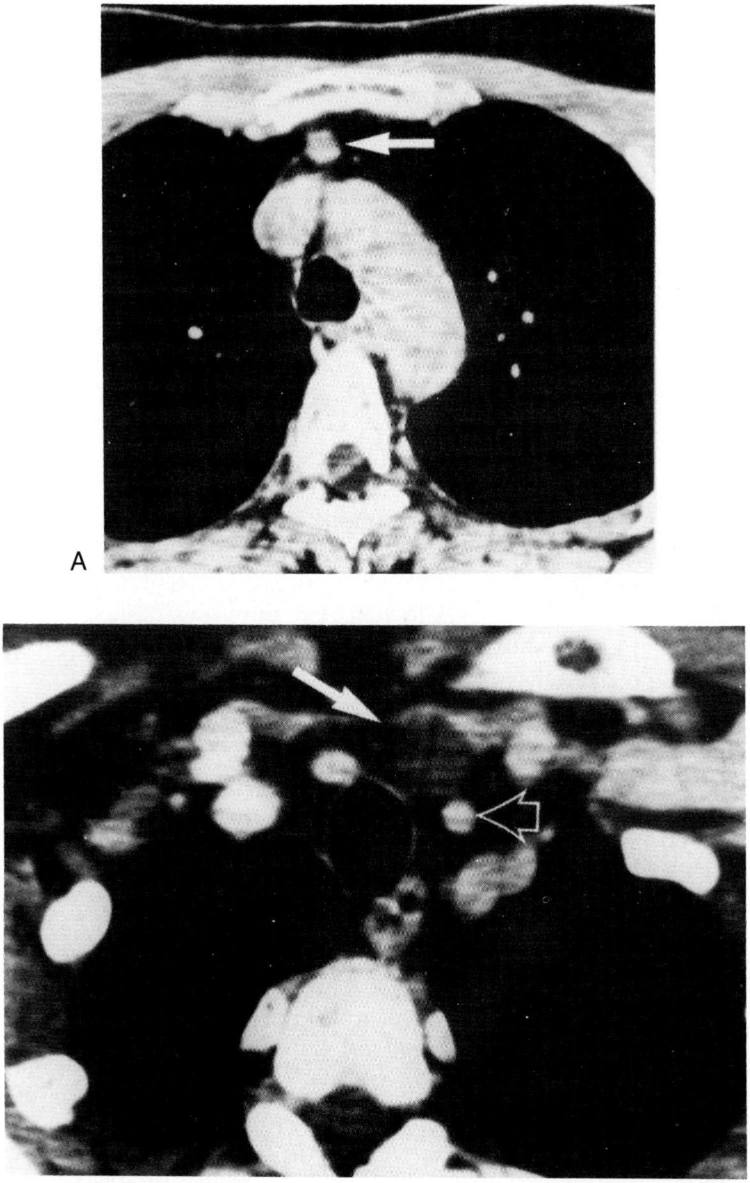

Fig. 4-7 Localization of parathyroid tissue by computed tomography. **(A)** Computed tomographic scan of mediastinum shows 2 cm mass (arrow) in superior mediastinum, which proved at surgery to be an ectopically located 1500 mg parathyroid adenoma. **(B)** High-resolution computed tomographic scan shows cyst (solid arrow) just anterior to the left common carotid artery (open arrow). (From Winzelberg,[23] with permission.)

either arteriography or selective venous catheterization is heavily dependent upon the skill of the angiographer. They are also time-consuming, tedious, and expensive procedures. On the other hand, they hold the promise of specific localization and, in this regard, should be reserved for those patients in whom it is vitally important to know beforehand the exact location of the abnormal parathyroid tissue. This consideration is particularly applicable to patients who have undergone several unsuccessful operations.

Guidelines for Parathyroid Surgery

In the days when primary hyperparathyroidism was more frequently associated with target organ involvement, the case for parathyroid surgery was straightforward. It is now not so clear.[25] The diagnosis of primary hyperparathyroidism is made most commonly in patients who have mild hypercalcemia without any other manifestations of the disease. Complicating the therapeutic dilemma are the following additional points. We do not know and cannot predict who among the asymptomatic will develop complications of primary hyperparathyroidism. We lack effective nonsurgical approaches to the disorder.[26] Finally, although newer methods to detect parathyroid bone disease in this asymptomatic population are showing evidence for parathyroid action on bone, we do not yet know whether this information can be related to the future course of the disease.

Suggested guidelines for surgery include a serum calcium level consistently greater than 1 mg/dl above the upper limits of normal, any complications of primary hyperparathyroidism (e.g., overt bone disease, nephrolithiasis); an episode of acute primary hyperparathyroidism; and relative youthfulness. These indications are not absolute and are subject to individualization both with respect to the physician and the patient. Some physicians advocate surgery whenever the diagnosis is made. Others believe that surgery should be reserved for those who are symptomatic. With respect to the patient, some will simply refuse surgery while others with coexisting medical problems may not wish to face the greater risk that would be associated with surgery. In addition, there are patients who have undergone multiple previous unsuccessful operations. Without the use of successful localization procedures, these patients also may not be regarded as surgical candidates.

Medical Management

The management of the patient with acute, parathyroid-hormone-dependent hypercalcemia is based upon the same principles for any severely hypercalcemic individual (see below). For chronic management of the mildly hypercalcemic individual, adequate hydration and ambulation are always encouraged. If possible, diuretics should be avoided because of the risk of dehydration and other electrolyte problems. Thiazide diuretics, in particular, are to be avoided because they may actually worsen the hypercalcemia. The diet should be adequate in calcium. High-calcium diets, which have been considered reasonable because of their possible suppressive effects on parathyroid hormones, could conceivably worsen the hypercalcemia, especially in those patients with elevated levels of 1,25 dihydroxyvitamin D. The rationale for a low calcium intake is based upon the notion that less calcium will be made available for absorption. On the other hand, low-calcium diets could conceivably predispose patients to a further increase in levels of parathyroid hormone. Until the pathophysiology of primary hyperparathyroidism is more completely understood, it seems wise to advise patients to maintain a normal calcium intake.

A number of more specific approaches to the medical management of primary hyperparathyroidism have been considered. H_2 receptor antagonists and beta-adrenergic inhibitors are not effective despite in vitro data suggesting that their respective agonists may stimulate parathyroid hormone secretion.[27] Calcitonin, an agent theoretically useful to counteract the actions of parathyroid hormone on bone, is not efficacious either as a chronic therapy. Oral phosphate will lower the serum calcium in primary hyperparathyroidism by approximately 1 mg/dl when a dosage of 1 to 2 g daily is used. Long-term use of phosphate, however, is associated with the potential for ectopic calcification due to deposition of calcium–phosphate complexes in soft tissues and a further increase in parathyroid hormone levels.[28] Recently, estrogen therapy has been studied in women whose primary hyperparathyroidism becomes evident in the early postmenopausal period.[29,30] The rationale for this approach is the antagonism by estrogen of parathyroid-hormone-mediated bone resorption. In these postmenopausal women, the calcium has declined in conjunction with estrogen therapy by approximately 1 mg/dl. Finally, newer diphosphonate agents that are potent inhibitors of bone resorption are being developed. In view of the early promising effects of dichloromethylene diphosphonate,[31] an agent no longer available in the United States, newer diphosphonates may prove to be useful in primary hyperparathyroidism.

Hypercalcemia Associated with Malignancy

Malignancy is an important consideration in the differential diagnosis of hypercalcemia. It constitutes, along with primary hyperparathyroidism, the most common cause of hypercalcemia.[32] The diagnosis of malignancy is usually readily made because the tumor is rarely occult and clinical manifestations are often present. Facilitating the clinical distinction between malignancy and primary parathyroidism is the parathyroid hormone level. As noted above, patients with malignancy, independent of the mechanism of the hypercalcemia, do not demonstrate elevations in parathyroid hormone by most available radioimmunoassays for the hormone. The parathyroid hormone level is actually suppressed in most assays (Fig. 4-4). Thus, in the patient with hypercalcemia, the level of the parathyroid hormone establishes or rules out a hyperparathyroid state. If primary hyperparathyroidism is not present, the odds are great that the patient will be shown to have a malignant disorder. The other causes of hypercalcemia are considered only after malignancy and hyperparathyroidism have been ruled out or unless the history or physical examination suggests that another explanation for the hypercalcemia is likely.

The hypercalcemias associated with malignancy are best considered from the viewpoint of pathophysiologic mechanisms. One mechanism of hypercalcemia appears to be related to direct invasion of bone by the tumor leading to local osteolysis and release of calcium into the extracellular space.[33,34] The most common tumors that act via this mechanism are multiple myeloma and breast cancer but virtually any tumor that metastasizes to bone can cause hypercalcemia, presumably by the same or a similar mechanism. The histologic picture is of striking osteoclast hyperactivity. In multiple myeloma, the osteoblast is characteristically inactive. It is not known why the signal to stimulate osteoblast action, a normal consequence of osteoclast activation, is absent in myeloma. It is currently believed that the tumor in bone is responsible for the elaboration of local factors that in turn activate the osteoclast. The original description of this factor was called *osteoclast activating factor* (OAF[35]) but it is now appreciated that there are a number of bone-resorbing principles that could be responsible for osteoclast activation. Leading candidates are tumor necrosis factor alpha, lymphotoxin, interleukin-1, and prostaglandin E_2.[36] In in vitro models, each agent has been shown to stimulate bone resorption. One of the factors responsible for the hypercalcemia of multiple myeloma is likely to be lymphotoxin.[37] It is possible that a given tumor may be responsible for the elaboration of more than one factor, either directly or by stimulating the production of lymphokines and monokines. Any one might not be present in sufficient concentration to cause osteoclast activation but together there might be a synergistic effect sufficient to lead to bone resorption.

Another mechanism responsible for malignancy-associated hypercalcemia is the production by the tumor, not resident in bone, of a factor that stimulates osteoclast-mediated bone resorption. This is an old hypothesis, orginally proposed by Albright,[38] that has taken over four decades to be tested directly. Humoral hypercalcemia of malignancy (HHM) appears to be an important mechanism of hypercalcemia in squamous cell carcinomas (lung, esophagus, head and neck), renal and bladder tumors, and in ovarian cancer. These patients manifest certain biochemical characteristics of primary hyperparathyroidism, such as hypophosphatemia and elevated urinary cAMP.[39] In fact, for many years it was believed that these tumors were producing parathyroid hormone ectopically. It has been unequivocally established, however, that these tumors do not produce the native parathyroid hormone. An array of radioimmunoassays for parathyroid hormones used to measure circulating material as well as tumor-derived activity has shown conclusively that parathyroid hormone levels are suppressed in HHM. In addition, there is no detectable mRNA encoding for parathyroid hormone in the malignant tissue.[40] There are other differences between HHM and primary hyperparathyroidism in that fractional urinary calcium excretion is elevated and 1,25 dihydroxyvitamin D levels are suppressed in HHM.[34,39] However, the HHM factor, like parathyroid hormone, does stimulate adenylate cyclase activity in renal and skeletal tissues and can be inhibited by antagonists of parathyroid hormone.[34] The inference that the factor in HHM is similar, in part, to parathyroid hormone has recently been confirmed by several laboratories.[41–43] The first 15 amino acids of the factor share with parathyroid hormone close sequence homology (with only a few conservative substitutions) but the remainder of the molecule diverges extensively and shares no other primary features of the parathyroid hormone molecules. Homology at the extreme N-terminal end of the molecule explains its PTH-like bioactivity. Divergence beyond position 15 is likely to account for its poor cross-reactivity with PTH-specific antisera that are virtually exclusively directed at sites beyond position 20.

Another family of factors that may ultimately be shown to be important in the syndrome of HHM is transforming growth factor (TGF[44]). The TGFs of the alpha and beta classes have in vitro bone-resorbing properties. Molecules with features similar to the TGFs have been extracted from tumors associated with HHM.

In malignancy-associated hypercalcemia, yet another class of molecules may be responsible for hypercalcemia.[45–46] In histiocytic lymphomas, elevated levels of 1,25 dihydroxyvitamin D have been measured in the circulation. It is believed that the tumor produces the active form of vitamin D by converting the substrate 25-hydroxyvitamin D to 1,25 dihydroxyvitamin D. This is similar to the demonstration of 1,25 dihydroxyvitamin D-producing activity in a wide variety of granulomatous diseases. It is not clear whether the hypercalcemia seen in human-immunodeficiency-associated lymphoma is also caused by the same mechanism.

Uncommon Causes of Hypercalcemia

The long list of causes of hypercalcemia includes a large number that are uncommon or rare. In the aggregate, they account for a very small minority of patients with hypercalcemia. Nevertheless, when the common causes of hypercalcemia (primary hyperparathyroidism or malignancy) have been excluded, the longer differential diagnosis of hypercalcemia should be recalled and considered. For the purposes of organization, this discussion considers them in terms of system and pathophysiologic groups although Table 4-1 more practically presents them in terms of uncommon and rare causes. The therapeutic approach to hypercalcemia of all causes is considered separately (see below).

Vitamin Toxicity

Vitamin D toxicity can be associated with hypercalcemia of life-threatening proportions. When vitamin D toxicity occurs, it is usually in conjunction with its therapeutic role in the hypoparathyroid states or among those who ingest excess quantities as a result of misguided "health diets." The course of vitamin D toxicity is somewhat dependent upon the form of the vitamin ingested. When the parent compound is used, hypercalcemia can be prolonged because vitamin D is stored in fat tissues and may be released over a period of weeks to months. In this case, hypercalcemia can persist for months. The duration of hypercalcemia is shorter if vitamin D toxicity is due to preparations of 25-hydroxyvitamin D or to the active metabolite, 1,25 dihydroxyvitamin D.

The diagnosis of vitamin D toxicity is relatively straightforward if there is a history of vitamin ingestion but can be obscure if a history is not obtained. In toxicity due to vitamin D, 25-hydroxyvitamin D is markedly elevated but the 1,25 dihydroxyvitamin D level may be only minimally so.[47] This is due to the exquisite control of 1,25 dihydroxyvitamin D production in the kidney, preventing overproduction of the active hormone, but relatively poor control of the hepatic conversion step. If toxicity is due to overadministration of 25-hydroxyvitamin D or to 1,25 dihydroxyvitamin D itself, the ingested compound will be measured in excess amounts in the circulation. In all cases, the hypercalcemia is due to increased absorption of calcium from the gastrointestinal tract and to calcium mobilization from bone. A clue to the presence of vitamin D toxicity is the elevated phosphorus level that may accompany the hypercalcemia.

Hypercalcemia due to **vitamin A** toxicity is most unusual.[48] In excess of 50,000 international units daily, over many months, must be injested before hypercalcemia develops. Usually, other manifestations of vitamin A toxicity (hepatic dysfunction, dermatitis, dementia) are also present. The hypercalcemia is due to excessive calcium mobilization from bone. Occasionally, the periosteal changes of vitamin A excess are seen in radiographs of long bones. Measurements of total vitamin A levels and its retinyl esters help to confirm the diagnosis.

Hypercalcemia in Association with Other Endocrinopathies

Thyrotoxicosis is associated with mild hypercalcemia in 5 to 10 percent of patients. Although the pathophysiologic basis for the elevated serum calcium is not clear, it is believed that excessive osteoclast activity is induced by the thyrotoxic state. With return of thyroid function to normal, the hypercalcemia remits.

Pheochromocytoma may be accompanied by hypercalcemia, usually in association with coexisting primary hyperparathyroidism in multiple endocrine neoplasia, type II.[49] The possible production by the pheochromocytoma of a humoral substance that causes osteoclast-mediated bone resorption, in a manner similar to the HHM syndrome, has been suspected in rare instances.[50] It is highly unlikely, although theoretically possible, that the catecholamine(s) produced by the tumor induces the secretion of excess parathyroid hormone via their beta-adrenergic actions. The proper therapeutic approach to the patient with a pheochromocytoma and hypercalcemia is first to remove the adrenal tumor for reasons of safety and also for the remote possibility that the hypercalcemia will return to normal.

Adrenal Insufficiency is a rare cause of hypercalcemia. The elevated serum calcium level is due to loss of the antagonist properties of glucocorticoids on calcium absorption and on bone mobilization as well as to dehydration that always is seen in untreated adrenal insufficiency. The coexistence of tuberculosis, which used to be the most common cause of Addison's disease, should also be considered as a cause of the hypercalcemia.

Vasoactive Intestinal Polypeptide (VIP)-producing tumors of pancreatic islet cells are not infrequently associated with hypercalcemia.[51] In some cases, the hypercalcemia has been reported to normalize after removal of the VIP-oma. More commonly, the hypercalcemia is seen in association with the multiple endocrine neoplasia syndrome, type I.

Drug-Induced Hypercalcemia

Thiazide Diuretics may cause hypercalcemia in the absence of any intrinsic abnormality in mineral metabolism. Actions of the thiazides to reduce glomerular filtration, to enhance tubular reabsorption of calcium, and perhaps also to alter sensitivity of target tissues to parathyroid hormone are all possible explanations for the hypercalcemia that may occur. It is important to be mindful of a history of thiazide use in the hypercalcemic patient suspected of having primary hyperparathyroidism. A number of patients whose hypercalcemia becomes evident on thiazide therapy will continue to be hypercalcemic after the medication is discontinued. The diagnosis of primary hyperparathyroidism is eventually made. Thiazide-associated hypercalcemia is one of the causes of hypercalcemia that may be associated with elevated levels of parathyroid hormone. The diagnosis of primary hyperparathyroidism cannot be established definitively unless the patient remains hypercalcemic with elevated parathyroid hormone levels 2 to 3 months after thiazide therapy has been discontinued.

Lithium Carbonate can be associated with hypercalcemia. It used to be thought that lithium alters the set point for regulation of parathyroid hormone secretion by calcium but more recent evidence has made this explanation doubtful.[52,53] Similar to the situation with thiazide diuretics, the diagnosis of primary hyperparathyroidism cannot be made with confidence until the drug has been discontinued. If hypercalcemia and elevated levels of parathyroid hormone persist, primary hyperparathyroidism can be confirmed. Often, however, the serum calcium level returns to normal.

Estrogens and Antiestrogens have been associated with hypercalcemia, particularly in patients being treated with these agents for breast cancer.[54] The hypercalcemia usually develops in patients who have obvious skeletal metastases. This cause of hypercalcemia usually does not present any difficulty with the differential diagnosis of hypercalcemia because it occurs in a known setting.

Theophylline has also been reported to be responsible for hypercalcemia when the drug is circulating in toxic amounts.[55]

Hypercalcemia Associated with Granulomatous Diseases

The list of known granulomatous diseases that have been associated with hypercalcemia is long (Table 4-1). The best known examples are sarcoidosis and tuberculosis but more unusual ones include histoplasmosis, coccidioidomycosis, leprosy, berylliosis, candidiasis, eosinophilic granuloma, and even the granulomas that may be induced after silicone implantation.[56] In all cases, the mechanism for the hypercalcemia is likely to be due to production by the granuloma itself of 1,25 dihydroxyvitamin D. These patients, especially those with sarcoidosis, tend to be exquisitely sensitive to small amounts of vitamin D compounds. In the patient whose hypercalcemia is a diagnostic problem, elevated 1,25 dihydroxyvitamin D levels can become a clue to the presence of a granulomatous disorder. This is particularly true if primary hyperparathyroidism has been excluded and if the other disorders that can be associated with elevated 1,25 dihydroxyvitamin D levels (vitamin D toxicity, lymphoma) are also excluded.

Familial Hypocalciuric Hypercalcemia

Familial hypocalciuric hypercalcemia (FHH) is an autosomal dominant disorder with high penetrance and can be confused with primary hyperparathyroidism.[57,58] Similar to the common presentation of primary hyperparathyroidism, patients with FHH are asymptomatic. In contrast to primary hyperparathyroidism, this is not a disorder of the parathyroids. The parathyroid glands are virtually always normal histologically, and the parathyroid hormone level is within normal limits. Surgery, short of total parathyroidectomy, does not cure the hypercalcemia. Clues to the diagnosis are the family history and the low urinary excretion of calcium, usually a ratio below 0.01 of calcium clearance to creatinine clearance. Although this disorder holds great interest with respect to its underlying pathophysiology, and for its association with neonatal primary hyperparathyroidism and/or familial cystic parathyroid adenomatosis, both of which are clear disorders of the parathyroid glands, FHH itself is rare.

Immobilization Hypercalcemia

Although negative calcium balance occurs regularly in any individual subjected to prolonged immobilization, hypercalcemia occurs only in young patients or in those who harbor an underlying disorder of mineral metabolism such as Paget's disease of bone or malignancy (with or without overt skeletal metastases). On histologic examination of bone in this setting, immobilization is associated with enhanced osteoclast activity and diminished osteoblast activity.[59] Levels of parathyroid hormone, nephrogenous cyclic AMP, and 1,25 dihydroxyvitamin D are all suppressed.[60] It should be emphasized that despite the negative calcium balance that regularly occurs in immobilization, it is distinctly unusual for an otherwise healthy individual to become hypercalcemic when bed-ridden. In primary hyperparathyroidism, mild hypercalcemia can be worsened rapidly leading to a parathyroid crisis when the patient is immobilized.

Situational Hypercalcemias

Several distinctive clinical situations may be associated with hypercalcemia and are obvious in terms of the setting in which they occur. In the patient receiving long-term parenteral nutrition, hypercalcemia is seen usually in association with a syndrome of osteomalacia. There are interesting pathologic similarities between this syndrome and the osteomalacia associated with aluminum toxicity in patients maintained on dialysis.[61] Another form of situational hypercalcemia occurs during the recovery phase of acute renal failure.[62] It is believed that the hypercalcemia is most likely due to a rebound phenomenon of the elevated parathyroid hormone and 1,25 dihydroxyvitamin D levels that were induced in the early stages of the renal failure. In a contrasting picture, the patient with posttransplantation hypercalcemia develops an exuberant production of 1,25 hydroxyvitamin D by the new kidney. Finally, the milk alkali syndrome describes a setting of hypercalcemia that used to be observed when patients were treated with large amounts of absorbable antacids and milk for peptic ulcer disease.[63] It is rarely seen today.

MANAGEMENT OF HYPERCALCEMIA

Clinical Features

Hypercalcemia is associated with a set of signs and symptoms that are independent of its cause. The absolute level as well as the rate of rise of the serum calcium are both important when assessing the patient for features of symptomatic hypercalcemia. The serum albumin concentration should also be considered, in view of the fact that an ionized calcium level is not always readily available. If the serum albumin concentration is reduced, the ionized calcium level will actually be higher than the estimate based upon the total calcium concentration. Thus, for a given concentration of calcium, the patient with a reduced serum albumin level is likely to be more symptomatic. Mild hypercalcemia (below 11.5 mg/dl) is rarely associated with specific symptoms, whereas higher levels are more likely to cause symptoms. Symptoms are invariably present at levels greater than 13.5 mg/dl. In very rare situations, marked elevations in total serum calcium level in the absence of symptoms is due to a myeloma protein that binds calcium.[64] In these patients, the ionized calcium level is normal.

A list of signs and symptoms of hypercalcemia is presented in Table 4-3. Superimposed upon generalized weakness, a number of specific organ systems

Table 4-3. Clinical Features of Hypercalcemia

General	
	Weakness
	Dehydration
	Metastatic calcification
Central nervous system	
	Impaired concentration
	Increased sleep requirement
	Altered states of consciousness (confusion, lethargy, stupor, coma)
Gastrointestinal tract	
	Polydypsia
	Anorexia
	Nausea
	Vomiting
	Constipation
	Pancreatitis
	Peptic ulcer
Renal	
	Polyuria
	Decreased function
	Decreased concentrating ability
	Nephrolithiasis
	Nephrocalcinosis
Cardiovascular	
	Hypertension
	Electrocardiographic changes (shortened QT interval)
	Increased sensitivity to digitalis

may be involved. Gastrointestinal signs include anorexia, which may lead to nausea and vomiting, if the hypercalcemia is severe. Constipation is common. Polydypsia may accompany polyuria as a consequence of impaired renal concentrating ability. Other renal manifestations include nephrolithiasis, nephrocalcinosis, and generally decreased glomerular function. Specific cardiovascular signs of hypercalcemia are an elevated blood pressure, shortened QT interval on electrocardiogram, and increased sensitivity to digitalis. Finally, the central nervous system is affected by hypercalcemia. Altered states of consciousness, from confusion to coma, are all potential complications of the hypercalcemic state.

Therapy

The condition underlying the hypercalcemia should influence both the decision to treat and the aggressiveness of therapy. If the diagnosis is unclear or is known to be a curable disorder, such as acute primary hyperparathyroidism, vigorous intervention is appropriate. On the other hand, severe hypercalcemia in a comatose patient with a terminal malignancy is not always best considered in an aggressive light.

General measures to treat hypercalcemia are useful for all hypercalcemic conditions and are designed to reduce the serum calcium level independent of the underlying pathophysiology (Table 4-4).[65] Rehydration is always an initial mainstay of general therapy. The administration of saline is also useful to

Table 4-4. Management of Hypercalcemia

General	Specific
Rehydration	Plicamycin (Mithramycin)
	Diphosphonates
Saline administration	Calcitonin
Diuresis with furosemide	Glucocorticoids
Dialysis (if necessary because of renal failure)	Phosphate
Mobilization	Therapy of underlying condition

induce a saliuresis, which in turn is accompanied by an obligatory loss of urinary calcium.[66] Fluid and saline should be tailored to the degree of dehydration and need not be overvigorous, especially in an elderly patient whose cardiovascular tolerance for salt and water is marginal. If there are concerns in this regard, a loop diuretic such as furosemide can facilitate the calciuresis. The patient's overall status and potential loss of other electrolytes with aggressive use of loop diuretics should be considered. If furosemide is to be used, hydration should always be accomplished first. Thiazide diuretics should never be used for this purpose because they may actually worsen the hypercalcemia. Although mobilization is not usually possible in the early course of hospitalization in the symptomatic hypercalcemic patient, it should be attempted as soon as possible. A last general measure to consider in the patient with severe hypercalcemia, who is refractory to other approaches, is dialysis. Dialysis is usually not instituted unless the more specific approaches to the management of hypercalcemia have been attempted without success.

Specific measures to treat hypercalcemia are designed to inhibit the mechanisms responsible for the abnormality and are thus somewhat dependent upon the cause of the hypercalcemia. For the most common causes of hypercalcemia, (primary hyperparathyroidism and malignancy) excessive calcium mobilization from bone due to osteoclast-mediated bone resorption is the underlying pathophysiologic mechanism. Thus, the most efficacious agents, overall, are those that alter osteoclast function.

Plicamycin (Mithramycin) is a major specific approach to treating life-threatening hypercalcemia. It is an osteoclast inhibitor and acts reliably and predictably to lower the serum calcium within 24 to 48 hours after administration.[67] The dosage is 15 to 25 μg/kg given as a daily 4 hour infusion for up to 5 days. The calcium level will begin to fall after the first or second administration. Continued daily use of mithramycin increases the risks of side effects such as nephrotoxicity, hepatotoxicity, and platelet dysfunction.

The diphosphonates represent another class of agents that reduce the serum calcium level by interfering with osteoclast function. In the United States, only ethane hydroxy 1,1 diphosphonic acid (EHDP) is available for parenteral use.[68] However, several other diphosphonates, including dichloromethylene diphosphonate, are available in other countries.[69] The diphosphonates will lower the serum calcium with a time course similar to that of mithramycin. They have not been reported to be associated with any significant side effects when used in the acute setting.

Calcitonin should theoretically be an ideal anticalcemic drug because it not only inhibits osteoclast-mediated bone resorption but also increases the urinary excretion of calcium. Unfortunately, the use of calcitonin for the management of hypercalcemia has been disappointing. At most, only a mild reduction in the serum calcium level, in the range of 1 to 2 mg/dl, can be expected. Some investigators have reported it to be more efficacious when calcitonin is used in combination with glucocorticoids.[70] It is best, however, not to rely upon calcitonin when the serum calcium level is markedly elevated.

Phosphate will also lower the serum calcium level by inhibiting bone resorption. Other mechanisms include interference with gastrointestinal absorption of calcium and inhibition of the renal formation of 1,25 dihydroxyvitamin D. Unfortunately, parenteral phosphate, which is the only preparation to be considered in the acute setting, may be associated with ectopic deposits of calcium–phosphate complexes in vital organs, the vasculature, and the extracellular space. This potentially dangerous side effect of phosphate therapy should be balanced against its potential to reduce the serum calcium. It should be reserved for patients with persisting hypercalcemia after all other measures have failed.

Two additional anticalcemic agents, WR2721 and gallium nitrate, act, in part, by inhibiting bone resorption.[71,72] Investigational experience with each compound is too limited to know how effective they will be in the management of symptomatic hypercalcemia.

Although the vast majority of patients with symptomatic hypercalcemia are best treated with agents that block accelerated bone resorption, the differential diagnosis does include a number of settings associated with vitamin D sensitivity. The pathophysiology of the hypercalcemia in these instances (vitamin D toxicity, granulomatous diseases, and some lymphomas) is due, at least in part, to the specific actions of vitamin D. The anti-vitamin-D properties of glucocorticoids can help to reduce the serum calcium levels in these disorders. Glucocorticoids are also useful in multiple myeloma and in some kinds of breast cancer. Classically, they are ineffectve in the treatment of primary hyperparathyroidism.[73]

An important specific therapy in the management of the acutely hypercalcemic individual relates to the underlying disorder. Obviously, definitive management depends upon being able to treat the disorder responsible for the hypercalcemia. However, even when this is feasible, the hypercalcemia is preferably first reduced by instituting some of the general and specific measures described in this section. Rarely, an emergency operation for uncontrollable hypercalcemia due to acute primary hyperparathyroidism can be a life-saving procedure.

HYPOCALCEMIC DISORDERS

Only those hypocalcemic disorders associated with absent (or inadequate) levels of parathyroid hormone or resistance to parathyroid hormone are considered in this chapter. These hypoparathyroid states are to be differentiated from

Table 4-5. The Hypoparathyroid States

Following neck surgery
Idiopathic
Isolated
Multiple end-organ endocrine failure
Familial
Hypomagnesemia, severe
Infiltrative
Hemochromatosis
Thalassemia
Wilson's disease
Metastatic carcinoma
Following neck irradiation
DiGeorge's syndrome
Neonatal hypocalcemia
Pseudohypoparathyroidism

those disorders in which the primary problem responsible for hypocalcemia is associated with a normal, compensatory increase in parathyroid hormone (see Chapters 2, 5, and 8).

The differential diagnosis of hypoparathyroidism is shown in Table 4-5. Hypocalcemia is virtually always present in untreated hypoparathyroidism. With the exception of the pseudohypoparathyroid states, the hypoparathyroid patient demonstrates low or undetectable levels of parathyroid hormone. The combination of hypocalcemia and frankly low or relatively low parathyroid hormone levels is necessary to define the condition as hypoparathyroidism.

Idiopathic Hypoparathyroidism

Hypoparathyroidism may occur spontaneously at any age in patients without any other endocrinopathy. It is also seen in association with a syndrome of multiple end-organ endocrine failure. The most distinctive combination is the hypoparathyroidism that occurs in association with hypoadrenalism and mucocutaneous candidiasis.[74] Gonadal failure, hypothyroidism, and diabetes mellitus may also be seen in this syndrome. Nonendocrine abnormalities, besides mucocutaneous candidiasis, such as pernicious anemia, chronic active hepatitis, alopecia, vitiligo, or malabsorption may be present or may develop over time. The clinical presentation of this form of idiopathic hypoparathyroidism (type I polyglandular syndrome) varies with respect to the sequence of glandular involvement and also to the number of different glands affected in the course of a patient's life. Antibodies directed against specific endocrine tissues and T-cell abnormalities suggest an autoimmune cause.[75,76] In the isolated form of hypoparathyroidism, antibodies that inhibit the secretion of parathyroid hormone, as opposed to the parathyroid gland itself, have been demonstrated.[77,78]

Finally, there is a familial form of isolated hypoparathyroidism expressed via several different inheritance patterns. Antibodies are absent. In recent molecular studies of several kindreds, the parathyroid hormone gene appears to be intact, suggesting a genetic-induced alteration in synthesis and/or secretion of the hormone.[79]

Postsurgical Hypoparathyroidism

Hypoparathyroidism occurs most commonly following surgery either for hyperparathyroidism or for another disorder requiring an operation on the anterior neck. The hypoparathyroid state that occurs regularly following successful parathyroid surgery is transient. When all parathyroid tissue is removed, however, permanent hypoparathyroidism ensues. In some patients, hypoparathyroidism does not develop until years after surgery. It is not clear why the time of onset can be so far removed from the time of surgery. It is possible that the vasculature supplying the remaining parathyroid glands was rendered marginal at the time of surgery and becomes further compromised over the years. Postsurgical hypoparathyroidism is not associated with the nonendocrine signs of idiopathic hypoparathyroidism such as mucocutaneous candidiasis, suggesting that these features are not due to the hypocalcemia per se.

Hypomagnesemia

A particularly interesting, reversible form of hypoparathyroidism is seen in patients with severe hypomagnesemia. When the magnesium deficiency is associated with alcohol abuse, it is due both to diminished oral intake of magnesium-containing foods and to alcohol-induced urinary losses of magnesium. Magnesium deficiency also occurs in a variety of gastrointestinal diseases and in some patients receiving cisplatinum or aminoglycoside antibiotics.[80] Two mechanisms are responsible for the hypocalcemia of hypomagnesemia.[81,82] When the serum magnesium level is extremely low (i.e., < 1 mg/dl), parathyroid hormone secretion is impaired. Operationally, therefore, these patients are hypoparathyroid because they demonstrate concomitant hypocalcemia and low levels of parathyroid hormone. When magnesium is administered to these patients, parathyroid hormone levels rise within minutes (Fig. 4-8). The serum calcium level, however, does not begin to rise for 24 to 48 hours after magnesium administration. Thus, the secretory block to parathyroid hormone secretion does not account completely for the syndrome. The second mechanism for the hypocalcemia of hypomagnesemia is a peripheral resistance to the actions of parathyroid hormone. The peripheral resistance takes longer to overcome, several days following restoration of normal parathyroid secretory function.

These pathophysiologic features of hypomagnesemia call for a special approach to its therapy. In view of fact that the hypocalcemia is not rapidly corrected after magesium is given to the patient, the hypocalcemia must be treated with parenteral calcium if the patient is symptomatic. Symptoms of hypocalcemia are thus relieved until sensitivity to parathyroid hormone is restored.

Unusual Causes of Hypoparathyroidism

As noted in Table 4-5, hypoparathyroidism can be caused by infiltration of the parathyroid glands. Heavy metal accumulation with iron (hemochromato-

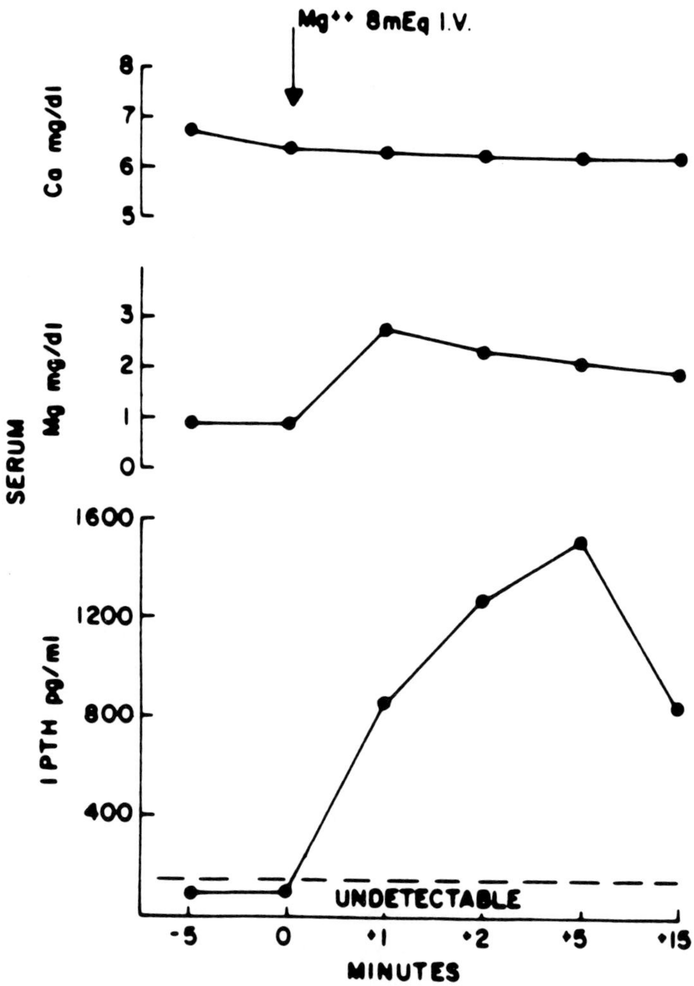

Fig. 4-8 The effect of an intravenous injection of 8 to 10 mEq magnesium on the serum concentration of calcium, magnesium, and parathyroid hormone (IPTH) in hypocalcemic magnesium-deficient patients with undetectable basal levels of IPTH. (From Rude et al.,[81] with permission.)

sis, thalassemia) or with copper (Wilson's disease) can lead, in rare instances to hypoparathyroidism. Infiltration of the parathyroid glands can also rarely be due to metastatic carcinoma. Hypoparathyroidism has been reported to be due to chemotherapy with doxorubicin or cytosine arabinoside. Hypoparathyroidism after exposure to ionizing radiation is most uncommon because the parathyroid glands are not generally sensitive to radiation.

Congenital hypoparathyroidism occurs as part of DiGeorge's syndrome. The thymus and parathyroids, which normally develop from the third and fourth branchial pouches, are absent in this disorder that is associated with death in the first few years of life. In another hypoparathyroid state of infancy, the offspring of mothers with primary hyperparathyroidism may demonstrate hypocalcemia in the first few weeks of life. Infantile hypoparathyroidism occurs because of suppression of the neonatal glands by maternal hypercalcemia. It is a transient condition until the neonatal parathyroid glands acquire responsiveness to normal serum calcium concentrations.

Relative Hypoparathyroidism

This category of hypoparathyroidism is associated with a normal, but inadequate, compensatory increase in parathyroid hormone concentration (Table 4-5). The parathyroid glands, per se, are not responsible for the hypocalcemia of these disorders. The hypocalcemia of acute pancreatitis is probably the most common example of relative hypoparathyroidism. In this setting, the hypocalcemia, which is due to deposition of calcium in conjunction with fatty acid release in severe pancreatitis,[83,84] does not lead to a vigorous increase in parathyroid hormone levels.[85] The true magnitude of the parathyroid response in acute pancreatitis needs reevaluation with the more sensitive, active species-specific radioimmunoassays for parathyroid hormone. Other causes of relative hypoparathyroidism are most unusual but include osteoblastic metastases (especially breast and prostatic carcinoma), multiple citrated blood transfusions, acute rhabdomyolysis, toxic shock syndrome, and chemotherapy for acute leukemia. In the last three examples, massive release of phosphate in association with cell lysis may precipitate the hypocalcemia.

Pseudohypoparathyroidism

Pseudohypoparathyroidism is one of the first described examples of hormone resistance. This genetic disease is associated with short stature, rounded facies, foreshortened neck, and shortening of the metacarpal and metatarsal bones[86–88] (Albright's hereditary osteodystrophy) (Fig. 4-9). Calcifications in soft tissues, cornea, and in the basal ganglia are common. These individuals have low-normal to frankly retarded intelligence.

In pseudohypoparathyroidism, biochemical characteristics are typical of any hypoparathyroid state, namely hypocalcemia and hyperphosphatemia. In contrast to classic hypoparathyroidism, however, parathyroid hormone levels are elevated by radioimmunoassay in this disorder. The fundamental pathophysiological abnormality in pseudohypoparathyroidism is resistance to the actions of parathyroid hormone. In these patients, the expected increase in urinary phosphate and cyclic AMP excretion following administration of parathyroid hormone is not seen[89] (Fig. 4-10).

The presentation of pseudohypoparathroidism is complicated by a number of variants. There is a form of parathyroid hormone resistance (pseudohypoparathyroidism, type II) that appears to occur at a step beyond the generation of a cyclic AMP.[90] In another variant, patients have the unmistakable appear-

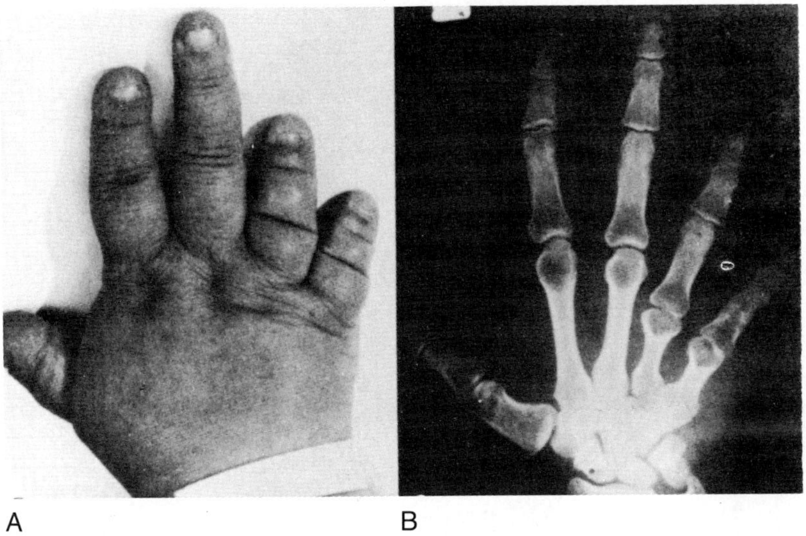

Fig. 4-9 Features of pseudohypoparathyroidism. **(A)** The metacarpal bones of the fourth and fifth digits are foreshortened giving this characteristic appearance to the knuckles. **(B)** Radiograph demonstrating the shortened metacarpal bones. (From Levine et al.,[87] with permission.)

ance of the disease but have neither hypocalcemia nor resistance to parathyroid hormone (pseudopseudohypoparathyroidism).[91] Genetic analysis of affected kindred indicates that pseudopseudohypoparathyroidism is probably part of the classic disorder because both forms can be found in the same families. Yet another form of pseudohypoparathyroidism has been described in which there are no phenotypic abnormalities but complete hormone resistance.[92] Occasionally, the parathyroid hormone resistance of pseudohypoparathyroidism is limited to the kidneys, leading to the unusual manifestation of hyperparathyroid skeletal disease (osteitis fibrosa cystica) in pseudohypoparathyroidism.[93]

The mechanism of resistance in pseudohypoparathyroidism may relate to the guanine nucleotide coupling protein, Gs. This coupling protein is an essential component of all receptor complexes that use cyclic AMP as a second messenger. In the classic disorder (type Ia), characterized by both phenotypical and biochemical abnormalities, there is a 50 percent reduction in Gs[94,95] (Fig. 4-11). The decrease in Gs is seen in all tissues, not just the target organs for parathyroid hormone, confirming the expectation of a disease transmitted in a genetic fashion. The reduction in Gs helps to explain other hormone-resistant states that are sometimes present in patients with pseudohypoparathyroidism.[94,96] Several problems, however, are noteworthy with respect to accepting a reduction in tissue Gs levels as the sole explanation for the hormone resistance of pseudohypoparathyroidism. First, at least three patients have been described with the classic disease in whom Gs levels are normal.[95] Second, the variant characterized solely by biochemical resistance (type Ib) does not show

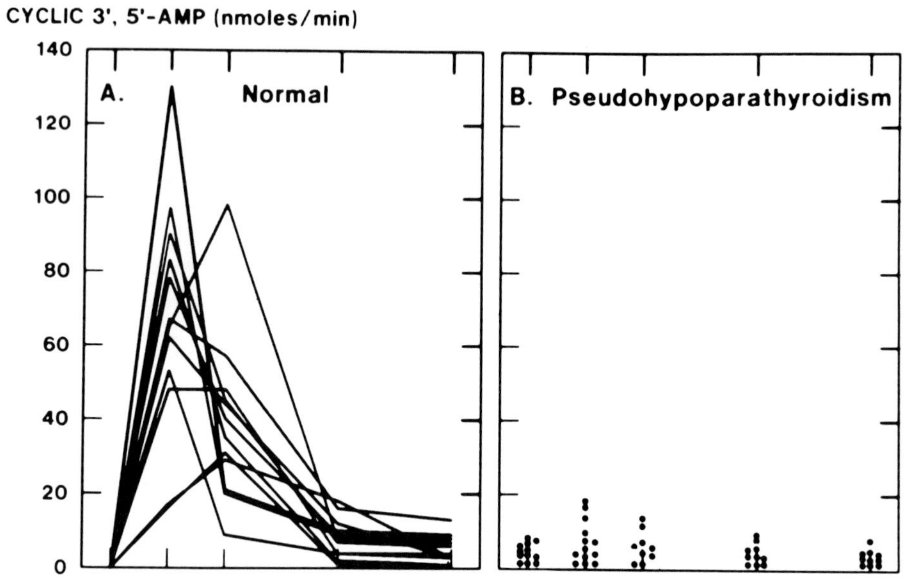

Fig. 4-10 Parathyroid hormone resistance in pseudohypoparathyroidism. **(A)** Normal patients respond to an infusion of parathyroid hormone with a rapid and marked increase in the urinary excretion of cyclic AMP. **(B)** In patients with pseudohypoparathyroidism, this response to parathyroid hormone is markedly blunted. (From Chase et al.,[89] with permission.)

reduced levels of Gs[95] (Fig. 4-11). Finally, in pseudopseudohypoparathyroidism, Gs levels are reduced despite normal sensitivity to parathyroid hormone.[97] It is apparent that pseudohypoparathyroidism cannot be explained easily or completely by reduced Gs levels. Other mechanisms may account for the parathyroid hormone resistance in some patients with pseudohypoparathyroidism. In this regard, the variant that shows parathyroid hormone resistance without phenotypical abnormalities (type Ib) may have a defect at the level of the parathyroid hormone receptor itself.[98]

Another proposed mechanism to account for the pathophysiology of pseudohypoparathyroidism is related to the parathyroid hormone molecule. By cytochemical bioassay, parathyroid hormone levels are reduced in pseudohypoparathyroidism. The discrepancy between reduced bioassay levels and elevated radioimmunoassay levels of parathyroid hormone raises the possibility of an inhibitor substance, perhaps related to parathyroid hormone, circulating in patients with pseudohypoparathyroidism.[99,100]

SIGNS AND SYMPTOMS OF HYPOCALCEMIA

The acute manifestations of hypocalcemia are related to neuromuscular irritability. Paresthesias, numbness, and tingling of the extremities can be fol-

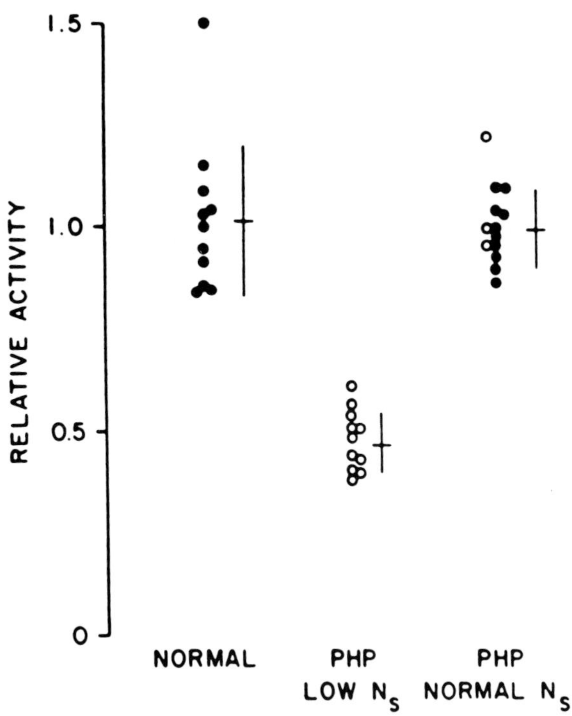

Fig. 4-11 N_s activity in pseudohypoparathyroidism. The data are expressed as activity relative to a standard pooled erythrocyte membrane preparation from normal individuals; for each group, the mean ± SD is shown. Open circles, patients with the phenotypic and biochemical defect. Closed circles, patients with normal body habitus but parathyroid hormone resistance. Normal subjects are also shown as closed circles in the left-hand lane. (From Downs et al.,[95] with permission.)

lowed by more serious complications such as carpal–pedal spasm, laryngospasm, and seizures. Early signs of symptomatic hypocalcemia are elicited by invoking Chvostek's sign: twitching of the ipsilateral facial muscles when the facial nerve is gently tapped. Another early sign is elicited by demonstrating carpal spasm after the blood pressure cuff is inflated above the systolic pressure for 2 minutes (Trousseau's sign).

As with the symptoms related to hypercalcemia, the symptoms of hypocalcemia are a function not only of the actual level of the serum calcium but also of the rate of fall. The electrocardiographic manifestation of hypocalcemia—prolonged QT interval—is also more often seen in connection with an acute fall in the serum calcium level.

Long-term consequences of chronic hypocalcemia are related, in part, to the coexistence of chronic hyperphosphatemia. Deposition of calcium–phosphate salts into soft tissue, cataracts, and basal ganglia calcification all may occur. Intestinal malabsorption, diarrhea, and papilledema may also occur in association with untreated hypocalcemia.

THERAPY OF HYPOCALCEMIA

Acute Management

The major aim of therapy is to alleviate the signs and symptoms of hypocalcemia or, if possible, to prevent their development. There is no urgent need to treat the patient with mild hypocalcemia who is asymptomatic. On the other hand, the patient with marked hypocalcemia poses a greater problem. Even if symptoms are not present, acute therapy should be instituted in a person who is at risk for seizures, especially in whom a convulsion is likely to lead to a vertebral compression fracture. Parenteral calcium salts should be administered slowly (e.g., 10 ml of 10 percent calcium gluconate [93 mg elemental calcium] infused over 10 minutes). In patients who are not in imminent danger, a slower infusion rate in a larger volume is appropriate (e.g., 10 mg/kg of elemental calcium over 6 to 8 hours in 500 ml of fluid). Anions such as phosphate or carbonate should not be coadministered because they will cause intravascular precipitation. Calcium chloride should not be used because extravasation is very irritating and may lead to irreversible precipitation in soft tissue.

Chronic Management

The chronic hypoparathyroid states require long-term therapy to maintain normal calcium levels. Vitamin D is a mainstay of treatment. Because these patients show impaired conversion of 25-hydroxyvitamin D to 1,25 dihydroxy vitamin D, the most rational preparation to use is the active metabolite itself, 1,25 dihydroxyvitamin D. One can use either the parent vitamin D compound or 25-hydroxyvitamin D effectively, but pharmacologic doses are required in contrast to doses of 1,25 dihydroxyvitamin D that are close to the physiologic amounts. For example, 50,000 to 100,000 international units of vitamin D (1.25 to 2.5 mg) are used typically for hypoparathyroidism (100 to 250 times the normal daily dose) whereas 0.25 to 0.50 μg of 1,25 dihydroxyvitamin D (1 to 2 times normal daily dose) are usually sufficient. Another reason for using 1,25 dihydroxyvitamin D instead of the precursor compounds is that the active metabolite is not stored in appreciable amounts in fat and thus is less likely to be associated with prolonged episodes of vitamin D toxicity. In the absence of vitamin D preparations, the calcium-conserving actions of thiazides have been reported to be efficacious[101] in treatment of the hypoparathyroid states.

If the diet does not contain at least 1 g of elemental calcium, patients will require supplemental calcium in addition to vitamin D. The exact form of calcium salt is more a matter of convenience than effectiveness. Any preparation can provide enough supplemental calcium. The more convenient preparations are those that contain a greater proportion of calcium than the accompanying salt. Thus, calcium carbonate is 40 percent calcium (60 percent carbonate) whereas calcium lactate is only 13 percent calcium (87 percent lactate).

REFERENCES

1. Bilezikian JP: Hyperparathyroidism. p.2123. In Stein JH (ed): Internal Medicine. 2nd Ed. Little, Brown, Boston, 1987
2. Heath H III, Hodgson SF, Kennedy MA: Primary hyperparathyroidism: incidence, morbidity, and potential economic impact in a community. N Engl J Med 302:189, 1980
3. Mallette LE, Malini S, Rappaport, Kirkland JL: Familial cystic parathyroid adenomatosis. Ann Intern Med 107:54, 1987
4. Shane E, Bilezikian JP: Parathyroid carcinoma: a review of 62 patients. Endocr Rev 3:218, 1982
5. Brown EM: Four-parameter model of the sigmoidal relationship between parathyroid hormone release and extracellular calcium concentration in normal and abnormal parathyroid tissue. J Clin Endocrinol Metab 56:572, 1983
6. Arnold A, Staunton CE, Gaz RD, HM Kronenberg: Monoclonality of parathyroid adenomas demonstrated by unique somatic gene rearrangement and by restriction fragment polymorphism analysis. J Bone Mineral Res 297A, 1987
7. Fialkow PJ, Jackson CE, Block MA, Greenwald KA: Multicellular origin of parathyroid "adenomas." N Engl J Med 297:696, 1977
8. Katz A, Braunstein GD: Clinical, biochemical and pathologic features of radiation-associated hyperparathyroidism. Arch Intern Med 149:79, 1983
9. Seeman E, Wahner W, Offord P, et al: Differential effects of endocrine dysfunction on the axial and appendicular skeleton. J Clin Invest 69:1302, 1982
10. Parfitt AM, Kleerekoper M, Rao D, et al: Cellular mechanisms of cortical thinning in primary hyperparathyroidism. J Bone Mineral Res 384A, 1987
11. Dempster DW, Shane E, Silverberg SJ, et al: Iliac crest bone biopsy in primary hyperparathyroidism: relationship to clinical presentation and biochemical indices. J Bone Mineral Res 105A, 1987
12. Patten BM, Bilezikian JP, Mallette LE, et al: The neuromuscular disease of hyperparathyroidism. Ann Intern Med 80:182, 1974
13. Scholz DA: Hypertension and hyperparathyroidism. Arch Intern Med 137:1123, 1977
14. Bilezikian JP, Aurbach GD, Connor TB, et al: Pseudogout following parathyroidectomy. Lancet 1:445, 1973
15. Mallette LE: Anemia in hypercalcemic hyperparathyroidism: renewed interest in an old observation. Arch Intern Med 137:572, 1977
16. Reinfrank RF: Primary hyperparathyroidism with depression. Arch Intern Med 108:162, 1961
17. Fitzpatrick LA, Bilezikian JP: Acute primary hyperparathyroidism. Am J Med 82;275, 1987
18. Marx SJ, Attie MF, Spiegel AM, et al: An association between neonatal severe primary hyperparathyroidism and familial hypocalciuric hypercalcemia in three kindreds. N Engl J Med 306:257, 1982
19. Lufkin EG, Kao PC, Heath H III: Parathyroid hormone radioimmunoassays in the differential diagnosis of hypercalcemia due to primary hyperparathyroidism or malignancy. Ann Intern Med 106:559, 1987
20. Broadus AE, Horst RL, Lang R, et al: The importance of circulating 1,25-dihydroxyvitamin D in the pathogenesis of hypercalciuria and renal-stone formation in primary hyperparathyroidism. N Engl J Med 302:421, 1980

21. Locascio V, Adami S, Galvanni, et al: Substrate-product relation of 1-hydroxylase activity in primary hyperparathyroidism. N Engl J Med 313:1123, 1985
22. Rossi RL, ReMine SG, Clerkin EP: Hyperparathyroidism. Surg Clin North Am 65:187, 1985
23. Winzelberg GG: Parathyroid imaging. Ann Intern Med 107:64, 1987
24. Mallette LE, Gomez L, Fisher RG: Parathyroid angiography: a review of current knowledge and guidelines for clinical application. Endocr Rev 2:124, 1981
25. Bilezikian JP: Surgery or no surgery for primary hyperparathyroidism. Ann Intern Med 102:402, 1985
26. Bilezikian JP: The medical management of primary hyperparathyroidism. Ann Intern Med 96:198, 1982
27. Heath H III: Biogenic amines and the secretion of parathyroid hormone and calcitonin. Endocr Rev 1:319, 1980
28. Broadus AE, Magee JS, Mallette LE, et al: A detailed evaluation of oral phosphate therapy in selected patients with primary hyperparathyroidism. J Clin Endocrinol Metab 56:953, 1983
29. Marcus R, Madvig P, Crim M, et al: Conjugated estrogens in the treatment of postmenopausal women with hyperparathyroidism. Ann Intern Med 100:633, 1984
30. Selby PL, Peacock M: Ethinyl estradiol and norethindrone in the treatment of primary hyperparathyroidism in post menopausal women. N Engl J Med 314:1481, 1986
31. Shane E, Baquiran DC, Bilezikian JP: Effects of dicloromethylene diphosphonate on serum and urine calcium in primary hyperparathyroidism. Ann Intern Med 95:23, 1981
32. Mundy GR, Martin TJ: Hypercalcemia of malignancy—pathogenesis and treatment. Metabolism 31:1247, 1982
33. Mundy GR: Pathogenesis of hypercalcaemia of malignancy. Clin Endocrinol 23:705, 1985
34. Godsall JW, Burtis WJ, Insogna KL, et al: Nephrogenous cyclic AMP, adenylate cyclase-stimulating activity, and the humoral hypercalcemia of malignancy. Rec Prog Horm Res 40:705, 1986
35. Mundy GR, Raisz LG, Cooper RA, et al: Evidence for the secretion of an osteoclast stimulating factor in myeloma. N Engl J Med 291:1041, 1974
36. Mundy GR, Ibbotson KJ, D'Souza SM, et al: The hypercalcemia of malignancy: clinical implications and pathogenic mechanisms. N Engl J Med 310:1718, 1984
37. Garrett IR, Durie BGM, Nedwin GE, et al: Production of lymphotoxin, a bone-resorbing cytokine by cultured human myeloma cells. N Engl J Med 317:526, 1987
38. Albright F: Case records of the Massachusetts General Hospital (#27461). N Engl J Med 255:789, 1941
39. Stewart AF, Horst R, Deftos LJ, et al: Biochemical evaluations of patients with cancer-associated hypercalcemia: evidence for humoral and non-humoral groups. N Engl J Med 303:1377, 1980
40. Simpson EL, Mundy GR, D'Souza SM, et al: Absence of parathyroid hormone messenger RNA in nonparathyroid tumors associated with hypercalcemia. N Engl J Med 309:325, 1983
41. Moseley JM, Kubota M, Diefenbach-Jagger H, et al: Parathyoid hormone-related protein purified from a human lung cancer cell line. Proc Natl Acad Sci USA 84:5048, 1987
42. Stewart AF, Terence W, Goumas D, et al: N-terminal amino acid sequence of two novel tumor-derived adenylate cyclase-stimulating proteins: identification of

parathyroid hormone-like and parathyroid hormone-unlike domains. Biochem Biophys Res Commun, 1987
43. Nissenson S, Leung S, Diep D, et al: Purification of a low molecular weight form of the tumor-derived parathyroid hormone-like protein. J Bone Mineral Res 388A, 1987
44. Mundy GR, Ibbotson KJ, D'Souza SM: Tumor products and the humoral hypercalcemia of malignancy. J Clin Invest 76:391, 1985
45. Breslau NA, McGuire JL, Zerwekh JE, et al: Hypercalcemia associated with increased serum calcitriol levels in three patients with lymphoma. Ann Intern Med 100:1, 1984
46. Rosenthal ND, Insogna KL, Godsall JW, et al: 1,25 Dihydroxyvitamin D-mediated humoral hypercalcemia in malignant lymphoma. J Clin Endocrinol Metab 60:29, 1985
47. Hughes MR, Baylink DJ, Jones PG, Haussler MR: Radioligand receptor assay for 25-hydroxyvitamin D_2/D_3 and 1-alpha-25-dihydroxyvitamin D_2/D_3. Application to hypervitaminosis D. J Clin Invest 58:61, 1976
48. Ragavan VV, Smith JE, Bilezikian JP: Vitamin A toxicity and hypercalcemia. Am J Med Sci 283:161, 1982
49. Miller SS, Sizemore GW, Sheps SG, Tyce GM: Parathyroid function in patients with pheochromocytoma. Ann Intern Med 82:372, 1975
50. Stewart AF, Hoecker J, Segre GV, et al: Hypercalcemia in pheochromocytoma: evidence for a novel mechanism. Ann Intern Med 102:776, 1985
51. Verner JV, Morrison AB: Endocrine pancreatic islet disease with diarrhea. Arch Intern Med 133:429, 1974
52. Brown E: Lithium induces abnormal calcium-regulated PTH release in dispersed bovine parathyroid cells. J Clin Endocrinol Metab 52:1046, 1981
53. Spiegel A, Rudorger M, Marx S, Linnoila M: The effect of short term lithium administration on suppressibility of parathyroid hormone secretion by calcium in vivo. J Clin Endocrinol Metab 59:354, 1984
54. Leha SS, Powell K, Buzdar AR, Blumenschein GR: Tamoxifen-induced hypercalcemia in breast cancer. Cancer 47:2803, 1981
55. McPherson ML, Prince SR, Atamer ER, et al: Theophylline-induced hypercalcemia. Ann Intern Med 105:52, 1986
56. Broadus AE, Stewart AF: Humoral Mechanisms of Hypercalcemia. Elsevier Biomedical, Amsterdam, 1984
57. Marx SJ: Familial hypocalcemia. p.217. In: Heath DA, Marx SJ (eds): Calcium Disorders. Butterworth Scientific, Boston, 1982
58. Law Wm Jr, Heath H III: Familial benign hypercalcemia (hypocalciuric hypercalcemia)-clinical and pathogenetic studies in 21 families. Ann Intern Med 102:511, 1985
59. Minaine P, Meunier P, Edouard C, et al: Quantitative histological data on disuse osteoporosis. Calcif Tissue Res 17:57, 1974
60. Stewart AF, Alder M, Byers CM, et al: Calcium homeostasis in immobilization: an example of resorptive hypercalciuria. N Engl J Med 306:1136, 1982
61. Ott SM, Maloney NA, Klein GL, et al: Aluminum is associated with low bone formation in patients receiving chronic parenteral nutrition. Ann Intern Med 98:910, 1983
62. Llach F, Felsenfeld AJ, Haussler MR: The pathophysiology of altered calcium metabolism in rhabdomyolysis-induced acute renal failure. N Engl J Med 305:117, 1981

63. Orwoll ES: The milk-alkali syndrome: current concepts. Ann Intern Med 97:242, 1982
64. Merlini G, Fitzpatrick LA, Siris ES, et al: A human myeloma immunoglobulin G binding four moles of calcium associated with asymptomatic hypercalcemia. J Clin Immunol 4:185, 1984
65. Bilezikian JP: Hypercalcemia. p.513. In Bayless TM, Brain MC, RM Cherniak (eds): Current Therapy in Internal Medicine. B.C. Decker, Inc., Philadelphia, 1984
66. Stewart AF: Therapy of malignancy-associated hypercalcemia. Am J Med 74:475, 1983
67. Perlia CP, Gubisch NJ, Cootter J, et al: Mithramycin treatment of hypercalcemia. Cancer 25:389, 1970
68. Jacobs T, Gordon AC, Silverberg SJ, et al: Neoplastic hypercalcemia; physiologic response to intravenous etidronate disodium. Am J Med 82(2A):42, 1987
69. Jacobs TP, Siris ES, Bilezikian JP, et al: Hypercalcemia of malignancy: treatment with intravenous dichloromethylene diphosphonate. Ann Intern Med 94:312, 1981
70. Binstok ML, Mundy GR: Effect of calcitonin and glucocorticoids in combination on the hypercalcemia of malignancy. Ann Intern Med 93:269, 1980
71. Goler DJ, Shaw L, Glick JH, et al: Treatment of hypercalcemia in parathyroid cancer with WR-2721. Ann Intern Med 103:55, 1985
72. Warrell RP, Bockman RS, Coonley CJ, et al: Gallium nitrate inhibits calcium resorption from bone and is effective treatment for cancer-related hypercalcemia. J Clin Invest 73:1487, 1984
73. Watson L, Moxham J, Fraser P: Hydrocortisone suppression test and discriminant analysis in differential diagnosis of hypercalcemia. Lancet 1:1320, 1980
74. Neufield RB, Maclaren N, Blizzard R: Two types of autoimmune Addison's disease associated with different polyglandular autoimmune syndromes. Medicine 60:355, 1981
75. Blizzard RM, Chee D, Davis W: The incidence of parathyroid and other antibodies in the sera of patients with idiopathic hypoparathyroidism. Clin Exp Immunol 1:119, 1966
76. Jackson RA, Haynes BF, Burch WM, et al: Ia^{+}T cells in new onset Graves' disease. J Clin Endocrinol Metab 59:187, 1984
77. Posillico JT, Wortsman J, Srikanta S, et al: Parathyroid cell surface autoantibodies that inhibit parathyroid hormone secretion from dispersed human parathyroid cells. J Bone Mineral Res 1:475, 1986
78. Brandi MR, Aurbach GD, Fattorossi A, et al: Antibodies cytotoxic to bovine parathyroid cells in autoimmune hypoparathyroidism. Proc Natl Acad Sci USA 83:8366, 1986
79. Ahn TG, Antonarakis SE, Kronenberg HM, et al: Familial isolated hypoparathyroidism: a molecular genetic analysis of 8 families with 23 affected persons. Medicine 65:73, 1986
80. Cronin RD, Knochel JP. Magnesium Deficiency. p. 509. Yearbook Medical Publishers, Chicago, 1983
81. Rude RK, Oldham SB, Sharp CF, Singer FR: Parathyroid hormone secretion in magnesium deficiency. J Clin Endocrinol Metab 29:842, 1978
82. Rude RK, Singer FR. Magnesium deficiency and excess. Annu Rev Med 32:245, 1981
83. Weir GC, Lesser PB, Drop LJ, et al: The hypocalcemia of acute pancreatitis. Ann Intern Med 83:185, 1975

84. Stewart AF, Longo W, Kreutter D, et al: Hypocalcemia due to calcium soap formation in a patient with a pancreatic fistula. N Engl J Med 315:496, 1986
85. Robertson GM, Jr., Moore EW, Switz DM, et al: Inadequate parathyroid response in acure pancreatitis. N Engl J Med 294:512, 1976
86. Albright F, Burnett CH, Smith PH, Parson W: Pseudohypoparathyroidism—an example of "Seabright-Bantam syndrome." Endocrinology 3:922, 1942
87. Levine MA, Parfrey NA, Feinstein RF: Pseudohypoparathyroidism. Johns Hopkins Med J 151:137, 1982
88. Drezner MK: Pseudohypoparathyroidism. p.1508. In Stanbury JB, Wyngaarden JB, Friedrickson DS, et al (eds): The Metabolic Basis of Inherited Disease. 5th Ed. McGraw-Hill, New York, 1983
89. Chase LW, Melson GL, Aurbach GD. Pseudohypoparathyroidism: defective excretion of 3′, 5′-AMP in response to parathyroid hormone. J Clin Invest 48:1832, 1969
90. Drezner M, Neelon FA, Lebovitz HE. Pseudohypoparathyroidism type II: a possible defect in the reception of the cyclic amp signal. N Engl J Med 289:1056, 1973
91. Albright F, Forbes AP, Henneman PH: Pseudopseudohypoparathyroidism. Trans Assoc Am Physicians: 65:337, 1952
92. Moses AM, Rao KJ, Coulson R, Miller M: Parathyroid hormone deficiency with Albright's hereditary osteodystrophy. J Clin Endocrinol Metab 39:496, 1974
93. Frame B, Hanson C, Frost HM, et al: Renal resistance to parathyroid hormone with osteitis fibrosa. Am J Med 52:311, 1972
94. Van Dop C, Bourne HR. Pseudohypoparathyroidism. Annu Rev Med 34:259, 1983
95. Downs RW, Sekura RD, Levine MS, Spiegel AM: The inhibitory adenylate cyclase coupling protein in pseudohypoparathyroidism. J Clin Endocrinol Metab 61:351, 1985
96. Verhoeen GFM, Wilson JD: The syndromes of primary hormone resistance. Metabolism 28:253, 1979
97. Levine MA, Jap T, Mauseth RS, et al: Activity of the stimulatory guanine nucleotide-binding protein is reduced in erythrocytes from patients with pseudohypoparathyroidism and pseudopseudohypoparathyroidism. J Clin Endocrinol Metab 62:497, 1986
98. Silve C, Santora A, Breslau N, et al: Selective resistance to parathyroid hormone in cultured skin fibroblasts from patients with pseudohypoparathyroidism type 1b. J Clin Endocrinol Metab 3:1105, 1981
99. Loveridge N, Fischer JA, Deuxchaisnes CN, et al: Inhibition of cytochemical bioactivity of parathyroid hormone by plasma in pseudohypoparathyroidism type I. J Clin Endocrinol Metab 5:1274, 1982
100. Mitchell J, Goltzman D: Examination of circulating parathyroid hormone in pseudohypoparathyroidism. J Clin Endocrinol Metab 61:328, 1985
101. Porter RH, Cox BG, Heaney D, et al: Treatment of hypoparathyroid patients with chlorthalidone. N Engl J Med 298:577, 1978

5 Disorders of Vitamin D Metabolism: Rickets and Osteomalacia

Marc K. Drezner

Rickets and osteomalacia are diseases characterized by defects of bone and cartilage mineralization in youths and bone mineralization in adults. The abnormal calcification of cartilage occurs at the growth plates (epiphyses) of children, while that of bone is restricted to the bone–osteoid (organic bone matrix) interfaces of remodeling tissue. The mineralization process depends upon the availability of sufficient calcium and phosphorus at mineralization sites. Other conditions necessary for normal calcification include (1) intact metabolic and transport functions of bone-forming cells; (2) presence of normal bone matrix; (3) phosphorylation or alternative metabolic modification of matrix constituents; (4) maintenance of an appropriate pH (approximately 7.6) at mineralization sites; and (5) low concentration of calcification inhibitors (e.g., proteoglycans) in bone matrix. An unsufficiency of calcium or phosphorus or an abnormality in any of the additional control steps may lead to a defect in mineralization.

Although vitamin D deficiency was by far the most common form of rickets/osteomalacia early in this century, the therapeutic use of vitamin D_2 has virtually eliminated this disease in humans. With the disappearance of this form of the disorder, attention became focused on the remaining subtypes of rickets/osteomalacia, which are in general characterized by a failure to respond to physiologic doses of vitamin D. In a patient with such a disease, Albright in 1937 first showed that very large doses of vitamin D resulted in healing of the rickets. This observation led to identification of vitamin-D-resistant rickets, a broad spectrum of diseases that were recognized then and later. These include various genetic and acquired disorders that bear a remarkable resemblance to each other (and vitamin D deficiency) but have a unique pathophysiology. Their occurrence is now recognized worldwide with ever-increasing frequency since a greater reliance has been placed on bone biopsy and quantitative histomorphologic studies to establish a diagnosis in patients with undefined osseous abnormalities.

This chapter presents an overview of various vitamin D deficiency rachitic/osteomalacic syndromes and several vitamin-D-resistant diseases. This information highlights the similarities and differences between the diseases and underscores the remaining knowledge gaps in our understanding of their pathophysiology and treatment.

RACHITIC/OSTEOMALACIC DISEASES

Vitamin D Deficiency

Diseases of Simple Vitamin D Deficiency

Since most foods contain only small amounts of vitamin D_3, we must rely upon endogenous production of cholecalciferol or dietary supplements of ergocalciferol for maintenance of an adequate vitamin D supply. Sunlight plays a critical role in the epidermal synthesis of vitamin D_3; thus, growing children and adults living in temperate zones are at risk for rickets and/or osteomalacia if foods are not fortified with vitamin D.[1]

Adequate exposure to sunlight and therapeutic use of vitamin D_2 by public health services, however, have virtually eliminated this disorder in humans, with several notable populations excepted. In Asian immigrants in Britain, for example, rickets and osteomalacia secondary to vitamin D deficiency are seen in neonates and infants, adolescents during pubertal growth, and less frequently among adults. Insufficient intake of vitamin D secondary to use of unfortified foods, racial pigmentation (which interferes with ultraviolet transmission through the skin), genetic factors, and social customs such as avoidance of sun exposure contribute to development of disease in these subjects. In the United States, a surprisingly frequent incidence of vitamin D deficiency osteomalacia has also been observed in alcoholics, institutionalized patients, and the elderly. Poor diet, in some cases including avoidance of milk due to lactose intolerance, and lack of sunlight exposure are among the factors predisposing these patients to vitamin D deficiency and consequent bone disease.

The clinical manifestations of the disease are primarily related to skeletal pain and deformity, bone fractures, slipped epiphyses, and abnormalities of growth. In addition, hypocalcemia when present may be sufficient to produce tetany, laryngeal spasm, and/or seizures. In infants and young children features include listlessness, irritability, and, in some cases, profound hypotonia and proximal muscle weakness. In addition, throughout early life classic skeletal deformities appear. By age 6 months a skull deformity manifested as frontal bossing with flattening at the back is evident. Later, a lateral collapse of both chest walls (Harrison's sulcus) and rachitic rosary may appear. If the disease remains untreated, progressive bone deformities result in bowing, particularly of the lower extremities, and fractures. In addition, dental eruption may be delayed and, in some forms of the disease, enamel defects may frequently occur.

In contrast, clinical signs of osteomalacia in adults are nondescript. Symptoms, when present, include diffuse skeletal pain and generalized muscular weakness. Pain may be especially localized about the hips and result in an antalgic gait. Fractures of involved bones may occur with minimal trauma and those of the vertebral bodies and long bones may lead to progressive deformities. The muscle weakness is primarily proximal and often associated with wasting and hypotonia. The persistent skeletal defects include rachitic rosary, frontal bossing, and bowed lower extremities.

Radiologic Features. The radiographic abnormalities in both rickets and osteomalacia reflect the histopathologic changes. In rickets the cardinal alterations are evident at the growth plate, which is increased in thickness, cupped, and displays an irregular hazy appearance at the diaphyseal line secondary to uneven invasion of the recently calcified cartilage by adjacent bone tissue. Additional radiographic changes include thinning of the diaphyseal cortices and bowing of the long bones. Successive periods of healing and recurrence of the rickets, secondary to inconsistent treatment, may also result in Harris lines of arrested growth in the bone shafts, as well as transverse regions of irregular structure.

Similar to the clinical presentation, the radiologic abnormalities of osteomalacia are not at all precise. In general, there is usually a mild decrease in bone density associated with a coarsening of trabeculae and a blurring of their margins. Occasionally subperiosteal resorption and bone cysts may be seen, which are indicative of hyperparathyroidism. A more specific radiographic abnormality characteristic of osteomalacia is the presence of Looser's zones, also called pseudofractures or Milkman fractures, in the shafts of long bones. These are ribbonlike zones of rarefaction ranging from a few millimeters to several centimeters in length and usually oriented perpendicular to the bone surface. Generally they occur symmetrically and most commonly are present at the medial aspect of the femurs near the femoral heads, in the metatarsals, or in the pelvis. Their origin is almost certainly a consequence of trauma, since the localization of these zones follows the distribution of various forms of stress fractures in normal skeletons and/or corresponds to sites where major arteries cross the bone, creating the mechanical stress of pulsating vessels. Further definitive radiographic abnormalities occur in cases of chronic long-standing osteomalacia. These include collapsing of vertebrae into a bioconcave shape and creation of a trefoil (or triangular) pelvis.

Laboratory Findings. Patients with vitamin D deficiency rickets/osteomalacia characteristically present with a low or marginally normal serum calcium level, a decreased serum phosphorus concentration, and secondary hyperparathyroidism.[2] In addition, serum 25(OH)D levels are low, generally <3 ng/ml. In contrast, the serum $1,25(OH)_2D$ concentration may not be overtly decreased secondary to the prevailing hyperparathyroidism. The increased parathyroid function may also result in a mild metabolic acidosis and generalized aminoaciduria. Alkaline phosphatase levels are invariably elevated secondary to the increased rate of bone remodeling. The development of overt clinical and laboratory evidence of vitamin D deficiency rickets/osteomalacia is generally preceded by a fall in circulating 25(OH)D levels. The availability of a sensitive and reliable assay for this vitamin D metabolite has served to identify populations at risk for the disease and facilitated early detection of the disorder.

Treatment. Treatment of vitamin-D-deficiency rickets/osteomalacia invariably results in healing of the bone disease. As a general rule, the disorder is best treated with vitamin D and restoration of normal dietary calcium and phosphate intake. The use of ergocalciferol (vitamin D_2) is preferred because it provides the missing substrate and allows physiologic control of vitamin D metabolite concentrations through normal regulatory mechanisms. Calcifediol [25(OH)D] and calcitriol [$1,25(OH)_2D$] may also heal nutritional rickets/osteomalacia but offer no significant advantages. Indeed, the potential for vitamin D intoxication is greater when these medicines are used.

The amount of ergocalciferol administered can vary widely: children with vitamin D deficiency respond to doses of 25 to 50 μg (in association with 1 g calcium orally). In contrast, adults show healing of nutritional osteomalacia in response to 10 to 100 μg ergocalciferol per day. The amount of vitamin D_2 administered determines only the rate at which healing occurs. Normal mineralization may be restored within 3 months at the higher doses but the risk of toxicity is enhanced. Thus, unless severe and symptomatic hypocalcemia, extensive muscle weakness, and/or inordinately frequent bone fractures complicate the clinical presentation, lower-dose treatment will suffice.

A therapeutic response is initially indicated by a rise in the serum phosphorus usually after 3 to 4 days of treatment. Concomitantly, a transient decrease of the serum calcium level may occur secondary to mineral deposition in bone. Indeed, a sustained increase of the serum calcium concentration in accord with an elevation of the previously decreased 24 hour urine calcium excretion does not occur until significant bone healing is manifest. These changes may be used as an indication to reduce the amount of vitamin D_2 administered. In any case, histologic evidence of complete bone healing requires at least one bone remodeling cycle (approximately 60 days).

Complications. Careful monitoring of plasma biochemical values is imperative to avoid iatrogenic complications. The potential for vitamin D (or calcium) intoxication is great if appropriate care is not taken to assess the adequacy of therapy. Therefore, therapy is started at low doses and titrated upward until a therapeutic effect is observed. As the osteomalacia heals, the dose may be reduced.

The clinical manifestations of vitamin D intoxication are nonspecific and in general reflect the effects of hypercalcemia and hypercalciuria. The occurrence of anorexia, nausea, vomiting, mental status changes, or hypertension in a vitamin-D-treated patient should suggest the possibility of vitamin D intoxication. In addition, both reversible and permanent changes in renal function may occur. Volume depletion and renal vasoconstriction caused by hypercalcemia result in a decreased glomerular filtration rate. Alternatively, chronic renal damage may result from long-term hypercalciuria, which may induce nephrocalcinosis or recurrent nephrolithiasis with obstruction and infection. In general, therefore, the serum calcium level should be maintained within normal limits while the urinary calcium to creatinine ratio should be kept less than 0.25 mg/kg body weight.

The treatment of vitamin D intoxication depends on its severity. In mild cases the hypercalcemia will respond to discontinuation of the vitamin D compound. The rate of reversibility depends on the biologic half-life of the vitamin D analog used. Because of extensive tissue stores, the time to reverse intoxication with ergocalciferol or calcifediol is prolonged; it may take 6 to 8 weeks for the effects to abate. Calcitriol has a much shorter half-life and less tissue storage; effects may persist up to 1 week following cessation of use of this analog. Severe intoxication should be treated initially with saline to correct the extracellular volume contraction that invariably coexists. After the volume deficit is restored, calciuresis can be enhanced by a saline diuresis induced by the administration of large volumes of isotonic saline plus intravenous furosemide. Urine volume and concentration of sodium and potassium must be monitored and replaced to maintain euvolemia and to avoid hyponatremia and hypokalemia.

Vitamin D Malabsorption

Mechanism and Features. Gastrointestinal malabsorption may result in decreased absorption of vitamin D and calcium and/or depletion of endogenous 25(OH)D stores secondary to abnormal enterohepatic circulation. The resulting deficiency of vitamin D or its metabolites is often associated with osteomalacia.[3] Indeed, the majority of patients may have asymptomatic disease, and many have only reduction in bone volume rather than overt evidence of defective bone mineralization. Intestinal bypass surgery, adult celiac disease, regional enteritis, and cholestatic diseases treated with cholestyramine (Questran) are common examples of disorders in which the suspicion for osteomalacia should remain high.[4] Vitamin D absorption, which normally occurs via chylomicrons, is impaired in those diseases causing steatorrhea, where emulsification of fat is disturbed. In contrast, patients with cholestatic liver disease or extraheptic biliary obstruction may have reduced vitamin D stores, secondary not only to malabsorption but also to decreased hepatic production of 25(OH)D and disruption of the enterhepatic circulation as well.

Patients who have had partial or total gastrectomy for peptic ulcer disease or other indications may also develop osteomalacia. Malabsorption of vitamin in this circumstance may be due to loss of gastrointestinal acidity and/or malfunction of the proximal small bowel. Indeed, factors other than failure to absorb vitamin D may contribute to the development of bone disease in patients with gastrointestinal disease.[5] These may include absence of sufficient absorbing surface or failure of intestinal mucosal cells to respond to vitamin D or its metabolites.

The clinical features of the disease are, of course, similar to those of simple vitamin D deficiency. However, these may be masked by various abnormalities directly attributable to the gastrointestinal disease. Laboratory and radiographic findings are likewise comparable to those of the vitamin-D-deficient disease.

Treatment. Treatment of documented disease generally requires pharmacologic amounts of vitamin D or its metabolites both to overcome the defective absorption and/or aberrant enterohepatic circulation and to offset end-organ resistance at the intestinal mucosa. Generally, the dose of vitamin D required varies from patient to patient and must be individualized. However, most subjects can be treated with calcium supplements (1 to 1.5 g/day) and ergocalciferol (50,000 to 200,000 units/day) or calcifediol (20 to 200 μg/day). Monitoring the serum 25(OH)D concentration is valuable to assess adequacy of the treatment regimen, since achieving normal circulating levels of this metabolite is the goal of therapy. If oral administration is impractical, parenteral administration of ergocalciferol (500,000 to 1,000,000 units intramuscularly) once per month is a reasonable alternative. More recently, calcitriol (1 to 2 μg/day) has been used successfully in the treatment of this disorder. While the onset of effects is faster and toxicity more quickly resolved, use of this drug removes serum 25(OH)D measurements as a simple means for monitoring therapy.

Magnesium deficiency may coexist in malabsorptive states, slowing the healing of osteomalacia. Thus, magnesium oxide (250 to 500 mg orally four times daily) may be a necessary adjunct treatment. Renal insufficiency reduces the dose required.

Impaired 25-Hydroxylation of Vitamin D

Liver Disease. Since vitamin D is hydroxylated in the liver to form 25(OH)D, severe hepatic disease has the potential to reduce production of this metabolite and cause bone disease.[6] However, patients with liver dysfunction rarely manifest biochemical and/or histologic evidence of osteomalacia. Indeed, the principal bone disease in affected subjects is osteoporosis. Furthermore, low levels of 25(OH)D, if present, are generally due to nutritional deficiency and/or interruption of the enterohepatic circulation. Thus, patients with severe cirrhosis manifest normal 25-hydroxylase activity if adequate amounts of vitamin D are provided. Nevertheless, in the rare instance when biopsy-proven osteomalacia is found in a patient with biliary cirrhosis (or another severe hepatic disease), therapy should be similar to that for malabsorption.

Anticonvulsant Osteomalacia. In recent years the occurrence of rickets and osteomalacia has been recognized in epileptic patients taking long-term, high-dosage dilantin and/or phenobarbital.[7] The pathogenesis of the bone disease is multifactorial and not completely understood, but is often associated with a decreased serum 25(OH)D concentration. The apparent defect in vitamin D metabolism is believed to be secondary to epileptic drug induction of hepatic microsomal enzymes that metabolize vitamin D and 25(OH)D to inactive metabolites. Despite these demonstrable abnormalities, the serum $1,25(OH)_2D$ concentration remains normal (or even elevated) in affected patients. Thus, alternative mechanisms may be operative in the genesis of anticonvulsant-induced osteomalacia.

In this regard, recent studies indicate that the anticonvulsant drugs may have direct effects on mineral and bone metabolism independent of their effects on vitamin D metabolism.[8] This is particularly true of dilantin, which has been shown to inhibit intestinal calcium transport by virtue of its effect on membrane-bound ATPase transport systems. Additionally, both dilantin and phenobarbital directly inhibit calcium mobilization from bone in response to parathyroid hormone, calcitonin, and $1,25(OH)_2D$. Thus, anticonvulsant drugs may produce their deleterious effects on mineral and bone metabolism through at least two mechanisms: (1) a dose-related stimulation of hepatic microsomal enzyme systems, resulting in increased catabolism of vitamin D, 25(OH)D and perhaps, its biologically active metabolite, a consequent decrease in intestinal calcium absorption, and decreased availability of mineral to calcify bone; and (2) direct inhibitory effects on intestinal calcium transport and bone metabolism.

In any case, detection of anticonvulsant-induced osteomalacia is particularly important. The associated hypocalcemia characteristic of this disorder (occurring in 20 to 25 percent of institutionalized patients with epilepsy) may increase the frequency of seizures and prompt increase in the anticonvulsant drugs. In addition, results of large surveys of noninstitutionalized populations indicate that treated patients routinely manifest a 10 to 30 percent reduction of bone mass compared to age-matched normal values. Thus, in the appropriate clinical setting (e.g., evaluation of fracture) the presence of osteomalacia should be sought. Treatment of clinically evident bone disease and/or hypocalcemia in adults should consist of an initial vitamin D dose of 50,000 to 75,000 units of vitamin D per week. In children doses should be proportionately reduced according to body area (50,000 units/m^2). When this regimen is used, the serum and urine calcium levels must be evaluated carefully so that the dose can be adjusted to individual requirements and vitamin D overdosage avoided.

Alternatively, prophylactic administration of vitamin D to all patients maintained on anticonvulsants long term has been advocated. While this approach has been challenged because of the cost of chronic vitamin D supplementation and the ever-present possibility of vitamin D overdosage, the potential for aggravating the naturally occurring osteopenia of aging may justify such an approach. Thus, prescribing 5,000 to 10,000 units vitamin D per week to all patients maintained on anticonvulsants for greater than 6 months may be warranted.

Vitamin-D-Resistant Diseases

"Vitamin-D-resistant rickets" is used imprecisely to describe a variety of rachitic/osteomalacic disorders that have as their characteristic feature an inadequate therapeutic response to physiologic (and often pharmacologic) amounts of vitamin D. In the majority of these syndromes, a poor understanding of their pathophysiologic basis, as well as an inadequate appreciation of their unique clinical features underlies such ineffective treatment. Recent studies of X-linked hypophosphatemic rickets/osteomalacia (XLH), the archetypal vitamin-D-resistant disease; tumor-induced osteomalacia (TIO), a prototypic form of hypophosphatemic vitamin-D-resistant osteomalacia; and vitamin-D-dependent rickets, a hypocalcemic vitamin-D-refractory rachitic disorder, have provided extensive information regarding the physiologic derangements resulting in the phenotypic expression of vitamin-D-resistant diseases. An enlightened insight into effective therapy of these disorders has resulted.

X-Linked Hypophosphatemic Rickets/Osteomalacia

The XLH syndrome is an X-linked dominant disorder characterized by hypophosphatemia, renal phosphate wasting, growth retardation, osteomalacia, and rickets in growing children. The clinical expression of the disease is widely variable, ranging from a simple chemical defect to severe bone disease. The mildest abnormality is asymptomatic hypophosphatemia, which generally is detected at birth. However, its presence may not become apparent until age 6 to 12 months. The most common clinically evident manifestation is short stature. In addition, affected children display evidence of rickets on x-ray examination, which reveals expanded areas of proliferating nonmineralized cartilage in epiphyseal regions and lateral curvature of the femora and tibia. These changes occur within the first year of life and are often associated with an elevated serum concentration of alkaline phosphatase, a biochemical marker of active rickets.

Early signs of the disease may also include late dentition, skull deformities, and "sitting" deformities of the legs. In severely affected children, abnormalities of the maxillofacial region, poor dental development, and spontaneous tooth abscesses often follow. Strikingly absent are common features of vitamin D deficiency osteomalacia such as muscle weakness, tetany, and convulsions.

Pathophysiology. The pathogenesis of XLH remains a subject of considerable controversy. However, investigators generally agree that the primary inborn error of this disorder results in an expressed abnormality in the renal proximal tubule (and perhaps the intestine) that impairs phosphate reabsorption (and absorption). This defect has been indirectly identified in affected patients and directly demonstrated in the brush border membranes of the proximal nephron in the *Hyp*-mouse, the murine homolog of the human disease. In spite of this agreement, it remains unclear whether the renal abnormality is primary or secondary to the elaboration of a hormonal factor.

More important is that this proposed defect, and the hypophosphatemia that develops as a consequence, do not account for the full spectrum of biochemical and skeletal abnormalities that constitute the X-linked hypophosphatemic syndrome. Most notably, treatment of patients with XLH with phosphorus (and/or vitamin D), while correcting phosphate deficiency, does not restore bone mineralization to normal, indicating that renal phosphate wasting and hypophosphatemia alone do not underlie the abnormal bone calcification in XLH. Therefore, several investigators have proposed that ancillary abnormalities may contribute to the pathogenesis of this disease. In this regard, a variety of recent studies indicate that abnormal vitamin D metabolism is a part of the XLH syndrome. Data supporting this conclusion include the presence in affected subjects of (1) a normal circulating level of the active vitamin D metabolite, $1,25(OH)_2D$, despite the prevailing hypophosphatemia[9–11]; (2) a significantly reduced increment of the serum calcitriol level in response to parathyroid hormone stimulation compared to that in age-matched controls[12]; and (3) a subnormal increase of the serum $1,25(OH)_2D$ concentration after dietary phosphorus deprivation.[13] While these data are in accord with the presence of an apparent defect in $1,25(OH)_2D$ production (and/or metabolism), they do not establish (1) if the abnormality represents a defect in enzyme [25(OH)D-1α-hydroxylase] function (which may be a primary or acquired derangement secondary to the abnormal renal phosphate transport); or (2) whether the defect contributes to the genesis of the disorder. However, recent studies in the *Hyp*-mouse and therapeutic trials in humans have provided data indicating that the abnormal renal phosphate transport and vitamin D metabolism may be interrelated.

Regulation of Vitamin D Metabolism in the *Hyp*-Mouse. In 1976 Eicher et al.[14] reported the discovery of an X-linked dominant mutation named "hypophosphatemia" (gene symbol *Hyp*) in the laboratory mouse. The mutant *Hyp* allele was transferred to the C57 BL6J inbred strain of mice by repeated matings of *Hyp*/+ females and C57 BL6J +/Y males. The mutation is X-linked dominant and detailed linkage studies indicate that the *Hyp* allele is at the distal end of the murine X chromosome. Since the disorder affecting the *Hyp*-mouse appears similar to that in humans with XLH, it is likely that the human and murine diseases are caused by a mutation on the X chromosome, affecting an homologous gene that has withstood evolutionary alteration. Thus, the *Hyp*-mouse has provided an excellent model in which to elucidate the basic defect(s) underlying the X-linked hypophosphatemic disorders.

Investigations of the *Hyp*-mouse have confirmed that aberrant regulation of renal 25(OH)D-1α-hydroxylase activity underlies abnormal 1,25$(OH)_2$D production in the X-linked hypophosphatemic syndrome. In this regard, Lobaugh and Drezner[15] reported a serum 1,25$(OH)_2$D concentration in *Hyp*-mice (45.0$\pm$4.1 pg/ml) that was not significantly different from that of normal littermates (39.5$\pm$3.9 pg/ml) but was significantly less than that of phosphate-depleted normal mice (72.2$\pm$7.0 pg/ml). The discordant values were not due to differences in vitamin D stores since serum 25(OH)D levels were similar in mutant, normal, and phosphate-depleted mice (24.4$\pm$1.2, 20.8$\pm$2.9, 22.69$\pm$1.6 ng/ml, respectively).

Moreover, assay of renal 25(OH)D-1α-hydroxylase activity in the kidneys of normal, phosphate-depleted, and mutant mice established that defective 1,25$(OH)_2$D production underlies this abnormality in part.[15] Renal homogenates from phosphate-depleted mice repeatedly had profoundly (259 percent) increased activity compared to that of normals. In contrast, enzyme activity in the *Hyp*-mouse kidney was far below that in the kidneys of phosphate-depleted mice. Indeed, the increment of enzyme activity in the *Hyp*-mouse kidney was fully fourfold less than that in kidneys of phosphate-depleted mice.

However, it remained unclear whether the abnormality represented altered enzyme response to hypophosphatemia alone or was indicative of a more generalized defect. In further studies, therefore, Nesbitt et al.[16] examined the effects of parathyroid hormone and calcium on 25(OH)D-1α-hydroxylase activity. In normal mice they observed a decrease in enzyme activity in response to parathyroidectomy and an increase upon calcium depletion (and the consequent elevation of circulating parathyroid hormone). In contrast, in *Hyp*-mice calcium depletion and/or parathyroid hormone administration did not normally stimulate enzyme function. Similarly, Tenenhouse[17] reported that *Hyp*-mice maintained for 6 weeks on a rachitogenic diet exhibited significantly diminished enzyme activity compared to that of normal mice fed the same diet.

Although these experiments provide evidence that the defect in 25(OH)D-1α-hydroxylase activity in *Hyp*-mice does not represent altered response to hypophosphatemia alone, such data proved insufficient to establish the ubiquity of the abnormality. In this regard, Akiba and associates[18] and Kurokawa et al.[19], using microdissected nephron segments, identified the presence of two distinct and uniquely regulated 25(OH)D-1α-hydroxylase systems located in the proximal convoluted and proximal straight tubules of the mammalian kidney. Since previous investigations had addressed only the regulation of enzyme activity in the PTH (phosphate)-sensitive proximal convoluted tubules, the status of enzyme function in the calcitonin-responsive proximal straight tubules remained unknown. However, Nesbitt et al.[20] have recently reported that calcitonin stimulation in *Hyp*-mice elicits a normal increment of renal 25(OH)D-1α-hydroxylase activity, paradoxic to the muted effects of phosphate deficiency and parathyroid hormone. These data suggest that the abnormal parathyroid hormone and phosphate-regulated activity in *Hyp*-mice (and affected patients) may be localized in the proximal convoluted tubule. In contrast, the normal calcitonin-responsive 25(OH)D-1α-hydroxylase is likely located in the proximal straight tubule. Moreover, since defective phosphate transport in *Hyp*-mice occurs in the proximal convoluted tubules, aberrant enzyme function at this site may result from the abnormal phosphate transport and/or consequent changes in the intracellular milieu. Under these circumstances, the enzyme dysfunction in *Hyp*-mice (and patients with XLH) may not be a genetically determined abnormality of 25(OH)D-1α-hydroxylase structure/function, but rather an acquired aberration secondary to the primary genetic abnormality.

These observations support a previously unrecognized role for renal phosphate transport in the regulation of vitamin D metabolism. Indeed, in further studies of normals and patients with XLH, tumor induced osteomalacia (TIO), and tumoral calcinosis, Lyles et al.[21] have observed that the renal tubular maximum for the reabsorption of phosphate per liter of glomerular filtrate (TmP/GFR) (an index of phosphate transport) bears a strong linear correlation with the plasma calcitriol levels (Fig. 5-1). These data suggest that the effects of phosphate depletion or loading on $1,25(OH)_2D$ production may be modulated by the compensatory inverse alteration of renal phosphate flux that occurs in response to these perturbations. In addition, the observations provide an explanation for the previously ill-understood and apparently paradoxic regulation of plasma calcitriol concentrations (relative to circulating levels of phosphorus) in patients with XLH, TIO, Fanconi's syndrome, and tumoral calcinosis.

More recently, Seino and associates[22] have found that *Hyp*-mice also exhibit a more rapid turnover of $1,25(OH)_2D$ than normals, possibly contributing to the relatively low circulating calcitriol levels in mutants. These observations indicate that the aberrant vitamin D metabolism in the hypophosphatemic syndrome may be exceptionally complex.

In any case, these investigations of vitamin D metabolism in *Hyp*-mice have provided the basis for a unified hypothesis that can account for the multiple derangements characteristic of XLH. In this regard, the concept seems attractive that the abnormalities of phosphate transport and $1,25(OH)_2D$ production are, in general, interrelated and, together, underlie the pathogenesis of XLH. Recent studies in humans support this possibility.

Treatment. In past years the cornerstone for treatment of XLH was pharmacologic doses of vitamin D_2 (10,000 to 25,000 units/d for infants and up to 300,000 units/day for older children and adults). However, long-term observations indicate that this therapy fails to cure the disease and poses the serious problem of recurrent vitamin D intoxication and renal damage. In general, institution of therapy has resulted only in incomplete healing of the rachitic disease, while hypophosphatemia and impaired growth are sustained without improvement. Treatment with $25(OH)D_3$ offers no substantive advantage over that with vitamin D_2 alone.

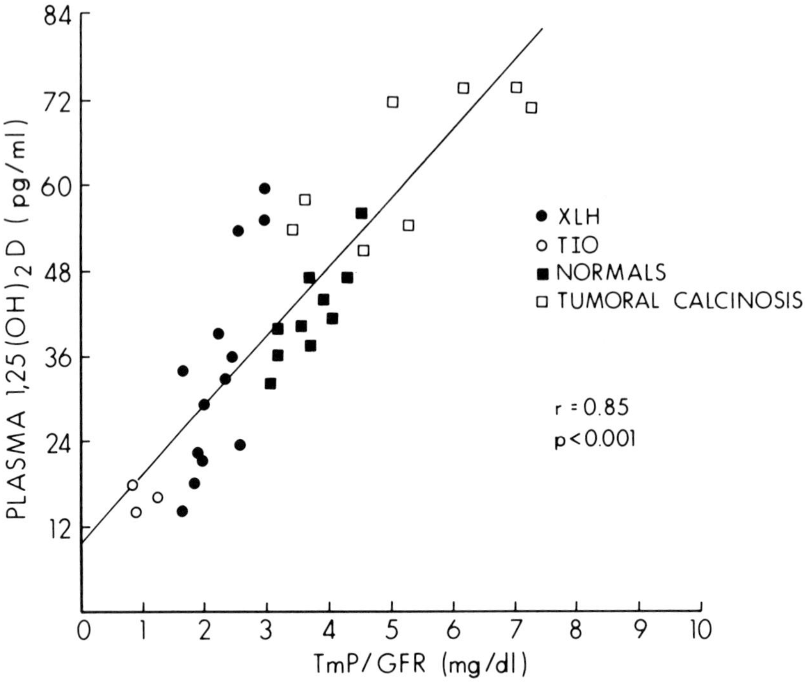

Fig. 5-1 Correlation between renal TmP/GFR and plasma 1,25$(OH)_2D$ levels in normals and patients with XLH, TIO, and tumoral calcinosis. Significant linear correlation is evident, suggesting a potential relationship between renal phosphate transport and the prevailing plasma levels of active vitamin D. (From Drezner MK: Understanding the pathogenesis of X-linked hypophosphatemic ricketts. A CPC Series, Cases in Metabolic Bone Disease 2(1): 1987 with permission of the Rogosin Institute; and modified from Lyles KW et al: Correlations of serum concentrations of 1,25 dihydroxyvitamin D, phosphorus, and parathyroid hormone in tumoral calcinosis. J Clin Endocrinol Metals 67, 1988, in press.)

More recently, choice of therapy in XLH has been markedly influenced by our understanding of the pathogenetic factors underlying this disease. With the recognition that the sequelae of XLH may be due to phosphate depletion, physicians aimed treatment strategies at providing oral phosphorus supplementation. On this regimen the serum phosphorus increased into or near the normal range. To prevent the secondary hyperparathyroidism attendant upon oral phosphorus administration, such therapeutic regimens often included pharmacologic amounts of vitamin D_2 (10,000 to 50,000 units/day).

Since this combination therapy results in radiographic healing of the rachitic lesions and accelerated growth in affected subjects, many investigators claimed that such treatment heals the bone disease of XLH. However, because radiographic examination of bone offers only an incomplete evaluation of therapeutic effect, the efficacy of this therapy has remained open to debate. In subsequent studies Costa et al.[23] and Lyles et al.[24] used histomorphometric analysis of bone biopsies to examine the effects of long-term (12 to 48 months) treatment with oral phosphate and vitamin D on bone healing in affected children and adults. Evaluation of bone biopsies revealed that long-term combination therapy does not eliminate the osteomalacic bone defect characteristic of this disease.

The failure to effect healing of the osteomalacia by combination therapy is due to a persistent defect in the dynamics of bone mineralization. The inordinately low mineralization front activity and mineral apposition rate in the bone biopsies of untreated patients indicate that the characteristic inadequate mineralization may be attributed to (1) a delayed onset of mineralization in newly synthesized osteoid; (2) prolonged and frequent pauses in the mineralization process; and (3) premature cessation of mineralization in osteoid seams. In treated patients the dynamics of mineralization are significantly improved: the defect in mineralization front activity is resolved while mineral apposition rate is enhanced, but to levels significantly less than those in normal subjects. These data indicate that the persistence of osteomalacia is most likely the result of a continuation of the prolonged and frequent pauses in mineralization. In contrast, attainment of normal mineralization front activity no doubt reflects normalization of the onset of mineralization in newly synthesized osteoid.

Although the observations of Costa et al. and Lyles et al. clearly establish that combination therapy does not heal the osteomalacic disease, they are paradoxic to the effects of phosphates and vitamin D_2 in curing the active rickets typical of XLH. These data suggest that the control of mineral accretion in epiphyseal and diaphyseal bone may be modulated independently. The explanation for phosphorus/vitamin D_2 treatment failure in patients with XLH remained enigmatic for a considerable time. However, appreciation that a relative $1,25(OH)_2D$ deficiency may contribute to the pathogenesis of the disease offered new hope for a successful therapy. Thus, several recent studies[25–27] have been directed at testing the efficacy of new combination drug regimens: $1,25(OH)_2D_3$ [or $1\alpha(OH)D_3$] and phosphorus. These treatment strategies directly attack the combined phosphorus and calcitriol deficiencies that have been documented in affected subjects. Indeed, several investigators have reported that administration of $1,25(OH)_2D_3$ or $1\alpha(OH)D_3$ and phosphorus results in improved mineralization. However, while the improvements in bone histologic findings were superior to the effects realized with conventional treatment regimens, complete healing of the osteomalacia was not achieved in any of the studied subjects, despite normalization of the serum phosphorus concentration.

The persistence of osteomalacia in these treated subjects may have been due to the relatively small doses of $1,25(OH)_2D_3$ [or $1\alpha(OH)D_3$] used. Since recent studies indicate that patients with XLH do not manifest an appropriately elevated serum calcitriol level, a pharmacologic dose of $1,25(OH)_2D_3$ (or its analog) may be necessary to influence phosphorus homeostasis adequately and/or overcome osteoblast resistance and thereby induce healing of the osteomalacia. Alternatively, the inadequacy of these drug regimens may be related to their relatively short duration (<9 months).

Harrell et al.[28] recently examined whether long-term treatment with $1,25(OH)_2D_3$ in pharmacologic amounts and phosphorus supplements is more effective in the management of XLH. In an ongoing study, 12 subjects, aged 4 to 36 years, received calcitriol (approximately 70 ng/kg/day) for an average of 11.2 months. Bone biopsies after therapy revealed reversal of the mineralization defect in all patients and consequent reduction of bone osteoid content to normal, which was evidence of the unprecedented complete healing of os-

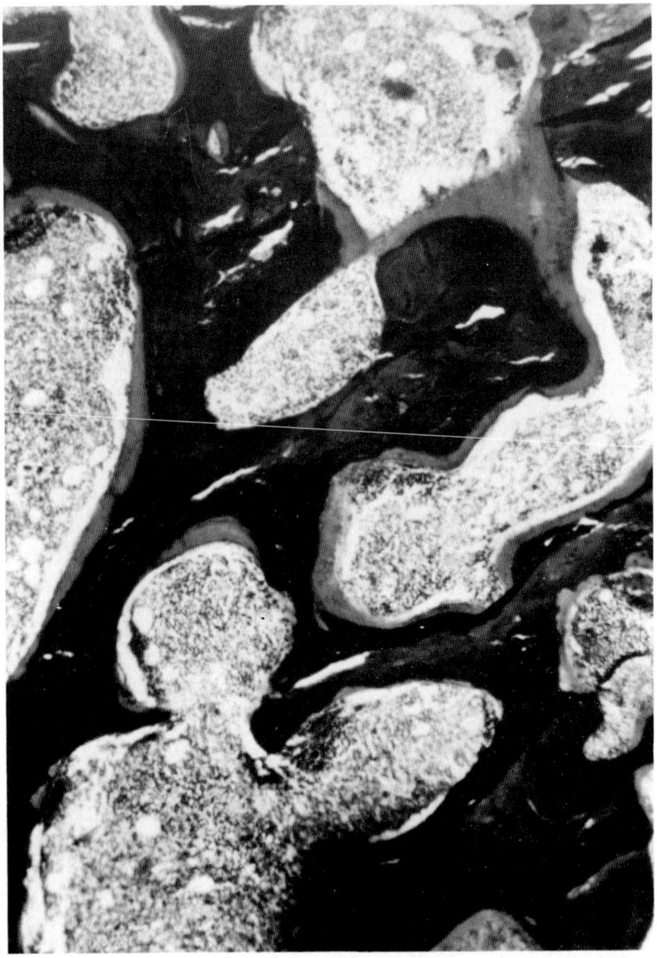

Fig. 5-2 (**A**) Goldner's-stained bone biopsy specimen from an untreated XLH patient showing an excessive amount of red osteoid on green stained mineralized bone surfaces. (*Figure continues.*)

teomalacia in XLH (Fig. 5-2). While these data indicate that high-dose $1,25(OH)_2D_3$ (and phosphorus) therapy is optimal for XLH, Harrell et al. have reported that complications of treatment (hypercalcemia/hypercalciuria or transient reduction of renal function) ensued in the majority of treated subjects within 1 to 7 months of bone healing. These events necessitated a reduction of the calcitriol dose to approximately 30 ng/kg/day. It is surprising that normal bone histologic characteristics persisted after 2 to 6 years of reduced-dose treatment.

Based on these observations, several investigators currently use an induc-

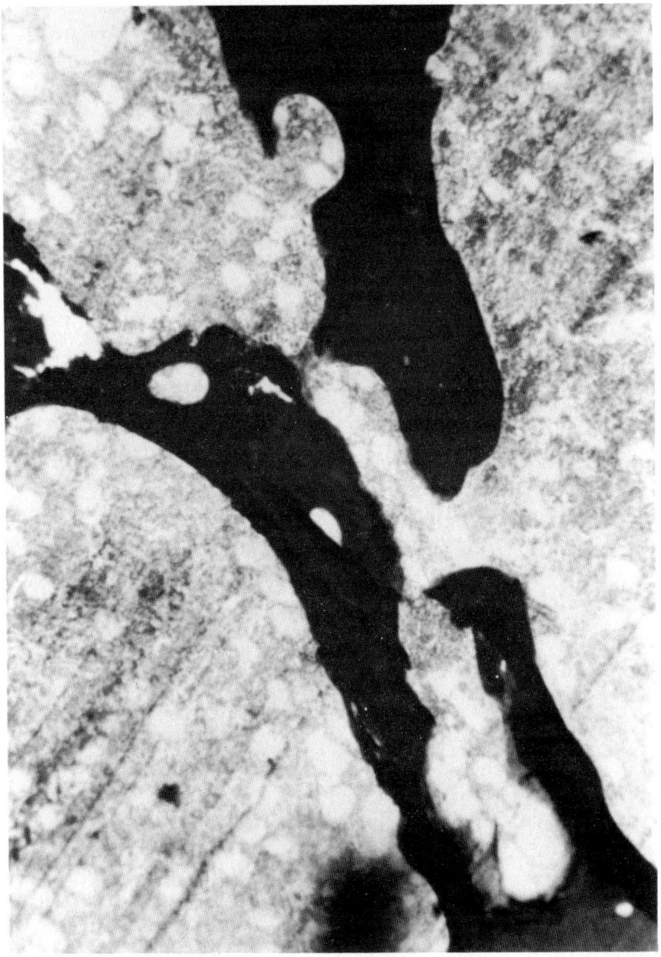

Figure 5-2 (*Continued*). (**B**) Goldner's-stained bone biopsy specimen from an XLH patient treated with high doses of calcitriol and phosphorus supplements. Red staining osteoid seams are scarce, consistent with normal histomorphology. (From Harrell RM, et al.,[28] with permission.)

tion/maintenance therapeutic strategy in patients with XLH. They prescribe high-dose $1,25(OH)_2D_3$ (and phosphorus) until bone healing has been documented, and reduce calcitriol at this juncture to maintenance levels in order to avoid hypercalciuria/hypercalcemia. The apparent requirement for pharmacologic amounts of calcitriol, as well as phosphate supplementation, to effect successful treatment of XLH indicates that the collective effects of hypophosphatemia and abnormal vitamin D metabolism underlie the phenotypic expression of this disease. Indeed, several lines of evidence further support this possibility. Included among these is the observation that differences in the manifestations of XLH and the recently described syndrome hereditary hypophosphatemic rickets with hypercalcemia (HHRH),[21] two diseases marked by renal phosphate wasting, can be attributed to the normal vitamin D metabolism maintained in the latter disease. Thus, the elevated serum $1,25(OH)_2D$ levels in patients with HHRH result in increased gastrointestinal absorption of calcium and phosphorus. In contrast, the defective vitamin D metabolism in patients with XLH abrogates the normal homeostatic response to phosphate depletion (increased gastrointestinal absorption) and alters the therapy required for healing of the bone disease.

Complications. Although the beneficial effects of a calcitriol/phosphorus regimen make it a potentially preferred form of treatment for XLH, little is known about the long-term side effects of this therapy. Only recently have preliminary data appeared regarding the global impact of this treatment regimen. Harrell et al.[29] have reported that after 25 months of maintenance treatment, each of 12 subjects displayed a significant increase in the serum parathyroid hormone concentration. Nine of the 12 patients, however, did not exhibit common ill effects from the elevated hormone level, but two did develop persistent hypercalcemia. Friedman et al. (unpublished observations, 1987) have also observed sonographic evidence of nephrocalcinosis in several treated patients. However, none of these subjects has exhibited compromised renal function.

Although these data are preliminary, they do serve to highlight that the universal effects of treatment in XLH have yet to be realized. Indeed, it remains possible to identify several additional complications/benefits that may be influenced by long-term treatment. For example, the presence of enthesopathic disease[30] in patients with XLH raises the possibility that treatment may accelerate the deposition of calcium in periarticular areas and intensify joint-related problems. Since 69 percent of affected subjects manifest this complication, the impact of accelerating this process would be substantial. In fact, one might foresee extensive disease in treated patients at an earlier time, since this is an age-dependent process.

Collectively these observations indicate that intense and persistent evaluation of treated subjects with XLH remains an essential requisite to assure effective therapy. Modifications of the current therapeutic strategy may yet be necessary to ensure successful and complication-free treatment.

Tumor-Induced Osteomalacia

The tumor-induced osteomalacia syndrome (TIO) is characterized by remission of unexplained osteomalacia (or rickets) after resection of a coexisting tumor. The disease has been recognized for nearly 30 years but its pathogenesis remains incompletely understood. Presenting symptoms are bone pain and/or muscle weakness with occasional recurrent long bone fractures. The duration of symptoms in patients aged 7 to 65 years has been 5 months to 16 years. Additional symptoms common to younger patients are fatigue, gait disturbances, slow growth, and skeletal deformities, including bowing of the lower extremities.

The biochemical findings characterizing this disorder include hypophosphatemia and an abnormally low renal tubular maximum for the reabsorption of phosphorus per liter of glomerular filtrate, indicative of renal phosphate wasting. In addition, subjects generally manifest gastrointestinal malabsorption of phosphorus. The renal phosphorus wasting and gastrointestinal malabsorption result in a negative phosphorus balance. Radiographic abnormalities include generalized osteopenia, pseudofractures, and coarsened trabeculae, as well as widened epiphyseal plates in children.

The tumors associated with TIO have been of mesenchymal origin in the large majority of patients. However, the frequent occurrence of Looser zones in the radiographs of moribund patients with carcinomas of epidermal and endodermal derivation[31] indicates that this disease may be secondary to a variety of tumor types. Indeed, the recent observation of TIO in association with breast carcinoma,[32] prostate carcinoma,[33] multiple myeloma, and chronic lymphocytic leukemia[34] supports this conclusion. The occurrence of osteomalacia in patients with widespread fibrous dysplasia of bone,[35] neurofibromatosis,[36] and linear nevus sebaceous syndrome[37] could also be tumor-induced. Proof of a causal relationship has been precluded by the multiplicity of lesions and the consequent inability to effect surgical cure. However, in one case of fibrous dysplasia, removal of virtually all of the abnormal bone did result in appropriate biochemical and radiographic improvement.

Pathophysiology. The mechanisms responsible for TIO have been only partially elucidated. Such incomplete understanding of the disorder undoubtedly relates to its infrequent occurrence and, consequently, the few physiologic studies of the disease. Nevertheless, most investigators agree that tumor production of a phosphaturic factor that may affect multiple functions of the proximal renal tubule and result in hypophosphatemia is a possible explanation for the pathogenesis of the TIO syndrome. This possibility has been supported by (1) the presence of phosphaturic activity in saline extracts of tumors from two patients with TIO[38]; and (2) the coincidence of glycosuria and aminoaciduria with renal phosphate wasting in selected affected subjects, indicative of complex alterations in proximal renal tubular function.[39]

More recently, abnormal vitamin D metabolism has been identified as an additional factor that may contribute to the pathogenesis of this disorder. Several observations support this possibility, including (1) the presence of a decreased circulating level of 1,25$(OH)_2$D in 17 of 18 reported patients who manifested the characteristic syndrome, in spite of a normal or elevated serum 25(OH)D concentration; (2) normalization of the serum 1,25$(OH)_2$D concentration promptly after surgical removal of the coincident tumor, and in association with resolution of the characteristic biochemical abnormalities of the syndrome; and (3) diminished renal 25(OH)D-1α-hydroxylase activity in heterotransplanted tumor-bearing athymic nude mice.[40]

The effectiveness of the presumed blockade in 1,25$(OH)_2$D production has recently been tested. Reid et al.[41] observed persistence of subnormal circulating calcitriol levels despite supramaximal stimulation of renal 25(OH)D-1α-hydroxylase activity, by not only marked hypophosphatemia but also hyperparathyroidism. The degree of inhibition was further illustrated by a sevenfold rise of serum 1,25$(OH)_2$D levels following tumor removal.

The interrelationship of abnormal renal phosphate transport and the proposed defect in vitamin D metabolism remains unknown. An innate heterogeneity of the pathogenesis of the syndrome cannot be excluded but studies are too fragmented and infrequent to allow us to be sure. Alternatively, the abnormal vitamin D metabolism and tumor secretion of phosphaturic substances may be interrelated factors that coordinately result in the phenotypic expression of TIO. Similar considerations have been entertained to allow us to understand better the pathogenesis of XLH (see Fig. 5-1). However, the ultimate understanding of the interplay between renal phosphate wasting and abnormal vitamin D metabolism in the expression of TIO requires further investigation.

Differential Diagnosis. The TIO syndrome has all the classic biochemical and radiologic criteria of hypophosphatemic osteomalcia. Diagnosis is dependent, therefore, upon a diligent search for tumors in all patients with vitamin-D-resistant rachitic/osteomalacic disease. Tumors may range from small to large and benign to malignant. Moreover, the tumor may be present for many years before the clinical appearance of bone disease. Thus, regardless of the temporal association between the onset of the osteomalacia and the clinical awareness of tumor, TIO should be considered. Indeed, where possible resection of any associated tumor should be attempted both to confirm the diagnosis and possibly to induce resolution of the syndrome.

When the tumor cannot be totally resected, diagnosis remains inferential. However, several observations can support the diagnosis: (1) a normal serum 25(OH)D level; (2) a selective deficiency of 1,25$(OH)_2$D, manifest by a decreased serum concentration; (3) demonstration of phosphaturic activity in tumor extracts; and/or (4) induction of the TIO syndrome in athymic nude mice upon heterotransplantation of tumor tissue from affected subjects.

In the absence of tumor and/or family history of disease, and after exclusion of common causes of osteomalacia, the possibility of adult-onset hypophosphatemic osteomalacia with or without Fanconi's syndrome must be considered. This syndrome may result from acquired or genetic causes and age of onset is extremely variable. Biochemical abnormalities are indistinguishable from those in patients with TIO. Careful follow-up for tumor occurrence must be maintained in patients with this disorder.

Treatment. The first and foremost treatment of TIO is complete resection of the associated tumor. However, recurrence of mesenchymal tumors, such as giant cell tumors of bone, or inability to resect completely certain malignancies, such as prostatic carcinoma, has resulted in the need for developing effective therapeutic intervention for the TIO syndrome. Historically, pharmacologic doses of vitamin D have been used in an effort to heal the bone disease. For the most part, the trials have been short and the results have not been assessed in detail. Nevertheless, it appears certain that this treatment does not cure the rachitic or osteomalacic components of the syndrome. Moreover, no resolution of the abnormal biochemistries ensues.

More recently, $1,25(OH)_2D_3$ alone or with oral phosphate supplementation has been used in an effort to overcome the supposed pathogenetic defects underlying TIO. In large measure trials have been conducted in single patients and the available data are fragmentary. However, Drezner et al.[40] have reported extensive studies of therapy in eight patients with TIO. They initiated therapy with $1,25(OH)_2D_3$ alone in each of the affected subjects. Throughout the therapeutic trial they monitored effects on the biochemical and bone abnormalities of the syndrome. The response of the biochemical abnormalities to pharmacologic doses of $1,25(OH)_2D_3$ (2 to 3 μg orally/day) was variable. In two subjects, one with a mesenchymal tumor (giant cell tumor of bone) and one with prostatic carcinoma, the serum phosphorus level increased from pretreatment levels of 1.5 ± 0.07 and 2.2 ± 0.10 mg/dl, respectively, to normal values of 3.2 ± 0.03 and 2.8 ± 0.08 mg/dl. Similarly, the renal TmP/GFR rose from an abnormally low level, 0.8 ± 0.03 and 1.9 ± 0.03 mg/dl, to normal, 3.0 ± 0.01 and 2.8 ± 0.09 mg/dl. Commensurately, evidence of bone healing was present in bone biopsies from these two subjects. Histomorphometric analysis revealed normalization of the amount of osteoid perimeter, the osteoid seam width, and mineralization front activity.

In contrast, in the remaining six subjects, two with mesenchymal tumors (osteoblastoma, chondroblastoma), three with prostatic carcinoma, and one with linear nevus sebaceous syndrome, $1,25(OH)_2D_3$ administered at a similar dose improved the abnormal biochemistry levels but did not normalize them. Similarly, analysis of bone biopsies in these treated patients revealed incomplete healing of the osteomalacia. Although mineralization front activity and mineral apposition rate increased significantly, an overabundance of unmineralized osteoid remained after 9 to 18 months of treatment. The variable responses to $1,25(OH)_2D_3$ therapy occur in spite of maintenance of a normal serum 25(OH)D level in all treated patients and a uniform increase of the serum $1,25(OH)_2D_3$ concentration from subnormal values to levels greater than normal. The variable response that Drezner et al. observed in response to $1,25(OH)_2D_3$ therapy is in accord with single observations of several investigators.[42]

In subsequent studies, however, several such patients responded well to combined therapy with pharmacologic amounts of $1,25(OH)_2D_3$ and phosphorus.[43] In these cases treatment normalized the biochemical abnormalities of the syndrome and resulted in healing of the osteomalacia. Similar therapeutic efficacy has been observed in patients with adult acquired hypophosphatemic osteomalacia. These data provide substantive evidence that patients with TIO or adult acquired disease may be benefited by a combined drug regimen.

Complications of Therapy. Little information is available regarding the long-term consequences of therapy in patients with TIO. The doses of medicines used, however, raise the possibility that nephrolithiasis, nephrocalcinosis, and hypercalcemia may frequently complicate the therapeutic course. Indeed, hypercalcemia secondary to parathyroid hyperfunction has been documented in five affected subjects, representing approximately 10 percent of the reported cases of TIO. All of these patients had received phosphorus (as part of a combination regimen with vitamin D_2 or $1,25(OH)_2D_3$), which may have stimulated parathyroid hormone secretion and ultimately led to parathyroid autonomy. Thus, careful assessment of parathyroid function during treatment of TIO may be required to ensure *safe* and efficacious therapy.

Vitamin-D-Dependent Rickets

Vitamin-D-dependent rickets is a rare disorder with the symptoms and signs of vitamin-D-deficiency rickets. To date, two subtypes of this disorder have been identified. The clinical, radiologic, and biochemical characteristics of the two forms are similar in most respects. However, the serum $1,25(OH)_2D$ level is decreased in patients with type I disease but increased in type II. Within each subtype there is genetic heterogeneity as manifest by age of onset, severity of rachitic lesions, and dosage of vitamin D required to treat the disorder effectively. The incidence of vitamin-D-dependent rickets is much lower than that of the hypophosphatemic vitamin-D-resistant rachitic diseases.

Type I. Inheritance of type I disease follows the pattern characteristic of an autosomal recessive trait. Clinical symptoms usually appear in the first year of life and include hypocalcemic tetany (manifest as laryngospastic crisis, carpopedal spasm, or seizures), muscular hypotonia and weakness, motor retardation, and stunted growth. In other cases, pathologic fractures may be the presenting feature. Radiographs reveal classic signs of vitamin-D-deficiency rickets. Thus, irregular fraying at the provisional zone of calcification and metaphyseal widening are apparent at the distal ends of the radius and ulna. In untreated youths, metaphyseal changes including coarse trabeculation may develop.

Hypocalcemia is the cardinal biochemical abnormality and occurs concomitantly with a high concentration of parathyroid hormone. In several recent studies serum 25(OH)D levels have been reported normal in untreated affected subjects.[44] In contrast, the serum $1,25(OH)_2D$ concentration is profoundly decreased. Many of these findings are also characteristically observed in nutritional vitamin D deficiency. However, the absence of either biochemical or radiographic improvement of the rickets following therapy with physiologic doses of vitamin D clearly differentiates vitamin-D-dependent rickets from the vitamin-D-deficient form.

Pathophysiology. The presence of a depressed serum $1,25(OH)_2D$ level suggests that a defect in 25(OH)D-1α-hydroxylase activity is manifest in subjects with this disease and may be the pathogenetic basis for the disorder. The presumed defect in 25(OH)D-1α-hydroxylase activity has been substantiated in several additional studies that have shown no increase in the serum $1,25(OH)_2D$ concentration in response to classic stimuli of enzyme action. Thus, serum $1,25(OH)_2D$ levels remain low in patients treated successfully with vitamin D or 25(OH)D[45] in spite of a normal serum concentration of calcium and phosphorus and an elevated serum 25(OH)D level. Moreover, administration of parathyroid hormone, a known stimulus of enzyme activity, results only in a minimal increase of the already low serum $1,25(OH)_2D$ level (Drezner, unpublished observations, 1982). The failure to increase the serum $1,25(OH)_2D$ level suggests that the 25(OH)D-1α-hydroxylase activity does not respond to normal regulatory controls.

More recently, investigation of the porcine homologue of the human disease confirmed that abnormal enzyme activity underlies this disease. In these studies Wilke et al.[46] conclusively demonstrated that renal preparations from the mutants exhibit a relative absence of 25(OH)D-1α-hydroxylase activity. In addition, enzyme function proved refractory to stimulation.

These observations indicate that the vitamin-D-dependent rickets type I represents a pseudo-vitamin-D deficiency state. Response to therapeutic intervention supports this conclusion.

Treatment. Vitamin-D-dependent rickets, type I, responds to vitamin D in pharmacologic amounts. Upon institution of such treatment the biochemical and clinical abnormalities of the disorder remit. Similarly, pharmacologic amounts of 25(OH)D are required to effect healing of the rickets. Since $1,25(OH)_2D$ levels do not increase after vitamin D or 25(OH)D treatment, it is likely that the positive effects of therapy are not modulated by this presumed active vitamin D metabolite. However, all treated patients do have an elevated serum 25(OH)D concentration. Moreover, affected subjects treated with 25(OH)D have documented increased serum $24,25(OH)_2D$ levels. Thus, while it remains uncertain what factors modulate the therapeutic response, it is likely that the pharmacologic circulating levels of 25(OH)D (or perhaps $24,25(OH)_2D$) contribute to the healing process.

In contrast, consistent with the hypothesis that defective 25(OH)D-1α-hydroxylase activity underlies the disease, physiologic doses of $1,25(OH)_2D$ promote complete healing of the bone disease. Fraser et al.[47] and Prader et al.[48] treated patients with $1,25(OH)_2D_3$, 1 μg/day, and observed both normalization of the hypocalcemia within a few days after initiation of treatment and healing of the bone disease after several weeks. Similar therapeutic benefit has been reported in response to administration of low-dose $1\alpha(OH)D_3$ (1 to 3 μg/day), an analog of $1,25(OH)_2D_3$. Delvin et al.[49] have reported the results of the only long-term trial of treatment yet recorded. In their study they observed beneficial results in nine patients in response to $1,25(OH)_2D_3$ (0.5 to 1 μg/day) for 4 to

24 months. Several patients required higher doses (2 to 3 μg/day), however, but reduction in the dosage was possible after the rickets had healed.

In response to such treatment the serum level of 1,25$(OH)_2$D increases to normal. In addition, the serum 25(OH)D concentration decreases while the circulating level of 24,25$(OH)_2$D initially increases. After continuous treatment, however, the serum 24,25$(OH)_2$D concentration gradually declines at a rate roughly correlated with the fall in plasma alkaline phosphatase activity and in association with healing of the bone. These observations leave open the question of whether the therapeutic response to 1,25$(OH)_2D_3$ is merely the result of replacing the deficient vitamin D metabolite or involves a complementary effect of 24,25 $(OH)_2D_3$ on bone mineralization.

In any case, therapy with vitamin D or its metabolites must be continued for life to prevent relapse of hypocalcemia and subsequent bone disease. However, patients have been observed with a syndrome clinically identical to vitamin-D-dependent rickets type I in whom no reappearance of biochemical or radiographic signs of rickets occurred following treatment.

Type II. Vitamin-D-dependent rickets, type II, describes the hereditary spectrum of disorders that exhibit resistance to 1,25$(OH)_2$D effects. General features of the syndrome include rickets or osteomalacia, alopecia, hypocalcemia, secondary hyperparathyroidism, and high serum 1,25$(OH)_2$D concentrations (before or during treatment with calciferols). Each of these general features has a wide spectrum of expression in individual patients.[50] In the mildest forms of disease there is normocalcemia, mild secondary hyperparathyroidism, and modest elevation of 1,25$(OH)_2$D levels. Most reported cases, however, have exhibited more severe dysfunction marked by overt hypocalcemia prior to treatment. Approximately one-half of the affected subjects manifest a calcemic response to high doses of calciferol while the remainder display apparent total resistance to 1,25$(OH)_2$D effects. In general, the most severely affected patients are those who develop alopecia (or sparse hair) during the course of the disease.

Most cases recognized to date presented with rickets prior to age 3 years. Chemical disturbances, however, have been evident prior to age 6 months. Rarely, affected patients had no demonstrable rickets but presented with de novo osteomalacia at age 45 years or later. Subjects who presented late have been generally normocalcemic, and represent cases of the mildest form of the disorder.

Pathophysiology and Treatment. Although secondary hyperparathyroidism has been proposed as a factor contributing to the elevated levels of 1,25$(OH)_2D_3$ characteristic of vitamin-D-dependent rickets type II, the sustained increase in serum 1,25$(OH)_2D_3$ seen after treatment with vitamin D or 25$(OH)D_3$ (which corrected the hypocalcemia and secondary hyperparathyroidism) indicates that other factors are of greater significance in the pathogenesis of this disease. Indeed, more recently several investigators have proposed that resistance to 1,25$(OH)_2D_3$ at the level of the target organ results in the elevated circulating level of this metabolite.[51] Such resistance is clearly seen in the intestine, where 1,25$(OH)_2D_3$ is a major determinant of calcium absorption.

Several laboratories have reported that fractional intestinal absorption of calcium[47] is low in affected subjects despite the increased serum $1,25(OH)_2D$ concentration.

The nature of the defect in target tissues that causes resistance to the action of $1,25(OH)_2D_3$ is currently under investigation (Fig. 5–3). As with other steroid hormones, a multistep process at the cellular level is necessary before any metabolic effect of $1,25(OH)_2D_3$ can be demonstrated. At present defects affecting many of these steps have been identified. These abnormalities include[42,43] (1) a hormone-binding negative state, a defect likely due to focal abnormalities in the $1,25(OH)_2D_3$ binding domain of the seco-steroid receptor; (2) deficient hormone-binding capacity; (3) deficient hormone-binding affinity; (4) unmeasurable nuclear localization of hormones (in spite of normal

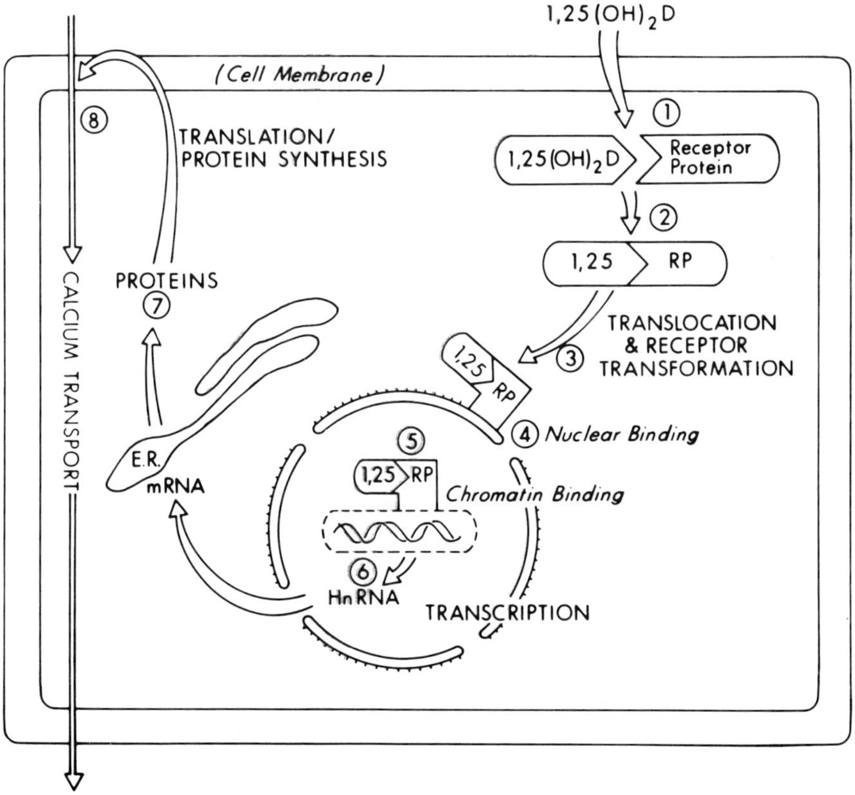

Fig. 5-3 Sites of potential abnormalities underlying vitamin-D-dependent rickets, type II are indicate by the circled numbers. These defects include (1) a decreased number of cytosolic receptors for $1,25(OH)_2D$; (2) altered affinity or stability of the cytosolic receptor; (3) abnormal translocation and/or transformation of the $1,25(OH)_2D$ receptor; (4,5) an altered nuclear and/or chromatin binding site; (6) abnormal transcription; and/or (7,8) defective protein synthesis or action thereby precluding expression of $1,25(OH)_2D$ specific effects such as calcium transport. (From Lyles,[21] with permission.)

$1,25(OH)_2D$ binding); and (5) an abnormal DNA binding domain for the $1,25(OH)_2D$–receptor complex. Each of these abnormalities might reflect modification of a separate functional domain of the $1,25(OH)_2D_3$ receptor. Alternatively, some could result from mutations affecting other than the receptor gene. In any case, regardless of the defect, there is good correlation between the degree of resistance to $1,25(OH)_2D_3$ exhibited by cells in vitro and responsivity to high doses of calciferols in vivo. Thus, these studies have aided our understanding of the resistance phenomenon in vitamin-D-dependent rickets type II and provided evidence of genetic heterogeneity in this disorder. In responsive patients, successful treatment of D type II with vitamin D usually requires pharmacologic amounts. However, the required doses of the metabolite are distinctly higher than those necessary for treatment of type I. Doses have ranged from 0.1 to 30 mg (4,000 to 1,200,000 units) per day for vitamin D_3, 0.05 mg to 1.5 mg per day for $25(OH)D_3$, and 5 to 20 μg/day of $1,25(OH)_2D_3$. The familial cases of vitamin-D-resistant rickets type II are particularly resistant to vitamin D, as are type II patients with alopecia. Isuchiya et al. found that 7 million units of vitamin D_3 were required daily to normalize serum biochemistries in one alopecic child. In patients unresponsive to calciferols, a beneficial effect from intravenous administration of calcium has been observed.

REFERENCES

1. Loomis WF: Seasonal variations in the incidence of osteomalacia. Science 147:501, 1967
2. Fraser D, Kooh SW, Scriver CR: Parathyroid-dependent phosphaturia and aminoaciduria in the vitamin D deficient rat. Am J Physiol 214:371, 1968
3. Baker LRI, Ackrill PP, Catell WR, et al: Iatrogenic osteomalacia and myopathy due to phosphate depletion. Br Med J 3:150, 1974
4. Morgan DB, Hunt G, Paterson CR: The osteomalacia syndrome after stomach operations Q J Med 39:395, 1970
5. Arnaud SB, Goldsmith RS, Lambert PW, et al: 25 hydroxyvitamin D_3: evidence of an enterohepatic circulation in man. Proc Soc Exp Biol Med 149:570, 1975
6. Long RG, Wills MR, Skinner RK, et al: Serum 25-hydroxyvitamin D in untreated parenchymal and cholestatic liver disease. Lancet 2:650, 1976
7. Rodbro P, Christiansen C, Land M: Development of anticonvulsant osteomalacia in epileptic patients on phenytoin treatment. Acta Neurol Scand 50:527, 1974
8. Koch HV, Kraft D, von Herrath D, et al: Influence of diphenylhydration and phenobarbital on intestinal transport in the rat. Epilepsia 13:829, 1972
9. Drezner MK, Haussler MR: Serum 1,25-dihydroxyvitamin D in bone disease. N Engl J Med 300:435, 1979
10. Delvin EE, Glorieux FH: Serum 1,25-dihydroxyvitamin D concentration in hypophosphatemic vitamin D resistant rickets. Calcif Tiss Int 33:173, 1981
11. Lyles KW, Clark AG, Drezner MK: Serum 1,25-dihydroxyvitamin D levels in subjects with X-linked hypophosphatemic rickets and osteomalacia. Calcif Tiss Int 34:125, 1982
12. Lyles KW, Drezner MK: Parathyroid hormone effects on serum 1,25-dihydroxyvitamin D levels in patients with X-linked hypophosphatemic rickets: evidence for

abnormal 25-hydroxyvitamin D-1-hydroxylase activity. J Clin Endocrinol Metab 54:638, 1982
13. Insogna KL, Broadus AE, Gertner JM: Impaired phosphorus conservation and 1,25-dihydroxyvitamin D generation during phosphorus deprivation in familial hypophosphatemic rickets. J Clin Invest 71:1562, 1983
14. Eicher EM, Southlard JL, Scriver CR, et al: Hypophosphatemia: mouse model for human familial hypophosphatemic vitamin D-resistant rickets. Proc Natl Acad Sci USA 73:4667, 1976
15. Lobaugh B, Drezner MK: Abnormal regulation of renal 25-hydroxyvitamin D-1α-hydroxylase activity in the X-linked hypophosphatemic mouse. J Clin Invest 71:400, 1983
16. Nesbitt T, Drezner MK, Lobaugh B: Abnormal parathyroid hormone stimulation of 25-hydroxyvitamin D-1-hydroxylase activity in the hypophosphatemic mouse: evidence for a generalized defect of vitamin D metabolism. J Clin Invest 77:181, 1986
17. Tenenhouse H: Abnormal renal mitochondrial 25-hydroxyvitamin D_3-1α-hydroxylase activity in the vitamin D and calcium deficient X-linked Hyp-mouse. Endocrinology 113:816, 1983
18. Akiba T, Endou H, Koseki C, et al: Localization of 25-hydroxyvitamin D_3-1α-hydroxylase activity in the mammalian kidney. Biochem Biophys Res Commun 94:313, 1980
19. Kawashima H, Torikai S, Kurokawa K: Calcitonin selectively stimulates 25-hydroxyvitamin D_3-1α-hydroxylase in the proximal straight tubule of the rat kidney. Nature (Lond) 291:327, 1981
20. Nesbitt T, Lobaugh B, Drezner MK: Calcitonin stimulation of renal 25-hydroxyvitamin D-1-hydroxylase activity in hypophosphatemic mice: evidence that the regulation of calcitriol production is not universally abnormal in X-linked hypophosphatemia. J Clin Invest 79:15, 1987
21. Lyles KW, Drezner MK: Diseases of abnormal phosphate metabolism. In Becker KL (ed): Principles and Practice of Endocrinology and Metabolism. JB Lippincott, Philadelphia, 1988
22. Seino Y, Yamaoka K, Ishida M, et al: Plasma clearance for high doses of 1,25-dihydroxy [23,23(n)-^{3}H] cholecalciferol in X-linked hypophosphatemic mice. Biomed Res 3:683, 1982
23. Costa T, Marie PJ, Scriver CR, et al: X-linked hypophosphatemia: effect of calcitriol on renal handling of phosphate, serum phosphate and bone mineralization. J Clin Endocrinol Metab 52:463, 1981
24. Lyles KW, Harrelson JM, Drezner MK: The efficacy of vitamin D_2 and oral phosphorus therapy in X-linked hypophosphatemic rickets and osteomalacia. J Clin Endocrinol Metab 54:307, 1982
25. Rasmussen H, Anast C: Familial hypophosphatemic rickets and vitamin D-dependent rickets. p.1743. In Stanbury JB, Wyngaarden JB, Frederickson DS, et al (eds): The Metabolic Basis of Inherited Disease. 5th Ed. McGraw-Hill, New York, 1983
26. Glorieux FH, Marie PJ, Pettifor JM, et al: Bone response to phosphate salts, ergocalciferol, and calcitriol in hypophosphatemic vitamin D resistant rickets. N Engl J Med 303:1023, 1980
27. Costa T, Marie PJ, Scriver CR, et al: X-linked hypophosphatemia: effect of calcitriol on renal handling of phosphate, serum phosphate and bone mineralization. J Clin Endocrinol Metab 52:463, 1981
28. Harrell RM, Lyles KW, Harrelson JM, et al: Healing of bone disease in X-linked hypophosphatemic rickets/osteomalacia: induction and maintenance with phosphorus and calcitriol. J Clin Invest 75:1858, 1985

29. Harrell RM, Drezner MK, Bowie JD, et al: Complications of successful therapy in X-linked hypophosphatemic rickets. J Bone Min Res 1(suppl):197(abstr), 1986
30. Polisson RP, Martinez S, Khoury M, et al: Calcification of entheses associated with X-linked hypophosphatemic osteomalacia. N Engl J Med 313:1, 1985
31. Dent CE, Stamp TCB: Vitamin D rickets and osteomalacia. p.237. In Avioli LV, Krane SM (eds): Metabolic Bone Disease. Vol. I. Academic Press, New York, 1978
32. Bhattacharyya M, DeLuca HF: Subcellular location of rat liver calciferol-25-hydroxylase. Arch Biochem Biophys 160:58, 1974
33. Lyles KW, Berry WR, Haussler M, et al: Hypophosphatemic osteomalacia: association with prostatic carcinoma. Ann Intern Med 93:275, 1980
34. Rao DS, Parfitt AM, Villaneuva AR, et al: Hypophosphatemic osteomalacia and adult Fanconi syndrome due to light-chain nephropathy: another form of oncogenous osteomalacia. Am J Med 82:333, 1987
35. Dent CE, Gertner JM: Hypophosphatemic osteomalacia in fibrous dysplasia. Q J Med 45:411, 1976
36. Saville PD, Nassim JR, Stevenson FH, et al: Osteomalacia in von Recklinghausen's neurofibromastosis: metabolic study of a case. Br Med J 1:1311, 1955
37. Carey DE, Drezner MK, Hamdan JA, et al: Hypophosphatemic rickets/osteomalacia in linear sebaceous nevus syndrome: a variant of tumor-induced osteomalacia. J Pediatr 109:994, 1986
38. Aschinberg LC, Solomon LM, Zeis PM, et al: Vitamin D-resistant rickets associated with epidermal nevus syndrome: demonstration of a phosphaturic substance in the dermal lesions. J Pediatr 91:56, 1977
39. Drezner MK, Feinglos MN: Osteomalacia due to a 1,25-dihydroxycholecalciferol deficiency. Association with a giant cell tumor of bone. J Clin Invest 61:1046, 1977
40. Lobaugh B, Burch WM Jr, Drezner MK: Abnormalities of vitamin D metabolism and action in the vitamin D resistant rachitic and osteomalacic diseases. In Kumar R(ed): Vitamin D. Martinus Nijhoff, Boston, 1984
41. Reid IR, Teitelbaum SL, Dusso A, et al: Hypercalcemic hyperparathyroidism complicating oncogenic osteomalacia: effect of successful tumor resection on mineral homeostasis. Am J Med 83:350, 1987
42. Nortman DF, Brautbar N, Coburn JW, et al: Response of tumor associated osteomalacia to 1,25-dihydroxyvitamin D_3 (abstract). Clin Res 92A, 1979
43. Fukumoto Y, Ichihara K, Moriwaki K, et al: Tumor-induced vitamin D resistant hypophosphatemic osteomalacia: phosphaturic substance in tumor and urine of the patient. p.420. In Cohn DV, Talmage RV, Matthews JL (eds): Hormonal Control of Calcium Metabolism. Excerpta Medica, Amsterdam, 1981
44. Balsan S, Garabedin M, Leiberherr M, et al: Serum 1,25-dihydroxyvitamin D concentrations in two different types of pseudodeficiency rickets. p.1143. In Norman AW, Schaefer K, Herrath DV, et al (eds): Vitamin D: Basic Research and Its Clinical Application. Walter de Gruyter, New York, 1979
45. Reade TM, Scriver CR, Glorieux FH, et al: Response to crystalline 1α-hydroxyvitamin D_3 in vitamin D dependency. Pediatr Res 9:593, 1975
46. Wilke R, Harmeyer J, Grabe C, et al: Regulatory hyperparathyroidism in pig breed with vitamin D dependency rickets. Acta Endocrinol 92:295, 1979
47. Fraser D, Kooh SW, Kind HO, et al: Pathogenesis of hereditary vitamin D dependent rickets: an inborn error of vitamin D metabolism involving defective conversion of 25-hydroxyvitamin D to 1,25-dihydroxyvitamin D. N Engl J Med 289:817, 1973
48. Prader A, Kind GP, DeLuca HF: Pseudo-vitamin D deficiency (vitamin D depen-

dency). p.115. In Bricket H, Stern J (eds): Inborn Errors of Calcium and Bone Metabolism. University Park Press, Baltimore, 1976

49. Delvin EE, Glorieux FH, Marie PJ, et al: Vitamin D-dependency: Replacement therapy with calcitriol. J Pediatr 99:26, 1981
50. Eil C, Liberman UA, Rosen JF, et al: A cellular defect in hereditary vitamin D dependent rickets type II. N Engl J Med 304:1588, 1981
51. Marx SJ, Liberman UA, Eil C, et al. Resistance to 1,25-dihydroxycholecalciferol in man and in other species. p.107. In Norman AW, et al (eds): Vitamin D: Chemical, Biochemical and Clinical Update. 3rd Ed. Walter de Gruyter, Berlin, 1985

6 Paget's Disease of Bone

Janet E. Rubin
Bayard D. Catherwood

Sir James Paget first described, in 1877, a disease of bone that presented with fluctuating bone pain, deformity that included enlargement and distortion of weight-bearing bones, and a propensity to fractures. Because of the bone growth, the unusual asymmetric distribution of the lesions, and the chronicity of the disorder, Paget thought that a chronic inflammatory process was the cause and he coined the term "osteitis deformans."[1] In the century since Paget's initial discussion and particularly in the last 20 years we have learned much about bone physiology. This knowledge has led to an improved understanding of the pathogenesis and treatment of Paget's disease as well as of its causes.

We now realize that this disease is quite common. Necropsy studies and radiologic surveys have demonstrated evidence of Pagetic bone in 3 to 5.1 percent of the western European population over 45 years of age, with the incidence slightly less in North America. Demographic studies in England and Wales show a marked tendency toward geographic clustering.[2] In addition, there appears to be an increased incidence of the disease among family members of affected patients.[3] Most affected persons identified by these surveys do not have the debilitating, polyostotic disease but rather a subclinical form.

Active Paget's disease is characterized by an intense focal bone resorption consisting of increased Howship's lacunar spaces filled with giant osteoclasts. The osteoclasts appear morphologically abnormal: the number of nuclei is increased, and the cells contain unusual inclusion bodies.[3] The cytoplasmic membrane has significantly more folds than normal, indicating that the osteoclast is highly active.[4] Osteoclastic activity is thought to be influenced by several adjacent elements such as the neighboring osteoblast, the bone matrix proteins, and local cytokines as well as by systemic hormone such as parathyroid hormone and 1,25 dihydroxyvitamin D. Elements of the immune system may also exert both local and systemic control over osteoclastic activity. Since the osteoclast appears to be derived from the same precursors as cells of the macrophage–monocyte series,[5] these controls may have ontologic reasons. Nevertheless, changes in local or systemic factors associated with Paget's disease bone have not been identified so far. The osteoblast in pagetic bone appears morphologically normal but must work at an increased level to keep up with the excessive osteoclastic activity.[4] The deposition of new bone matrix and its subsequent mineralization by the osteoblast is disorganized and irregular in Paget's disease. Collagen fibers secreted by osteoblasts in the pagetic region are randomly arrayed in the pattern of woven bone. Instead of eventual replacement of this woven bone with a more organized structure, such as would occur after the initial formation of, for instance, a fracture callus, the woven pattern persists. Normal dynamic bone remodeling would require osteoclasts to resorb this hastily formed bone prior to a more leisurely deposition of lamellar bone by the osteoblasts. Thus, the persistence of the immature woven bone in Paget's disease may be due to a functional abnormality of the osteoclast, such as inability to recognize this new bone as abnormal. Overall, the coupling between accelerated osteoclasts and osteoblasts is present but disturbed.

CAUSES

Clues to the causes of Paget's disease have arisen during ultrastructural examination of the abnormal osteoclast. In 1974 Rebel[4] first described the presence of unusual inclusion bodies in the nucleus and cytoplasm of pagetic osteoclasts. Mills[6] described microcylindric filamentous inclusions in the osteoclasts of every one of the patients with Paget's disease that her group studied (Fig. 6-1). No other cells in the pagetic bone, nor osteoclasts activated by other processes such as primary hyperparathyroidism, contained these inclusion bodies. The inclusions seen in pagetic osteoclasts are either randomly bunched or packed in a paracrystalline array reminiscent of the nucleocapsids of the measles RNA virus. This RNA virus can cause disease that appears many years after the initial infection, such as subacute sclerosing panencephalitis. Rebel has shown that pagetic osteoclasts react with measles and respiratory syncytial virus antibodies.[4,7] Respiratory syncytial virus and measles are members of the RNA paramyxovirus family. It has been hypothesized, therefore, that Paget's lesion is the delayed activation of an infection by an altered or as yet uncharacterized paramyxovirus. If we assume that the virus initially lodges in the osteoclast precursors of the monocyte—macrophage lineage, depending on the rate of infection, pagetic abnormalities might arise later in osteoclast daughter cells. Perhaps an age–related disturbance in local immune surveillance allows a fixed number of virus–bearing precursors to begin proliferating, resulting in clones of abnormal osteoclasts. Inclusion bodies similar to those seen in the bone of patients with Paget's disease are also present in certain giant cell tumor variants, suggesting a relationship between the proliferating osteoclasts of Paget's and these mesenchymal tumors.[7]

Despite these indications, the viral cause of the disease has not been established and a viral agent has not been isolated. The lack of an adequate animal model of Paget's disease hinders research in this area. Nevertheless, a primary cell line has been isolated from a pagetic lesion that bears viral antigens to RSV and measles viruses.[8]

CLINICAL PRESENTATION

The five cases that Paget originally presented to illustrate his formulation were unusually debilitating and his examination of these devastating examples of bone involvement led him to believe that "osteitis deformans" was a rare disease. With the advent of radiology and the biochemical assessment of bone metabolism, it became apparent that Paget's disease was not at all rare. Most Paget's disease is subclinical, and the diagnosis is often suggested by radiographs obtained for unrelated reasons. Only about 5 percent of patients with identifiable Paget's disease actually present with the signs and symptoms of the clinical syndrome (see Table 6-1).

The pain that commonly brings the pagetic patient to the physician derives both from bone primarily affected by the disease and joints that are secondarily stressed. The pain attributable to the actual pagetic lesions characteristically occurs in weight-bearing bones while the patient is standing and is more severe during the lytic phase of the disease.[9] Affected bones can also cause pain if they are dependent during sleep. The most intense pagetic pain occurs when deformed vertebrae impinge on spinal cord or nerve roots. There is a lack of correlation between the intensity of pain and the severity of the disease and many patients with polyostotic disease never experience pain.[3]

Joint pain of degenerative arthritis also accounts for many patients' complaints. In fact, 91 percent of patients have preexisting osteoarthritis.[10] Joints that transmit weight from pagetic long bones, or are abnormally stressed due to abnormal weight bearing, frequently demonstrate acceleration of preexisting degenerative joint disease. The clinician should try to differentiate degenerative joint disease from primary bone pain since the former is best treated with standard anti-inflammatory therapy. In one large study, 37 percent of patients complained of back pain. In the majority of cases, the cause of the pain was related to osteoarthritis.[10] The differentiation between pain from Paget's disease and that from degenerative joint disease can be made by a careful examination of the joint physically and on the radiograph, where arthritis is evidenced by narrowing of the joint space and destruction of cartilage. Paget's disease rarely affects the articular cartilage directly.

Bone deformity with overlying warm skin is a frequent clinical presentation. The skull, clavicles, and long bones are often affected and show increased size, cortical thickening, and abnormal contours (Fig. 6-2). Extensive vertebral disease may cause decreased height due to collapse. Nearly half of the patients with skull involvement have a measurable loss of auditory acuity consisting of conductive as well as sensorineural hearing loss.[3] Infrequently other nerve

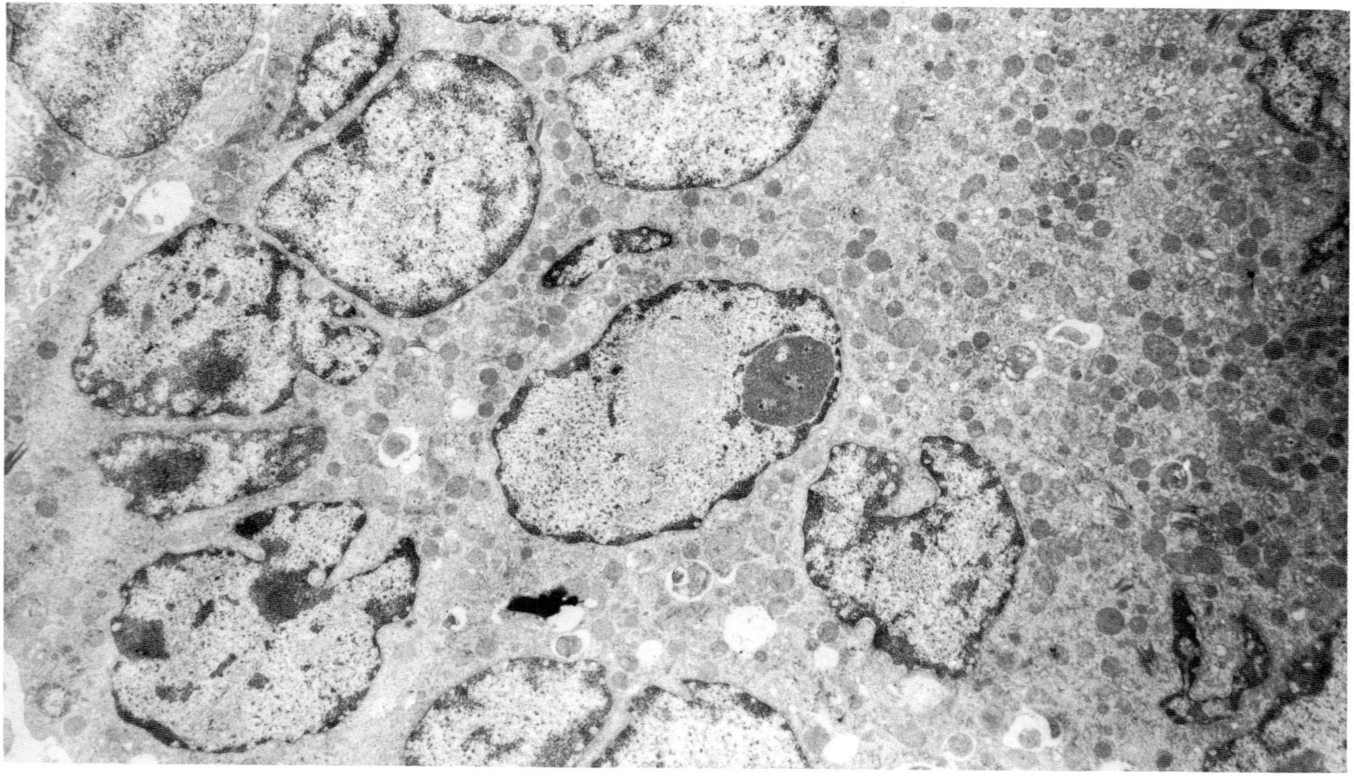

A

Fig. 6-1. (**A**) Electron micrograph of a portion of an osteoclast from a patient with Paget's disease. Note the large number of nuclei. The central nucleus contains a large inclusion typical of the disease (× 6,000). (*Figure continues.*)

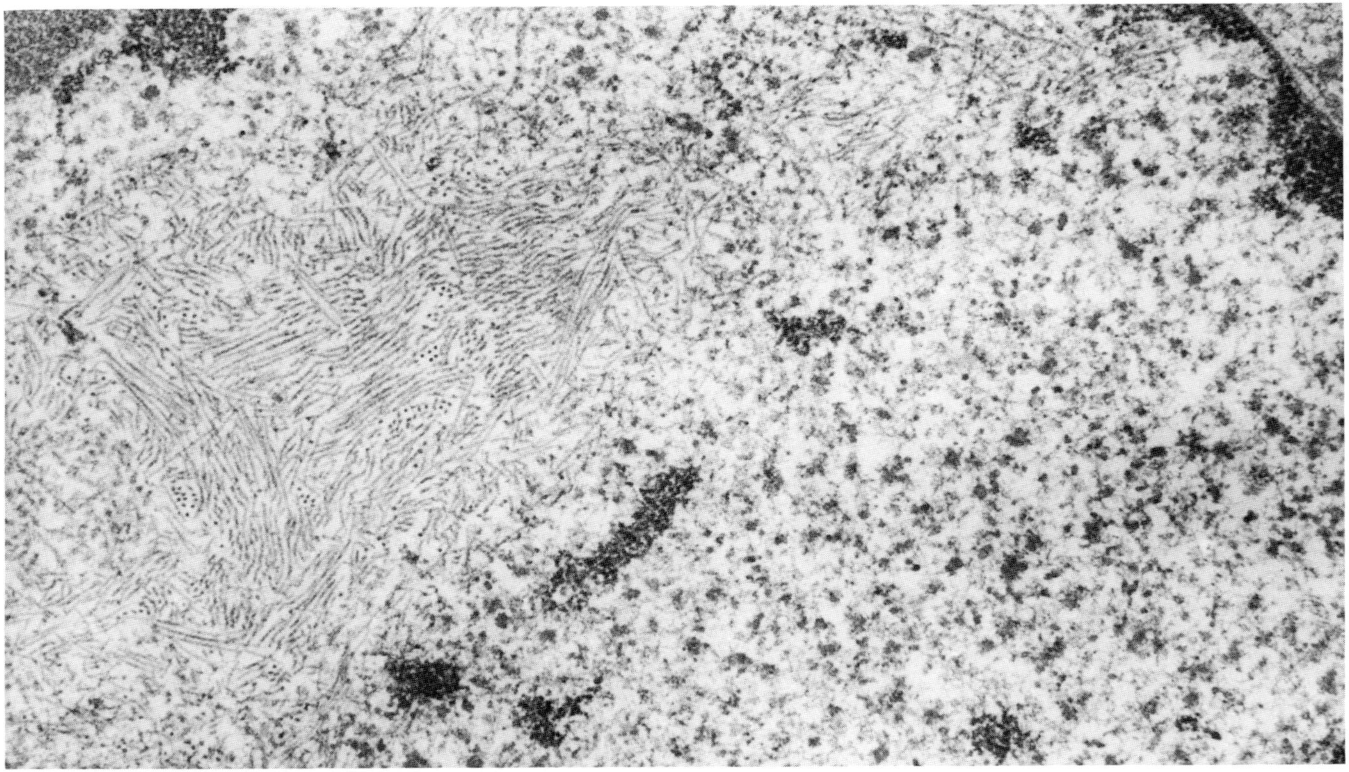

B

Fig. 6-1 (*Continued*). (**B**) Higher magnification of the nuclear inclusion illustrates the architecture of the microtubules forming the inclusion. They are randomly oriented, closely packed or loosely scattered in the nucleoplasm (× 36,000). (Courtesy of Dr. Barbara G. Mills.)

Table 6-1. Clinical Signs and Symptoms of Paget's Disease

Bone pain: back, hip, knee
Joint pain
Headache
Decreased auditory acuity
Bone deformity: enlargement, bowing
Pathologic fracture
Nerve impingement syndromes
High-output cardiac failure

compression syndromes including long tract signs from platybasia of the skull or spinal cord compression occur.

The abnormal woven bone characteristic of the pagetic lesion often results in fractures, which can occur with minimal trauma. These occur most frequently in the pelvis, spine, and long bones, especially during the lytic phase of the disease. Fracture nonunion is common in the untreated patient, as is refracture. Surgical repair of fractures is fraught with difficulty, including bleeding, hypercalcemia caused by immobilization, and poor healing. The surgical aspects of therapy are discussed below.[11]

Other rheumatic manifestations assocaited with Paget's disease have been

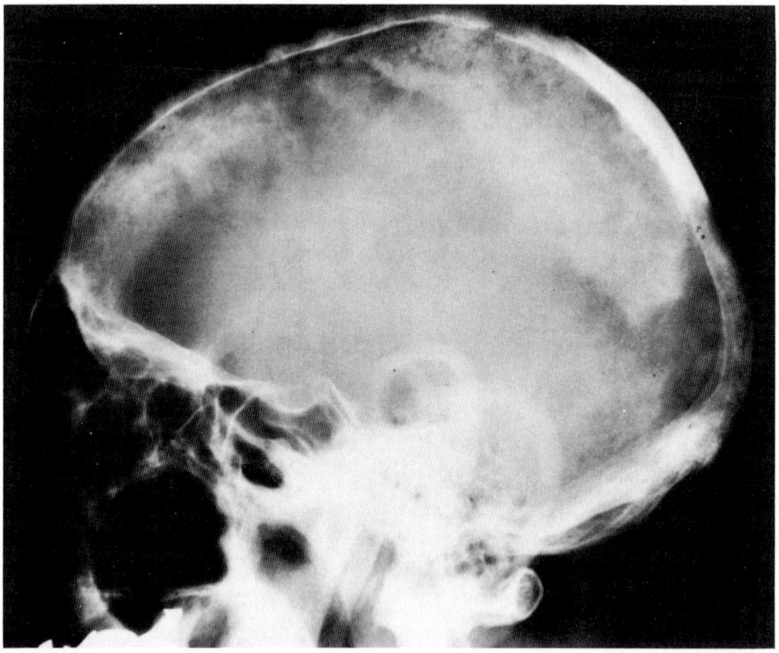

Fig. 6-2. Paget's disease presenting with osteoporosis circumscripta of the skull. In areas of previously resorbed bone, new sclerotic bone is visable. (Courtesy of Dr. Frederick J. Singer.)

also described by Franck.[12] There is an increased frequency of hyperuricemia and gouty arthritis, with the serum uric acid level correlating with the extent of the pagetic involvement. Rheumatoid arthritis and ankylosing spondylitis may also be seen in increased incidence, as well as calcific periarthritis.

Increased blood flow to affected extremities can cause other local signs and symptoms. It is surprising that most of the increased cardiac output appears to be flowing through dilated skin vasculature; warm skin localized over an involved bony area is a hallmark of this disease. A study examining extremity blood flow using patients as their own controls (one pagetic limb compared with a normal limb) showed a nearly sixfold increase in blood flow to the affected limb. This increased flow was largely attributable to cutaneous vasodilation, with only a modest increase in flow to the affected bone itself.[13] These results suggest that the underlying bone exerts reflex neural control of adjacent blood flow. As the bone lesion improves with therapy, the blood flow to the limb returns to normal. It is rare to see Paget's disease causing high-output cardiac failure, but it does occur. If more than 15 percent of bone is involved, cardiomegaly with disturbed ventricular performance may be seen.[14]

Malignant degeneration is a serious complication of Paget's disease and occurs in approximately 1 percent of symptomatic patients. The most common tumors are sarcomas, including osteogenic sarcoma, fibrosarcoma, osteoclastic sarcoma, giant cell histiocytoma, and chondrosarcoma.[7] These tumors are highly malignant, presenting with rapidly worsening pain and soft tissue masses. It is unclear how a disease predominantly affecting osteoclasts goes on to cause abnormal proliferation of bone cells that have a mesenchymal rather than monocytic origin. It may be that a longstanding disturbance in the local immune system allows this dedifferentiation. Another lesion that is associated with Paget's disease is the benign giant cell reparative granuloma that generally arises in the skull or jaw and invades locally but does not metastasize. This lesion is treated by dissection or irradiation, with a good prognosis.[15]

The extent of Paget's disease is best monitored by biochemical parameters, which reflect bone turnover. Since bone formation is tightly coupled to bone resorption, the pagetic resorption is immediately followed by osteoblastic activation and subsequent new bone formation. Markers of both resorption and formation rise in Paget's disease. Aklaline phosphatase is released by osteoblasts laying down new bone and nearly 40 percent of the enzyme in serum is normally derived from bone. This fraction rises during pagetic activity. Serum alkaline phosphatase levels can remain high during healing of a treated pagetic lesion, reflecting the continued osteoblastic activity. Urinary hydroxyproline excretion is the best way of assessing osteoclastic bone resorption. Hydroxyproline is released from collagen broken down during periods of osteoclastic activity, as well as from breakdown of dermal collagen, and is excreted by the kidney. The fraction of hydroxyproline that originates from bone is difficult to determine; yet there is evidence that this fraction rises during bone resorption and follows the "activity" of Paget's disease.[16] This measurement, albeit helpful, is difficult to perform and requires a 24 hour urine collection. For general assessment of pagetic activity, the alkaline phosphatase level mirrors the urinary hydroxyproline level closely enough to be a reliable marker of disease. Interest has arisen recently in the measurement of serum levels of bone gamma-carboxyglutamate-containing protein (bone gla protein or osteocalcin) as a marker of bone turnover. Serum levels are frequently elevated in states where the bone is metabolically active. Levels of this bone matrix protein, a specific product of the osteoblast, frequently rise prior to the elevation of serum alkaline phosphatase leves in primary hyperparathyroidism. In Paget's disease, however, bone gla protein elevation may be much less striking than that of alkaline phosphatase, suggesting that an abnormality in secretion of this protein might exist. During the first 10 days of treatment with bisphophonate the levels of bone gla protein increase, even while hydroxyproline and alkaline phosphatase levels are falling.[18] The reason for this increase is unknown.

Despite the rapid efflux and influx of calcium and phosphate into the metabolically active bone of Paget's disease the levels of these minerals in blood are normal reflecting a tight coupling of bone breakdown and bone formation. The equilibrium can, however, be disturbed by abrupt decreases in either resorption or formation. Immobilization due to fracture or other causes results in hypercalcemia.[16] The stress of weight bearing exerts a positive influence on osteoblastic activity and bone formation; once this trophic effect is removed the resorption–formation coupling must dynamically reset itself. During immobilization, pagetic resorption continues to proceed but formation is slowed, resulting in hypercalcemia. Hyperparathyroidism represents an alternative cause of the infrequent hypercalcemia in active Paget's disease. There is histologic evidence that elevated parathyroid hormone (PTH) levels, caused by a subclinical negative calcium balance,[18] have an effect on the uninvolved skeleton. Hypercalcemia can also occur during the initiation of therapy for Paget's disease because initially the bone calcium accretion rate continues unchanged, and this can transiently elevate PTH and 1,25 dihydroxyvitamin D levels.[19]

After the clinical history is obtained and biochemical parameters measured, the assessment of Paget's disease is greatly aided by radiographs of the skeleton. Radiologic changes consist of lytic lesions and sclerotic changes, frequently appearing concurrently. The lytic change is the earliest detectable. In the long bones this lesion appears as a V-shaped resorption front that advances distally at a rate of about 1 cm per year (Fig. 6-3). The osteoblastic phase of Paget's appears as enlarged bone with loss of the corticomedullary junction. The femur or tibia may be bowed and frequently small fractures are observed: these may be pseudofractures caused by dilated perforating arteries or may be true fissure fractures. The skull radiograph shows osteoporosis circumscripta during the lytic phase of the disease, with later thickening of the calvarium (Fig. 6-2). Sclerotic lesions on radiographs are frequently asymptomatic, and if they do not take up increased amounts of technetium bisphosphonate will almost certainly cause no clinical complaints.[20]

The bone scan has been widely used to assess the extent of bone involvement. Technetium diphosphate bone scans can be very helpful, especially in mono-ostotic disease when the diagnosis of Paget's disease is suspected but biochemical parameters are normal.[21] Since technetium bisphosphonate binds

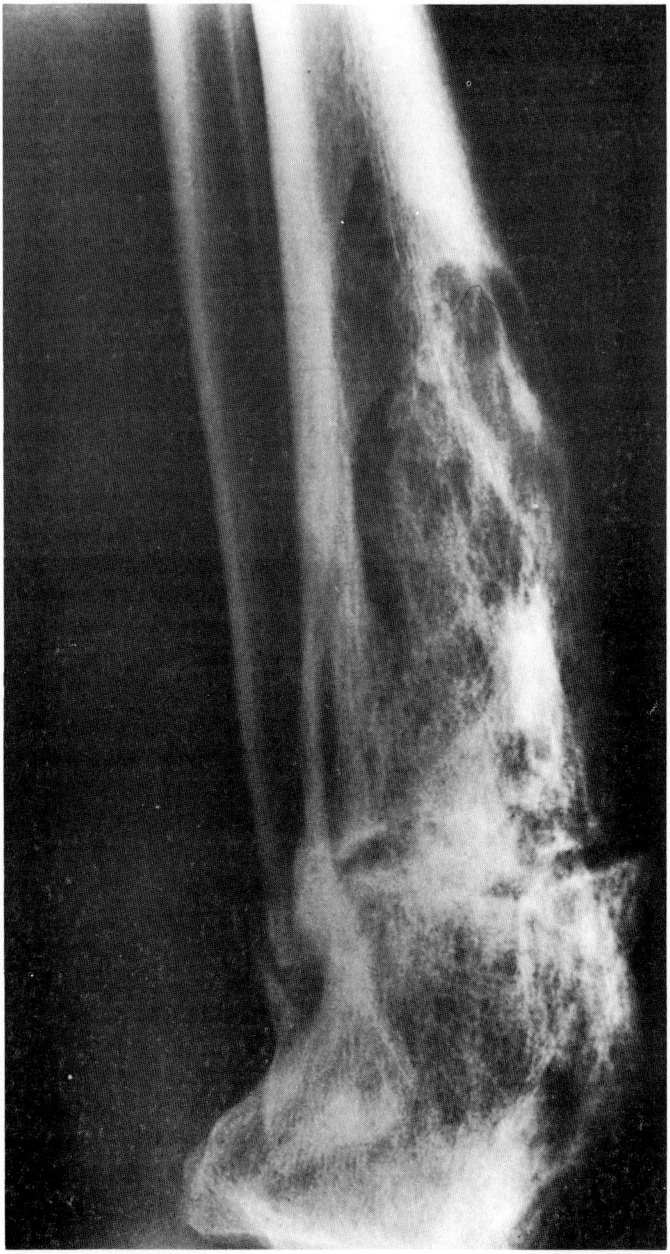

Fig. 6-3 Paget's disease extending distally in a tibial shaft. The primary resorption front is visable as a V-shaped decrease in bone density followed by a secondary expanding front with remodeling. There is also a healed pathologic fracture. (Courtesy of Dr. Frederick J. Singer.)

to actively forming bone increased uptake can represent either active disease or bone in the healing phase. A "positive" bone scan can appear similar to scans seen with the skeletal metastases of prostate cancer, and this diagnosis must be carefully ruled out. It spite of its value in the initial assessment of pagetic skeletal involvement, the bone scan has not been very helpful as a marker of response to therapy since the healing lesion will also scan "positively." Gallium bone scanning has been attempted as a better measure of response of the disease to therapy since the concentration of gallium in tissue depends on cellular activity. Decreased bone uptake of gallium might reflect an attenuation of pagetic activity. In one study gallium scanning correlated more closely with symptomatic improvement than did the diphosphonate bone scan.[22]

The histologic diagnosis of Paget's disease is made by bone biopsy, but this is more frequently used as an investigative tool. Under light microscopy, a single bone biopsy may show all phases of the pagetic lesion from the increased osteoclast numbers and resorptive activity to the woven bone surrounding marrow replaced by fat cells.[3] The characteristic microfilamentous inclusions seen in the osteoclasts by electron microscopy do not disappear with therapy of the disease.

CALCITONIN THERAPY

Exciting advances have developed in the therapy of this disease. Two types of agents effective in suppressing osteoclastic activity are available: calcitonins and bisphosphonates. The use of these agents has led to a better understanding of pathophysiology, as well as hope for symptomatic control of debilitating disease.

Salmon calcitonin is a 32-amino-acid peptide with effects on bone osteoclasts and kidney. Its effects on the osteoclast appear to be of major therapeutic importance in Paget's disease. Calcitonin has an acute effect on cultured human osteoclasts to decrease their activity and adherence.[23] A slower and more prolonged effect, when calcitonin is administered chronically, is a progressive decrease in osteoclast numbers. This action may occur at the level of the precursor cells to slow their fusion into osteoclasts.[24] The peptide also pharmacologically increases calcium and sodium excretion by the kidney, and its calcium-lowering effect results in enhanced production of $1,25(OH)_2D$, presumably mediated by PTH.[25]

Calcitonin has become a cornerstone in the treatment of Paget's disease. Its effects on bone are potent and purely antiosteolytic while its side effects are minimal. A single subcutaneous injection of either human calcitonin (0.5 mg) or salmon calcitonin (50 to 100 units) decreases serum calcium as much as 2.5 mg/dl in Paget's patients. In addition, it decreases acutely the urine hydroxyproline excretion.[25] In fact, within 30 minutes of injection osteoclasts are observed to detach from trabeculae and lose their ruffled borders.[23] Osteoblasts continue to use calcium from the blood for bone apposition: the serum calcium level thus acutely decreases until a new mechanism brings the exchangeable calcium pool back to equilibrium via the actions of PTH and 1,25$(OH)_2$D. Continuing calcitonin as a daily injection causes further decrease of hydroxyproline excretion and a decrease in alkaline phosphatase to about 50 percent of the pretreatment values. The nadir is reached at several months and an increase in dosage will have no further effect. Long-term treatment with daily subcutaneous injections of calcitonin has been shown to relieve bone pain, improve neurologic impairment including stabilization of hearing loss, and reverse increases in cardiac output. Most importantly, during calcitonin therapy lytic lesions of bone improve by radiologic and histologic examination.[25] A randomized study with a no-treatment group and a group receiving 50 units day of calcitonin showed a 50 percent decrease in alkaline phosphatase as well as an increase in bone mineral content measured by radial photon absorption in the calcitonin-treated group after 3 years. The favorable biochemical changes in the treated group compared with a decrease of alkaline phosphatase of only 8 percent in the untreated group and a progressive decrease of bone mineral content.[26] Side effects of calcitonin include flushing, nausea, polyuria, and a metallic taste sensation. These, however, can be minimized by starting with no more than 0.25 mg of human or 25 units of salmon calcitonin per day until the adverse symptoms subside. For lytic disease 0.5 mg of human or 50 to 100 U of salmon calcitonin administered at bedtime are recommended each day, and for bone pain without lytic disease, 0.5 mg of human calcitonin or 50 U of salmon calcitonin three times a week will generally give gratifying clinical results.

Salmon calcitonin, while 30 to 50 times more potent than the human hormone, results in antibody formation in nearly two-thirds of patients. Resistance, frequently on the basis of antibody production, is seen in 5 to 40 percent of patients. In a 1980 study, 26 percent of patients showed a return to their initial high alkaline phosphatase values at 1 year, and of these patients nearly all had neutralizing antibodies that were shown to inhibit the effects of calcitonin in a bioassay.[25] Because of the problem with immunologic resistance human calcitonin has significant advantages over salmon calcitonin. Human calcitonin, used at 0.5 mg subcutaneously provides 50 to 100 units of action, and should not cause antibody formation. In one study human calcitonin was shown to be efficacious in a majority of patients who had previously demonstrated resistance to salmon calcitonin and etidronate (5gm/kg/day) (Fig. 6-4).[27] The cost is comparable to salmon calcitonin. Other routes of administration of calcitonin are currently being investigated in an attempt to eliminate the need for subcutaneous administration. Intranasal calcitonin spray and rectal administration both require high daily doses (200 to 400 units) but have been able to improve the pagetic bone lesion.[28]

The improvement seen in Paget's patients in terms of clinical and biochemical parameters remains stable in most patients while calcitonin is continued. Calcitonin is particularly efficacious during the acute phase of the disease to cause healing of resorptive lesions, improvement of nerve impingment syndromes, and to relieve debilitating pagetic pain quickly. Calcitonin is also useful for treating the hypercalcemia that may occur with immobilization in these patients. Finally, calcitonin is a useful agent in preparing the patient's bone for

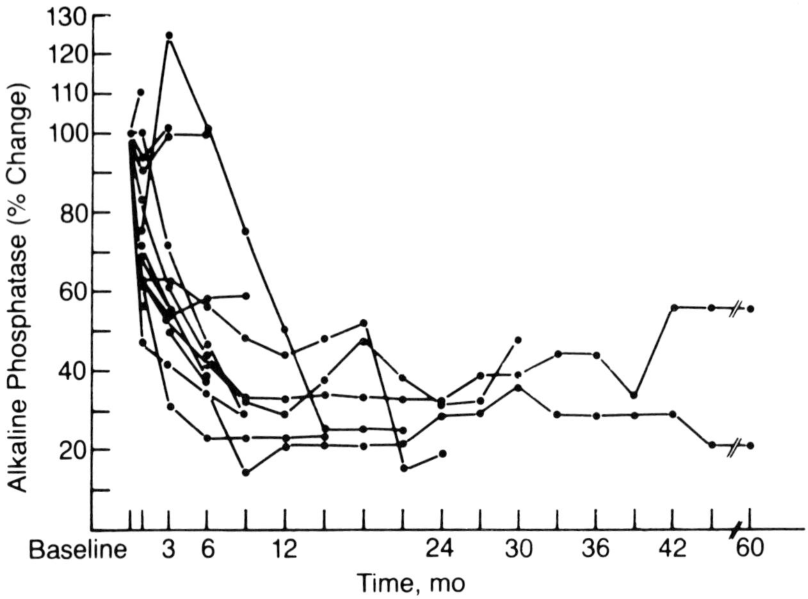

Fig. 6-4 Human calcitonin is efficacious in controlling Paget's disease refractory to other treatment. Eleven patients who had demonstrated resistance to salmon calcitonin as well as to EHDP (5mg/kg/d) were treated with human calcitonin, 0.5 mg/day. Along with clinical improvement a fall in serum alkaline phosphatase was seen; it leveled out at five times normal. (From Altman et al., [27] with permission.)

surgery—for instance, mechanical fixation of nonhealing pagetic fractures or total hip replacement. Calcitonin decreases the likelihood of intraoperative bleeding, postoperative hypercalcemia, and nonunion.[11] However, despite clinical responses during calcitonin use, if the drug is stopped the disease will return to its pretreatment level of activity in most cases within 3 to 9 months. Moreover, previously healed lesions may again become lytic. The lack of sustained remission after discontinuing calcitonin necessitates the chronic use of this agent, or, substitution with a biphosphonate after a patient has reached the plateau phase of treatment with calcitonin, and bone healing has occurred.

BISPHOSPHONATE THERAPY

Bisphosphonates developed over the last 15 years now offer a new era of therapy in the treatment of Paget's disease. At least four drugs of this class are being tested, but only one is in clinical use in North America. The chemical structure of the bisphosphonates derives from that of inorganic pyrophosphate, an inhibitor of calcium phosphate crystalization with affinity for hydroxyapatite. Replacement of the central oxygen atom by carbon makes the compounds biologically unhydrolyzable (Fig. 6-5).

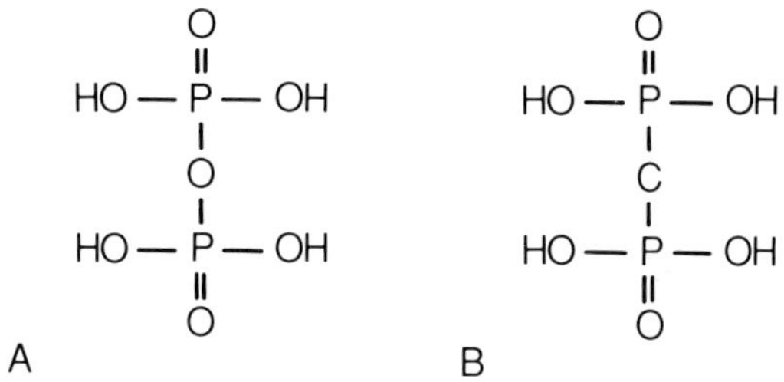

Fig. 6-5 (**A**) Inorganic pyrophosphate. (**B**) Bisphosphonic acid.

When pyrophosphate is given to animals subcutaneously, the formation, aggregation, and dissolution of bone hydroxyapatite are diminished.[16] Bisphosphonate substitution allows these compounds to be given orally without hydrolysis, while continuing to inhibit ectopic calcification and bone resorption. It appears, however, that the mode of action of bisphosphonate, is not via an extracellular inhibition of bone mineral dissolution, but through a cellular action.

The basic P–C–P structure of bisphosphonate allows for variations in the side chains that modulate biologic activity (Fig. 6-6). 1-Hydroxy ethylidene-1,1-bisphosphonate (disodium etidronate or EHDP) has been approved for use in the U.S. since 1977. 3-Amino-1-hydroxypropylidine-1,1-bisphosphonate (APD) appear to be the most promising clinically, and dicloromethylidine bis-

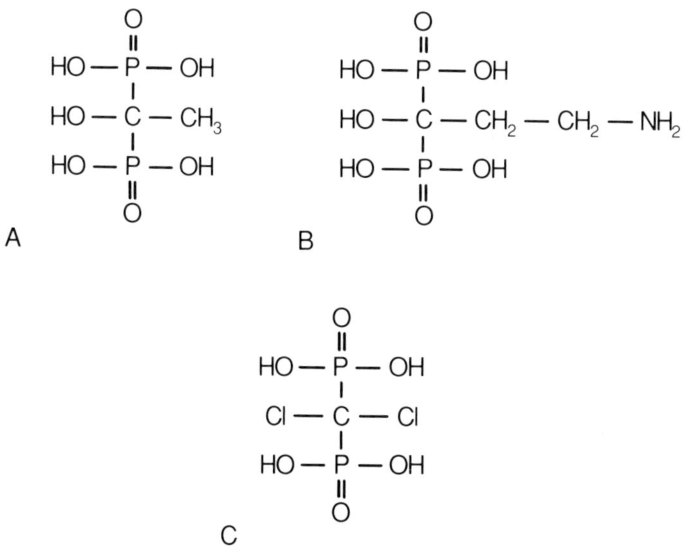

Fig. 6-6 (**A**) 1-Hydroyethylidene-1, 1-bisphosphonic acid (EHDP, etidronate). (**B**) 3-amino-1-hydroxypropylidine-1, 1-bisphosphonate (APD). (**C**) Dichloromethylidene bisphosphonate (Cl_2MDP)

phosphonate (Cl_2MDP) is also being used in Europe. All three of these compounds inhibit the precipitation of calcium–phosphate from solution and inhibit aggregation and dissolution of hydroxyapetite crystals. They are effective in preventing soft tissue calcification.[29] One might then infer that mineralization of bone would also be impaired, and this is, indeed, a problem with the less potent disodium etidronate. Cl_2MDP and ADP are effective inhibitors of bone resorption without impairing mineralization.

The inhibitory effect of the bisphosphonates on bone resorption in vivo appears to derive from direct cellular effects separate from their mineral-binding properties. In fact, there is no correlation between the ability of bisphosphonates to inhibit crystallization and to inhibit bone resorption in vivo. Bisphosphonate-induced inhibition of bone resorption may derive from several effects of the drug. It is clear that osteoclasts cannot successfully resorb bone covered with P–C–P. In addition there appears to be a direct effect of the bisphosphonate on the osteoclast itself, causing alteration of the morphology and function of these cells in vitro. Bone resorption due to other causes including hyperparathyroidism, malignant hypercalemia, and experimental retinoid therapy is also inhibited by these drugs.[29]

Low doses of bisphosphonate cause only inhibition of bone resorption by osteoclasts. Higher doses cause decreased longitudinal bone growth as well as inhibition of mineralization. The rate of new bone apposition by osteoblasts initially continues unchanged, taking 3 weeks to decelerate in rats, and 3 to 5 months in humans.[30] This sequence of events correlates with change in biochemical parameters. The urine hydroxyproline excretion drops off precipitously during the first 10 days, and the curve then becomes more shallow (see Fig. 6-7). Alkaline phosphatase levels fall at a slower rate until about 4 months, when the decline of the two parameters is parallel.

The differential effect of the bisphosphonates on resorption and formation parameters may be related to the biology of the corresponding cell types. The osteoclast is a short-lived cell, with a population half life of 2.5 to 10 days, while the half life of the osteoblast population may be about 50 days.[31] The biphosphonate initially halts the activity of existing osteoclasts; this action is responsible for the early phase of rapid fall off in urinary hydroxyproline. Osteoblasts that were initially active will continue to live out their normal life span, but will not be replaced by as many newly differentiated cells because the coupling signals arising from bone resorption are diminished by the bisphosphonate inhibition. The slow decline in osteoblastic activity is then responsible for the steady fall off of alkaline phosphatase values. The secondary kinetics of hydroxyproline decline (Fig. 6-7) probably reflects another action of diphosphonates on the osteoclast; that is, a decrease in further differentiation, fusion, or activation of osteoclast precursors. If the bisphosphonate therapy is stopped before the alkaline phosphatase begins to normalize, there is still a subsequent fall in alkaline phosphatase. As in the case of calcitonin, this dissociation between bone formation and resorption in favor of formation results in transient hypocalcemia and the observed compensatory rise in $1,25(OH)_2D$ and parathyroid hormone.

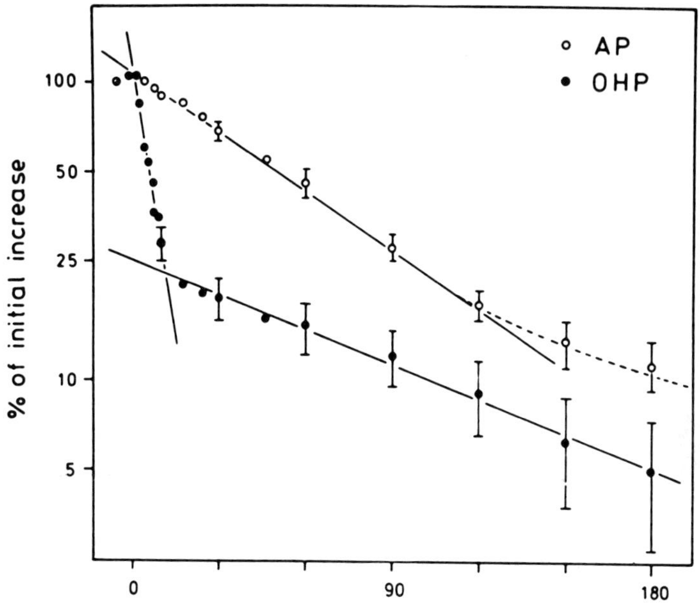

Fig. 6-7 Reductions in mean percentage of initial increase (+/−SE) of alkaline phosphatase (open circles) and urinary hydroxyproline (closed circles). Results pertain to 51 patients without prior bisphosphonate therapy treated for at least 6 months with 600 mg/day oral aminobisphosphonate. (From Harink et al.,[31] with permission.)

Initial therapy with APD causes a transient 2 to 5 day increase in body temperature, a decrease in zinc levels, an increase in acute phase reactants, and a decrease in peripheral lymphocyte counts. These all reflect activation of inflammatory mechanisms. In vitro, APD applied to cultures of human mononuclear cells causes a decrease in the number of esterase-positive (i.e., macrophage–like) cells. APD also decreases the lymphocyte proliferative response caused by mitogens.[30] Bijvoet theorized that APD might somehow reequilibrate the local immune system via these positive and negative controls, such that some abnormal pagetic immune stimulus to osteoclast activation is turned off. An exact correlation of the mechanism of APD's therapeutic effect with its ability to modulate cells of the immune system has not yet been achieved.

Experience with the clinical application of bisphosphonate therapy has been very rewarding. Disodium etidronate at 5 to 7.5 mg/kg/day decreases urinary hydroxyproline and serum alkaline phosphatase levels at 6 months in 60% of patients.[32] The intestinal absorption of bisphosphonates is both quite poor and variable (about 5 percent of the ingested dose). Failure of absorption may account for some treatment failures. Increasing the dose appears to suppress the disease overwhelmingly but higher doses of disodium etidronate do result in osteomalacia. Of those patients showing an initial response, up to 40 percent may have prolonged clinical and chemical improvement in spite of stopping treatment after one 6-month course. These individuals are usually those with initially less active disease. Forty-five percent of responders in a large study required retreatment at the end of a year, and 15 percent developed resistance to the 5 mg/kg/day dose.[32] In this author's experience with nearly 100 pagetic patients, if the initial alkaline phosphatase level was greater than 10 times normal, resistance was more likely to occur, and if the alkaline phosphatase was four times normal after 4 years of therapy, resistance had developed.

Higher doses of disodium etidronate are associated with less relapse after initial dosing. The ability to give very high doses over a short period should also theoretically reduce the osteomalacia caused by long-term inhibition of mineralization. Meunier has shown that all patients treated with 4.3 mg/kg/day intravenously for 10 days without a continuing maintenance dose exhibited reduction in biochemical parameters but a return to pretreatment levels at 90 days. Following the intravenous therapy with low-dose oral disodium etidronate resulted in a sustained remission.[33] Disodium etidronate given orally at 20 mg/kg/day for 1 month also caused significantly more improvement than treatment with 5 mg/kg/day orally for 6 months.[34] The trend in clinical research appears to be turning toward use of disodium etidronate at higher doses for shorter time periods. However, intravenous etidronate is not yet approved by the FDA for treatment of Paget's disease. A proviso is necessary in the use of EHDP. Because of etidronate's inhibition of mineralization, if it is administered daily for 6 months, a 2 to 3 month drug-free period is required for prevention of osteomalacia. Even with the use of only 5 mg/kg/day with this precaution, this complication may still (rarely) occur, and it is characterized by diffuse bone pain and a rise in alkaline phosphatase levels.

In contrast to etidronate, APD has no inhibitory effect on bone mineralization. Administered intravenously, it is approximately 20 times more potent than etidronate. In patients treated with APD (10 days of either 600 mg/day orally or up to 30 mg/day intravenously which was followed by oral APD if the urinary hydroxyproline had not normalized) 90 percent demonstrated normalization of biochemical parameters by one year.[31] The drug was discontinued at this point with resultant in sustained biochemical remission in 50 percent of patients at 2 years. This group also found that treatment failures on "low-dose" oral regimens routinely responded to high-dose intravenous therapy. Along with the improvement in biochemical parameters the radiologic progression of disease is halted with APD therapy, and at least half of patients show clear improvement in their lesions without osteomalacia. Bone histomorphometry also shows improvement, even at 10 days.

Cl_2MDP is only slightly more potent than etidronate, but like APD does not cause osteomalacia. Five days of 300 mg/day intravenous therapy caused a striking reduction in biochemical parameters that was sustained for at least 6 months. This was equivalent to the result obtained by dosing with 1.6 g Cl_2MDP orally for 6 months.[35]

The use of the bisphosphonates along with calcitonin is possible. A study of sequential 6 month courses of etidronate at 7.5 mg/kg/day and 0.5 mg human calcitonin/day showed interesting results.[36] Patients treated with 6 months of calcitonin and switched to EHDP showed continued reduction to 64 percent of initial alkaline phosphatase values. Those who were on EHDP at 5 mg/kg/day had a decrease in alkaline phosphatase levels to 54 percent of initial alkaline phosphatase values at 6 months. They were then switched to calcitonin, on which treatment they had a further decrease in this biochemical parameter (36 percent). This study implies that EHDP is not as effective following calcitonin therapy as it is alone. However, we have had experience with individual patients who obtained dramatic further reduction in disability from addition of etidronate to calcitonin after the latter had achieved maximal therapeutic benefit.

PLICAMYCIN (MITHRAMYCIN) THERAPY

In the past, this cytotoxic agent was used to treat severe Paget's disease that was unresponsive to other agents. When given to hypercalcemic patients intravenously it rapidly causes a decrease in calcium secondary to its inhibition of bone turnover. Prolonged symptomatic relief has been associated with an initial dosing schedule of 10 to 25 μg/kg each day for 10 days, followed by the same dose once weekly.[19] Histologic improvement of affected bone also results. The side effects of plicamycin can be serious, including bone marrow suppression, and hepatic and renal toxicity. With the advent of human calcitonin and the newer bisphosphonates, it should rarely be necessary to use plicamycin as a second-line therapy. Patients refractory to calcitonin and etidronate should be referred to a center having experience with these other agents.

NONSTEROIDAL ANTI-INFLAMMATORY DRUGS

The nonsteroidal anti-inflammatory drugs are still very useful in the treatment of patients with Paget's disease. As we have noted earlier, much of the pain in patients with Paget's is osteoarthritic in nature, and a smaller percentage is due to rheumatic disease such as hyperuricemia, gouty arthritis, rheumatoid arthritis, and calcific periarthritis.[12] It is important to diagnose the cause of the presenting pain syndrome. If it appears more arthritic in nature, (i.e., referable to the joint), a nonsteroidal agent such as ibuprofen or indomethacin may serve as the first-line drug. Active Paget's disease occurring in the bone adjacent to the affected joint will have to be concurrently evaluated, of course, but can be considered as a separate problem even though as it may be the likely cause of the accelerated joint degeneration.

SURGERY

Certain conditions arise in Paget's disease that are best treated by surgery. Fracture of involved long bones, especially the femur and tibia, frequently requires surgical repair, and may occur with only minor trauma. The tendency toward nonunion, as well as the brittle quality of the bone make surgical repair difficult, and require an experienced orthopedic surgeon. Bowing of the tibia may require osteotomy to relieve pain. Hip or knee replacement can be required to relieve pain and increase mobility when the joint is severely degenerated.

Neurosurgical consultation must be obtained when there is a suspicion that platybasia of the skull is causing a foramen magnum syndrome or hydrocephalus that may require occipital decompression. Laminectomy is indicated for spinal stenosis with cord compression.

Pretreatment of the patient, when possible, with 2 to 3 months of calcitonin therapy should increase the likelihood of a good surgical result, both perioperatively with respect to bleeding and long-term healing. The surgeon must also carefully assess the unusual strains and fracture patterns in the abnormal bone, and take these into consideration when planning surgery.

SUMMARY

Our understanding of the pathogenesis and treatment of Paget's disease of bone has been greatly advanced in the last 15 years. This is a primary disease of the osteoclast causing excessive resorptive activity. The initial lesion in this disease may be infection of the osteoclast or its progenitors with a paramyxovirus whose paracrystalline structure can be visualized in pagetic osteoclasts. Familial aggregation suggests that the hypothesized initial infection could occur early in life, after which small numbers of the putative virion may lie in a latent state until as yet unknown age-related factors allow its proliferation.

The clinical presentation is almost always bone pain, often associated with deformity. Levels of serum alkaline phosphatase and urinary hydroxyproline excretion are elevated and, along with bone scanning for areas of increased technetium diphosphonate deposition, provide simple clinical tools for following disease activity.

Treatment of the clinical syndrome involves first evaluating the arthritic component of the pain and treating this with nonsteroidal anti-inflammatory agents. The pagetic lesion itself is best treated with the osteoclast-inhibiting hormone calcitonin when the disease is in a lytic phase or there are fractures. Nonlytic Paget's disease can be treated with the bisphosphonate disodium etidronate, and a sustained improvement in disease activity can be expected in most cases, although true remissions of the disease are still rare. Second-generation bisphosphonates show promise for safer and even more effective control.

REFERENCES

1. Paget J: On a form of chronic inflammation of bones. Med Chir Trans 60:27, 1877
2. Collins D: Paget's disease of bone—incidence and subclinical forms. Lancet 2:51, 1956

3. Singer F: Paget's disease. p.1483. In Felig P(ed): Endocrinology and Metabolism. McGraw-Hill, New York, 1987
4. Rebel A, Basle M, Pouplard A, et al: Viral antigens in osteoclasts from Paget's disease of bone. Lancet 1:344, 1980
5. Owen M: The origin of bone cells in the postnatal organism. Arthritis Rheum 23:1073, 1980
6. Mills B, Singer F: Nuclear inclusions in Paget's disease of bone. Science 194:201, 1976
7. Mirra J: Case records of MGH. N Engl J Med 314:105, 1986
8. Mills B, Holst P, Stabile E, et al: A viral antigen bearing cell line derived from culture of Paget's bone cells. Bone 6:257, 1985
9. Woodhouse N: Paget's disease. Clin Rheum Dis 7:647, 1981
10. Altman R: Musculoskeletal manifestations of Paget's disease of bone. Arthritis Rheum 23:1121, 1980
11. Meyers M, Singer F: Osteotomy for tibia vara in Paget's disease under cover of calcitonin. J Bone Joint Surg [Am] 60:810 (1978)
12. Franck W, Bress N, Singer F, Krane S: Rheumatic manifestations of Paget's disease of bone. Am J Med 56:592, 1974
13. Heistad D, Abbovd F, Schmid P, et al: Regulation of blood flow in Paget's disease of bone. J Clin Invest 55:69, 1975
14. Arnalich F, Plaza I, Sobrino J, et al: Cardiac size and function in Paget's disease of bone. Int J Cardiol 5:491, 1984
15. Upchurch K, Simon L, Schiller A, et al: Giant cell reparative granuloma of Paget's disease of bone: a unique clinical entity. Ann Intern Med 98:35, 1983
16. Krane S: Skeletal manifestations of Paget's disease of bone. Arthritis Rheum 23:1087, 1980
17. Papapoulous SE, Frolich M, Mudde A, et al: Serum osteocalcin in Paget's disease of bone. J Clin Endocrinol Metab 65:89, 1987
18. Posen S, Clifton-Bligh P, Wilkinson M: Paget's disease of bone and hyperparathyroidism: coincidence or causal relationship? Calcif Tissue Res 26:107, 1978
19. Kanis J, Gary R: Long term followup observations on treatment in Paget's disease of bone. Clin Orthop Rel Res 217:99, 1987
20. Khairi M, Wellman H, Robb J, Johnston C: Paget's disease of bone: symptomatic lesions and bone scan. Ann Intern Med 79:348, 1973
21. Waxman A, Ducker S, McKee D, et al: Evaluation of 99 Tc diphosphonate kinetics in patients with Paget's before and after calcitonin treatment. Radiology 125:761, 1977
22. Waxman A, McKee D, Siesen J, Singer F: Gallium scanning in Paget's disease of bone Am J Radiol 134:303, 1980
23. Singer F, Melvin K, Mills B: Acute effects of calcitonin on osteoclasts in man. Clin Endocrinol 5:333S, 1976
24. Takahashi N, Mundy G, Kuehl T, Roodman G: Osteoclast-like cell formation in fetal and newborn long-term baboon marrow cultures is more sensitive to 1,25-dihydroxyvitamin D than adult long-term marrow cultures. J Bone Mineral Res 2:311, 1987
25. Singer F, Fredericks R, Minkin C: Salmon calcitonin therapy for Paget's disease of bone. Arthritis Rheum 23:1148, 1980
26. Toh S, Claunch B, Brown P: Effect of calcitonin treatment on the natural course of bone demineralization in Paget's disease. J Clin Endocrinol Metab 56:405, 1983
27. Altman RD, Collins-Yudiskas B: Synthetic human calcitonin in refractory Paget's disease of bone. Arch Intern Med 147:1305, 1987

28. Nagant C, Deogelaer J, Huaux J, et al: New modes of administration of salmon calcitonin. Clin Orthop Rel Res 217:56, 1987
29. Fleisch H: Experimental basis for use of bisphosphonates in Paget's disease of bone. Clin Orthop Rel Res 217:72, 1987
30. Bijvoet O, Frijlink W, Jie K, et al: APD in Paget's disease of bone. Arthritis Rheum 23:1193, 1980
31. Harinck H, Bijvoet O, Blanlesma H, Dahlinghaus P: Efficacious management with APD in Paget's disease of bone. Clin Orthop Rel Res 217:79, 1987
32. Altman R: Long term followup of therapy with intermittent etidronate disodium in Paget's disease of bone. Am J Med 79:583, 1985
33. Meunier P, Chapuy M, Delmas P, et al: Intravenous disodium etidronate therapy in Paget's disease of bone and hypercalcemia of malignancy. Am J Med 82(2A):71, 1987
34. Preston C, Yates A, Beneton M, et al: Effective short term treatment of Paget's disease with oral etidronate. Br Med J 292:79, 1986
35. Yates A, Gary R, Urwin G, et al: intravenous clodronate in the treatment and retreatment of Paget's disease of bone. Lancet 1:1471, 1985
36. Perry H, Drake D, Avioli L: Alternate calcitonin and etidronate disodium therapy for Paget's disease of bone. Arch Intern Med 144:929, 1984

7 Osteoporosis

Elizabeth Shane

Osteoporosis describes a group of skeletal disorders characterized by a reduction in bone mass per unit volume with a normal ratio of mineralized to unmineralized bone. Histologically, the bone cortices are thinned and porous and the trabeculae are reduced in number and in size[1] (Fig. 7-1). The clinical importance of osteoporosis relates to the increased risk of fracture in patients. Fractures are the culmination of a long period of asymptomatic bone loss and have devastating potential in terms of morbidity, mortality, and cost of health care.

Primary osteoporosis includes those forms of the disorder in which the cause is unknown, the most common forms of which are postmenopausal and senile. Secondary osteoporosis is due to a known cause such as certain drugs, endocrine, genetic, or other diseases (Table 7-1). The bone loss resulting from the secondary osteoporoses is superimposed upon the age-related bone loss that occurs in all individuals and the postmenopausal bone loss that occurs in all estrogen-deficient women. This classification provides a useful framework for recalling the multiple illnesses of which osteoporosis may be a presenting or complicating feature.

PRIMARY OSTEOPOROSIS

Epidemiology

Osteoporosis is now recognized as a public health problem of major proportions. Postmenopausal women are most frequently affected although men also lose bone mass with advancing age[2] (Fig. 7-2). At least 1.2 million fractures occur in the United States alone each year.[2] The most common fracture is the vertebral fracture, accounting for approximately 538,000 cases yearly, with a

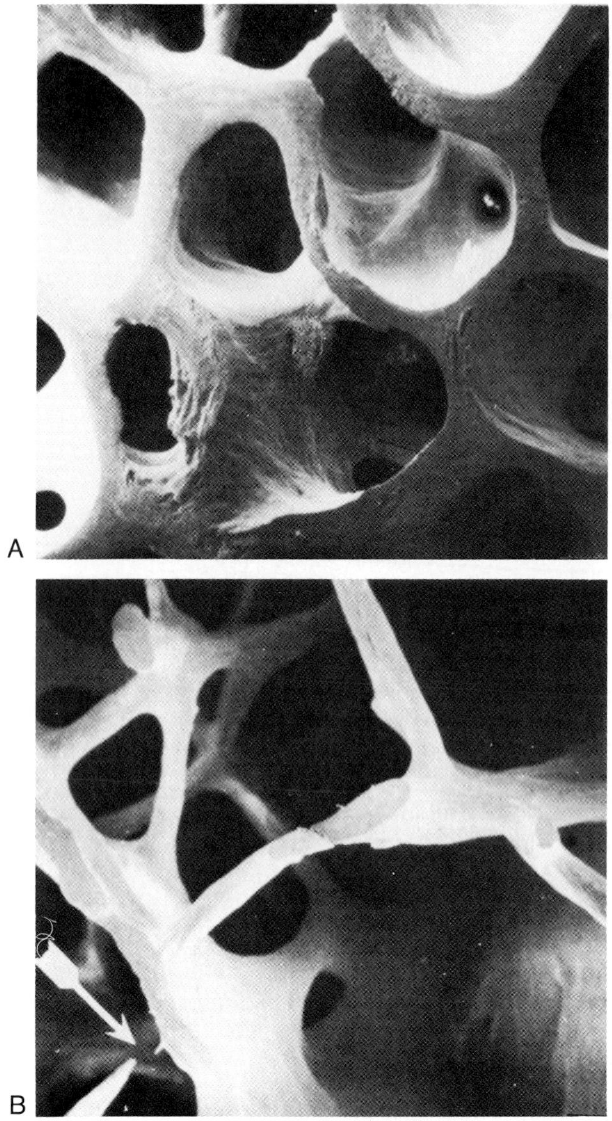

Fig. 7-1 Low-power scanning electron micrograph of iliac crest biopsies from a 44-year-old normal male (**A**) and a 47-year-old osteoporotic female (**B**) with multiple vertebral compression fractures. (From Dempster, et al,[1] with permission.)

female to male ratio of 10:1. It has been estimated that one-third of women over 65 will sustain a vertebral fracture.[2] About 210,000 hip fractures occur annually in the United States, over half in individuals over 65 years of age.[3,4] Women who suffer a hip fracture have a 12 to 20 percent excess mortality rate within the first year after the fracture.[4] Hip fractures are estimated to cost $7.2

Table 7-1. Classification of Osteoporoses

Primary (idiopathic) osteoporoses		
	Postmenopausal osteoporosis (type I)	
	Age-related or senile osteoporosis (type II)	
	Juvenile osteoporosis	
	Young adults	
	Male osteoporosis	
	Regional osteoporosis	
		Reflex sympathetic dystrophy
		Transient osteoporosis of the hip
		Regional migratory osteoporosis
Secondary osteoporoses		
	Congenital or inherited forms	
		Osteogenesis imperfecta
		Chromosome abnormalities
		Ehlers-Danlos syndrome
		Menke's syndrome
		Marfan's syndrome
		Homocystinuria
		Thalassemia
		Sickle cell anemia
		Glycogen storage diseases
		Hypophosphatasia
		Familial dysautonomia (Riley-Day syndrome)
	Endocrine Causes	
		Cushing's syndrome
		Thyroid disease
		Primary hyperparathyroidism
		Acromegaly
		Hypogonadism
		Hyperprolactinemia
		Diabetes mellitus
		Pregnancy and lactation
	Neoplasms	
		Myeloma
		Monocytic leukemias
		Diffuse bone carcinomatosis
	Gastrointestinal diseases	
		Malabsorption syndromes
		Gastric surgery
		Lactase deficiency
	Liver disease	
		Primary biliary cirrhosis
	Drug-related osteoporosis	
		Corticosteroids
		ACTH
		Methotrexate
		Heparin
	Immobilization: disuse	
		Bed rest
		Paraplegia
		Spina bifida
		Space flight
	Miscellaneous	
		Rheumatoid arthritis
		Cigarette smoking
		Alcoholism
		Chronic obstructive pulmonary disease
		Malnutrition
		Amyloidosis
		Hemochromatosis

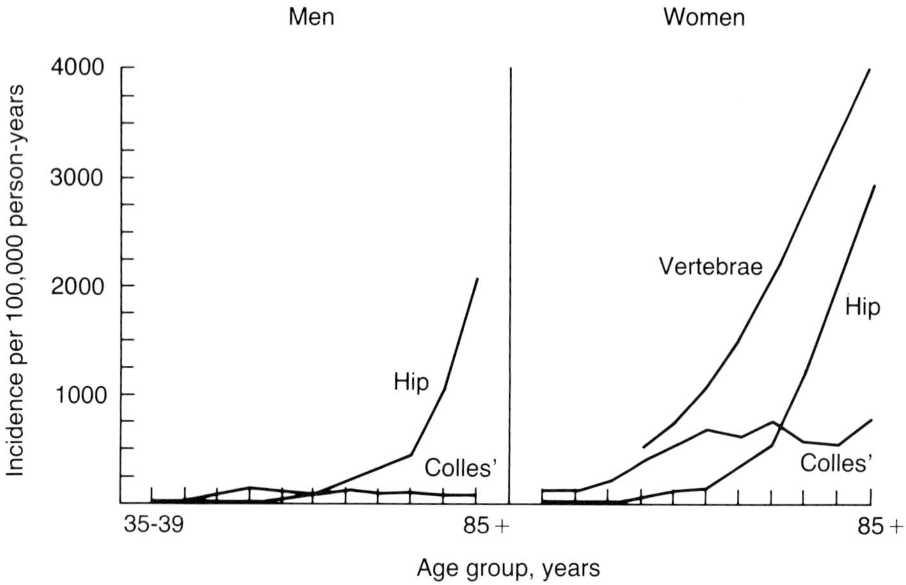

Fig. 7-2 Incidence rates for the three common osteoporotic fractures (Colles', hip, and vertebral) in men and women, plotted as a function of age at the time of the fracture. Data are from the population of Rochester, Minnesota. (From Riggs et al.,[2] with permission.)

billion a year (in 1984 dollars) in direct medical costs.[5] Fractures of wrist (Colles') and other limb sites are also very common among postmenopausal women. In the United States, the number of people over age 65 is currently 16 million and is projected to be 34 million by the year 2010.[6] Thus the toll of osteoporotic fractures, in both medical and personal costs, can be expected to increase dramatically over the coming decades.

Pathogenesis

The Concept of Peak Bone Mass

The development of osteoporosis appears to be related both to the bone mass achieved at maturity and to the rate of bone loss thereafter. Peak bone mass is reached between the ages of 20 to 35; it appears to be determined genetically[7] and to be influenced by sex, race and body habitus. Bone mass is greater in men than in women,[8] greater in blacks than in whites.[9] It correlates positively with body size. In addition, certain environmental factors, particularly dietary calcium intake[10] and physical exercise,[11-13] may also influence the development of peak bone mass.

It is becoming increasingly clear that failure to attain optimal skeletal mass during adolescence and young adulthood may contribute to the incidence of age-related fractures in later years. Thus, attention has been focused recently upon factors that enhance bone mass in the young adult. For example, calcium intake early in life may have great bearing upon adult bone mass. Although no prospective data are available on this issue, at least one retrospective study has demonstrated a positive correlation between calcium intake in youth and menopausal bone mass.[10] Exercise in the early years may also be of great importance in this regard. While no data are available regarding childhood physical activity levels, there is abundant evidence that increased weight-bearing exercise is associated with increased bone mass.[11–13] It is believed that dietary calcium intake and weight-bearing exercise may have greater influence on the achievement of peak bone mass than on prevention of bone loss later in life.

Patterns of Bone Loss

Loss of skeletal mass with aging occurs in all populations, regardless of race, sex, geographic location, or socioeconomic class.[3,4,14] The pattern of this age-related bone loss varies according to the type of bone, whether trabecular or cortical. Cortical bone is located mainly in the shafts of the long bones, whereas the vertebrae, pelvis, ribs, and ends of the long bones are composed predominantly of trabecular bone. In cortical bone there is a prolonged slow phase of bone loss that begins at about age 40 in both males and females. The initial rate of loss of 0.3 to 0.5 percent per year increases with age but declines or stops very late in life.[8,15] Superimposed upon the slow phase of cortical bone loss in women there is a more rapid phase of bone loss that begins at menopause and may achieve peak rates of 2 to 3 percent per year. The rapid rate of bone loss declines exponentially and ceases 8 to 10 years after menopause.[8,16]

The pattern of trabecular bone loss differs from that of cortical bone in several respects.[2] Both men and women begin to lose trabecular bone approximately a decade earlier than cortical bone, at age 30 to 35.[8,17–20] In women, premenopausal trabecular bone loss exceeds cortical bone loss. An accelerated phase of trabecular bone loss during the decade following menopause has been difficult to demonstrate consistently, but presumably occurs. This may reflect a problem in detection since postmenopausal trabecular bone loss may be more rapid but of shorter duration than cortical bone loss.[21]

Normal Bone Remodeling

To appreciate the contribution of various factors to the pathogenesis of age-related bone loss, an understanding of the process of bone remodeling is required. The normal adult skeleton undergoes a continous remodeling cycle in which old bone is replaced by new bone. In this sequence, bone resorption is coupled in space and in time to bone formation. According to the theory of Frost, bone remodeling occurs within packets of discrete cellular activity known as basic multicellular units (BMUs).[22,23] Osteoclasts, the bone-resorbing cells, develop from the monocyte–macrophage cell line. Osteoclasts are attracted to the specific area of bone surface to be resorbed by a signal, the precise nature of which is unknown. Once there, these giant multinucleate cells resorb a preprogrammed volume of bone (0.03 mm^3 in trabecular bone, 0.07 mm^3 in cortical bone). The osteoclasts then disappear to be replaced by osteoblasts, which lay down osteoid or unmineralized bone matrix that refills the resorption cavity. Mineralization of osteoid, which occurs next in the sequence and is also controlled by the osteoblast, completes the process. While this remodeling sequence occurs in both cortical and trabecular bone, the packets in the two types of bone differ in size and shape. The duration of the remodeling process of a given packet of bone is longer in cortical (14 weeks) than in trabecular bone (9 weeks). Of more significance clinically is the activation frequency of remodeling sites, which is greater in trabecular than cortical bone (900 sites/day versus 180 sites/day). This results in an annual turnover rate of 2 to 3 percent for cortical bone compared to 25 percent for trabecular bone. Thus, pathologic changes and responses to therapeutic maneuvers are more rapidly apparent in trabecular than in cortical bone.

In normal young adults, resorption and formation are coupled to each other and balanced so that bone mass is maintained. However, after the fourth decade, a gradual loss of skeletal mass occurs in both sexes. Such a reduction in bone mass implies that the amount of new bone tissue laid down by the osteoblast during each remodeling cycle is less than the old bone resorbed by the osteoclast.[24] It is currently not clear whether this is the result of excessive osteoclastic bone resorption, decreased formation of bone by osteoblasts, or an abnormality in the coupling mechanism such that resorption does not trigger or triggers only an inadequate formation response. It is likely that a combination of these events as well as a variety of alterations in endocrine or nutritional status may contribute to the progressive loss of bone mass that occurs with aging.

Pathogenesis of Age-Related Bone Loss

Several hypotheses have been proposed to provide a pathophysiologic basis for the loss of skeletal mass that occurs with aging. A defect in the renal production of 1,25 dihydroxyvitamin D [$1,25(OH)_2D$] with aging is the cornerstone of one major theory. This would result in malabsorption of dietary calcium, a compensatory increase in parathyroid hormone (PTH) secretion, and consequently accelerated bone resorption. An increase in the rate of activation of bone remodeling units associated with an underlying imbalance between resorption and formation could then lead to increased bone loss. This hypothesis is supported by the demonstrations of a fall in calcium absorption,[25–27] a decline in circulating $1,25(OH)_2D$ levels,[28,29] and a decrease in PTH-stimulated $1,25(OH)_2D$ formation[29–32] with aging. While only a minority of patients with clinical osteoporosis have frank elevations of PTH,[27,29,30] circulating PTH levels, as well as total and nephrogenous cyclic AMP excretion, do rise with age.[33–37]

Another theory implicates excessive calcium resorption from the skeleton and longstanding negative calcium balance as the primary causative factor in age-related osteoporosis. Careful balance studies have shown a negative calcium balance of 30 mg per day in postmenopausal women.[39] Such a deficit could lead to the gradual loss of 30 percent of skeletal mass over 30 years, sufficient to produce clinical osteoporosis. Excessive calcium resorption from the skeleton would suppress PTH secretion, resulting in diminished $1,25(OH)_2D$ synthesis, diminished calcium absorption, and further exacerbation of negative calcium balance in the aging individual. In support of this proposal, circulating PTH and $1,25(OH)_2D$ levels have been noted to be somewhat lower in osteoporotic subjects than in age-matched normal controls.[27,29,30]

There is also evidence for a decrease in osteoblast function with aging.[40] Beginning in the fourth decade, less bone is formed than resorbed at individual remodeling sites and the gap widens the age.[41] A defect in the osteoblast itself is unlikely to account for this observation since fracture healing in the elderly is not impaired. Impaired regulation of osteoblast activity by any of the hormones or local growth factors that act upon the osteoblast could explain this uncoupling phenomenon. Together, an increase in the rate of resorption and a decrease in the amount of bone deposited by the osteoblast could account for the inexorable decrease in bone mineral observed in all individuals.

Estrogen Deficiency

Estrogen deficiency, superimposed upon universal age-related bone loss, is the major cause of decreased skeletal mass in women.[42] Bone mineral density is lower in hypogonadal women regardless of its cause. At risk are women who have undergone menopause or oophorectomy at a young age,[16,21,42,43] those with primary ovarian failure or Turner's syndrome,[44] amenorrhea secondary to hyperprolactinemia[45,46] or anorexia nervosa,[47] and amenorrheic long-distance runners.[48,49] Natural menopause is also characterized by bone loss that is more rapid than that detected prior to or beyond a decade after cessation of menses.[8,16]

Fracture incidence also correlates with estrogen deficiency. In retrospective epidemiologic studies of postmenopausal women, estrogen replacement therapy is associated with a 50 percent reduction in the risk of fractures of the wrist and hip.[50–52] In addition, osteoporosis of the vertebral spine is more frequent in postmenopausal women who have not been treated with estrogens.[16,53] Moreover, a greater reduction in fracture risk is observed in women who have had therapy initiated close to the time of menopause and have been treated for longer periods.

Although all women have accelerated bone loss in the immediate postmenopausal period, it is thought that those who are the most estrogen deficient during this period have the most rapid bone loss. However, no difference in circulating estrogen concentrations has been demonstrated between women with established osteoporosis and age-matched normal women, which is perhaps not an unexpected finding considering that the measurements were made late in the course of the disease.[54–56] The relative protection from osteoporosis observed in obese women may be due to the lower levels of sex-hormone-binding globulin and consequent higher levels of free estrogens[57] as well as to the increased peripheral conversion of adrenal androgens to estrogen in adipose tissue.[58]

It is thought that estrogen withdrawal is associated with acceleration of the rate of bone remodeling, an increase in the ratio of bone resorption to bone formation, and a net loss of skeletal mass. However, the precise mechanisms by which estrogen deficiency predisposes to bone loss are unknown. Despite intensive efforts, it has not been possible for many years to demonstrate estrogen receptors in bone,[59,60] although recently two laboratories have reported preliminary evidence for their presence.[61,62] In addition, no effect of physiologic concentrations of estrogen upon osteoclast activity has been demonstrated.[63,64] This has suggested that the effect of estrogen withdrawal to increase bone resorption may be an indirect one mediated via another hormone. One theory postulates that estrogen withdrawal may lead to increased skeletal sensitivity to the actions of PTH, with a subsequent increase in bone resorption. Another possibility is that the lower calcitonin levels measured in women[65–67] may permit $1,25(OH)_2D$ and PTH to act in an unopposed fashion to stimulate excessive bone resorption. This is unlikely, however, in view of the demonstration that thyroidectomized patients with no calcitonin secretory reserve have normal bone mineral density.[68] Thus, the question of the mechanism of estrogen-deficient bone loss is far from clear. Since all menopausal women are estrogen deficient it is imperative to identify the other specific factors responsible for the bone loss in the subgroup of postmenopausal women who develop osteoporotic fractures.

Nutrition and Osteoporosis

While the current recommended daily allowance (RDA) for calcium is 800 mg/day, the average calcium intake of the adult American woman is only 500 mg/day and many women consume less than 300 mg/day.[33] Metabolic balance studies have demonstrated that the mean daily calcium requirement to maintain calcium balance for the premenopausal or estrogen-treated perimenopausal woman is 1 g, while that for the postmenopausal woman is 1.5 g.[39] Thus the population in general and the perimenopausal woman in particular may be relatively calcium deficient. When dietary calcium intake is insufficient to maintain the individual in calcium balance, calcium must be withdrawn from the skeleton.

Impaired absorption of calcium may exacerbate the deficiency of dietary calcium. Absorption capacity in a group of healthy white middle-aged women has been shown to be below levels needed to maintain calcium balance, even at elevated levels of calcium intake in some cases.[69] Since the normal response to a decline in calcium intake would be an increase in absorption efficiency,[70,71] attention has recently been focused upon the notion that subclinical vitamin D deficiency could play a role in calcium homeostasis in the elderly.[72] Indeed, it is possible that the observed decline in 25OHD levels[72] coupled with diminished responsiveness of the renal 1-alpha-hydroxylase enzyme[29–32] that occur with aging could exacerbate the deficiency of dietary calcium by superimposing upon it relative calcium malabsorption.

The available data regarding the effectiveness of calcium supplementation to suppress bone loss are conflicting and the subject of controversy.[33,73,74] We believe that adequate dietary calcium intake is necessary but not sufficient for maintaining skeletal mass. The evidence suggests that calcium can suppress bone loss due to deficiency of this nutrient.[33] It cannot, however, substitute for other deficiency states. For example, estrogen-related bone loss is probably not preventable by calcium supplementation.[74] Only that component of age-related or post-menopausal bone loss due to calcium deficiency is likely to be prevented by calcium.

Other nutritional factors are probably less important in the pathogenesis of osteoporosis.[2,33] Excess sodium intake is associated with significant hypercalciuria. There is some evidence for an increase in the dietary requirement for calcium associated with a high protein intake because of increased urinary calcium losses caused by acid radicals. High phosphorus intakes have long been thought to have harmful skeletal effects. Recent studies, however, have not shown any effect on calcium balance of wide variations in dietary phosphorus intake.[33] An association between negative calcium balance and excess caffeine intake has also been reported.[75]

Increased dietary fiber intake appears to lead to more negative calcium balance in short-term studies.[33] An increase in the fiber intake of 26 g has been reported to increase calcium requirements by 150 mg daily. While the effect of long-term fiber intake upon the skeleton is not clear, the recent recommendation to increase fiber intake for prevention of such disorders as colon carcinoma or diverticulosis are of concern in this regard. Excessive fiber intake may constitute a risk factor in certain individuals.

Other Risk Factors

In addition to female sex, estrogen deficiency, age, and dietary calcium intake, a number of other factors have been implicated as risk factors for the development of osteoporosis. They are summarized in Table 7-2, where they are arranged roughly in descending order of importance.[76]

Genetic and racial factors influence fracture risk in populations as well as individuals. Twin studies have demonstrated a genetic predilection for osteoporosis.[7,77] A positive family history thus is regarded as a risk factor. Whites and Orientals are more frequently affected by osteoporosis than blacks.[78] The importance of these genetic and racial factors could relate to their influence

Table 7-2. Risk Factors for Osteoporosis

Female sex
Early menopause (natural or surgical)
Caucasian or Oriental race
Positive family history
Small build or underweight
Chronic low dietary calcium intake
Lack of physical activity
Nulliparity
Alcohol abuse
Cigarette smoking
High caffeine intake
High sodium intake

upon peak bone mass. In addition, alterations of the vitamin D–endocrine system that have been reported in blacks could also be important in this regard.[79]

Considerable evidence suggests that physical activity affects bone mass.[11–13] Immobilization is associated with rapid bone loss due primarily to enhanced bone resorption.[80,81] Decreased gravitational pull associated with space travel has also been linked to reduction in bone density.[82] With resumption of weight-bearing activity, bone mass is restored, albeit at a slower rate and over a longer time. Several recent trials have suggested a positive effect of regular exercise upon bone mass in postmenopausal women.[83] Moreover, physically active women with anorexia nervosa have higher bone mineral density than sedentary anorectic women.[47] Whether there is any relationship between physical activity and fracture risk remains to be determined.

Cigarette smoking may be a risk factor for osteoporosis.[85–87] Possible mechanisms for this effect include an earlier age at menopause, reduction of estrogen levels at all ages, and lower body weight of women smokers. Moreover, a direct toxic effect on bone cells of the constituents of cigarette smoke as well as calcitonin resistance have been suggested in this regard.

Increased consumption of ethanol has been shown to be an independent risk factor for osteoporosis in men and is a contributing risk factor for all forms of osteoporosis.[86,88] Although the amount of ethanol required is likely to be subject to individual variation, one study demonstrated an increased risk of vertebral crush fractures with consumption of 3 ounces per day in men. While the mechanism for this effect in unclear, direct toxic actions of ethanol upon osteoblastic bone formation[89] and intestinal calcium transport[90] have been documented.

A variety of drugs, including glucocorticoids, heparin, loop diuretics, anticonvulsants, constant Gonadotropin releasing hormone (GNRH) infusions, high doses of thyroxine, and chemotherapeutic agents have been associated either with osteoporosis per se with alterations in calcium homeostasis.

The development of osteoporosis appears to be more common in men and women with hyperthyroidism, lactase deficiency, hemiplegia, rheumatoid arthritis, chronic obstructive pulmonary disease, primary biliary cirrhosis, and other types of chronic liver disease. Certain neoplasms, such as multiple myeloma, may present with osteoporosis. Type I insulin-dependent diabetes mellitus is associated with diminished bone mass. Type II diabetes, however, may be protective against osteoporosis.[92] A similar, and perhaps related, protective effect occurs in obesity.[57,58]

Many of the drugs and illnesses associated with an increased incidence of osteoporosis will be discussed in greater detail in the section on secondary osteoporosis. We agree with Riggs[2] that the bone loss that results from these drugs and medical conditions should be regarded as contributing to rather than independent of other major causes of osteoporosis in the elderly.

Finally, factors independent of bone mass may play a role in the increased incidence of fractures with aging.[2] These include diminished elasticity or tensile strength of bone, decreased dissipation of an applied force over bone by poorer muscle contraction and a greater tendency to fall in the elderly because of the increased prevalence of visual impairment, neurologic disease, and the use of sedative drugs.

Clinical Features of Age-Related and Postmenopausal Osteoporosis

Signs and Symptoms

The hallmark of osteoporosis is fracture. The most common form of the disease is encountered in postmenopausal women who present in their 50s and 60s with vertebral fractures. The vertebral fractures may be asymptomatic and noted incidentally on routine chest radiographs. Conversely, they may be accompanied by sharp pain over the involved area that develops after minimal or no trauma or during routine activities such as lifting heavy objects, opening windows, or bending. The pain may radiate anteriorly and is often exacerbated by movement and relieved by rest. Typically, the pain gradually subsides within 1 to 6 weeks regardless of therapy. Some women go on to suffer chronic, dull, diffuse pain that persists indefinitely, while others become symptom free. Whether asymptomatic or painful, successive vertebral crush fractures may lead to dorsal kyphosis and a "dowager's hump" or, rarely, to scoliosis. Moreover, the progressive loss of height associated with multiple vertebral compressions may cause the lower ribs to abut the iliac crest. This altered thoracoabdominal configuration may cause lower anterior rib pain, compression of intrathoracic and abdominal structures, shortness of breath, and gastrointestinal manifestations that include early satiety, bloating, and constipation. Pain or neurologic findings compatible with nerve root compression are unusual in osteoporosis and should prompt the physician to consider alternative diagnoses. The psychological effects of the chronic pain and the fear of further fractures has an extremely negative effect, causing many of these women to curtail work and social activities and to avoid exercise.

Hip fractures generally present later in life and occur in men and women over the age of 70. Although there is a great deal of overlap, those patients who sustain hip fractures may demonstrate proportionately greater loss of cortical bone; disproportionate loss of trabecular bone may be more prominent in those with vertebral and wrist fractures.

Riggs has proposed at least two distinct syndromes of involutional osteoporosis[2,93] (Table 7-3). Type I or postmenopausal osteoporosis affects primarily women within two decades of menopause. Clinically this form of the disorder involves skeletal sites with relatively large amounts of trabecular bone and is characterized by painful vertebral crush fractures, Colles' fractures, as well as increased tooth loss due to demineralization of the mandible. The rate of trabecular bone loss is three times greater than normal and exceeds the rate of cortical bone loss, which may be only slightly greater than normal. Type II or "senile osteoporosis" occurs in men and women over 70. Hip fracture and multiple wedge vertebral deformities are seen most commonly, as well as fractures of the proximal humerus, proximal tibia, and pelvis.

Riggs has suggested that the pathogenesis of these two forms of osteoporosis is different. Type I osteoporosis is primarily caused by factors related to ovarian failure. Estrogen deficiency leads to accelerated bone resorption, suppression of parathyroid hormone secretion, diminished conversion of 25(OH)D to $1,25(OH)_2D$, and impaired intestinal calcium absorption, which may further exacerbate negative calcium balance and aggravate skeletal loss. Type II osteoporosis affects both cortical and trabecular bone. The cause of this syndrome may simply be related to the age-related bone loss that occurs in the population at large. This notion is supported by the demonstration that bone mineral density measurements at various sites in the axial and appendicular skeleton are usually in the lower end of the normal range, adjusted for age and sex, in these patients. In this elderly population, impaired synthesis of $1,25(OH)_2D$ compromises intestinal calcium absorption. The resulting increase of parathyroid hormone enhances bone resorption. This, coupled with a decrease in osteoblast function with aging results in a slow erosion of skeletal integrity. The greater frequency of these fractures in women reflects the cumulative effects of menopause upon age-related bone loss. The presence of type I

Table 7-3. The Two Types of Involutional Osteoporosis

	Type I	Type II
Age (yr)	51–75	>70
Sex ratio (F/M)	6 : 1	2 : 1
Type of bone loss	Mainly trabecular	Trabecular and cortical
Rate of bone loss	Accelerated	Not accelerated
Fracture sites	Vertebrae (crush) and distal radius	Vertebrae (multiple wedge) and hip
Parathyroid function	Decreased	Increased
Calcium absorption	Decreased	Decreased
Metabolism of 25-OH-D to $1,25(OH)_2D$	Secondary decrease	Primary decrease
Main causes	Factors related to menopause	Factors related to aging

(From Riggs, et al,[2] with permission.)

osteoporosis may predispose patients to type II. While there is a great deal of overlap between these two syndromes, the classification is clinically useful.

Laboratory Findings

No biochemical changes are characteristic of osteoporosis. Total serum calcium and ionized calcium, phosphate, and alkaline phosphatase levels are normal; transient elevations in the serum alkaline phosphatase activity, however, may occur during fracture healing. Serum levels of parathyroid hormone and vitamin D metabolites are usually within the normal range although subtle abnormalities such as minimally increased PTH levels or depressed $1,25(OH)_2D$ levels might be found. Indices that reflect bone turnover, such as serum osteocalcin levels or urinary hydroxyproline excretion, are also within the normal range. Urinary calcium excretion is normal in postmenopausal or age-related osteoporosis although it may be elevated in other forms. There is some disagreement about calcitonin levels in osteoporosis[65–67]; this might reflect technical difficulties in the measurement of this hormone. Most recent data nevertheless suggest that although calcitonin levels are lower in women than in men, both basal and stimulated calcitonin levels in postmenopausal osteoporotic patients[67] are no different from those in normal women.

Radiologic Features

Routine skeletal radiography is an insensitive method of detecting osteoporosis. Approximately 25 to 30 percent of skeletal mineral must be lost before abnormal radiolucency is apparent. However, a standard set of lateral thoracic and lumbar spine films is useful to assess the number of fractured vertebrae and the efficacy of a therapeutic intervention in preventing further fractures. The films should be examined for several features.[94] An assessment of vertebral radiolucency (Fig. 7-3A) can be made by masking the cortical outline of the vertebrae and determining whether the trabecular portion of vertebral body is distinguishable from the surrounding soft tissue. Reduced density is also likely if the iliac crest can be seen through the fourth and fifth lumbar vertebrae. Accentuation of the vertical trabeculae (Fig. 7-3A) is a sign of early osteoporosis, since horizontal trabeculae are lost before vertical trabeculae. In younger patients, herniation of turgid intervertebral discs occurs, such that the disc protrudes into the vertebral body, to produce either a generalized pattern of vertebral biconcavity (''codfish'' vertebrae; Fig. 7-3B) or a more localized protrusion of the nucleus pulposus into the vertebral body to produce a ''Schmorl's node.'' This sign is appreciated less often in elderly individuals who have experienced more disc degeneration. Wedging (Fig. 7-3A) is present when the anterior height of the vertebrae is less than the posterior height and at least 15 percent smaller than the height of the anterior border of the neighboring vertebra. Posterior wedging is very rare and suggests a destructive lesion.

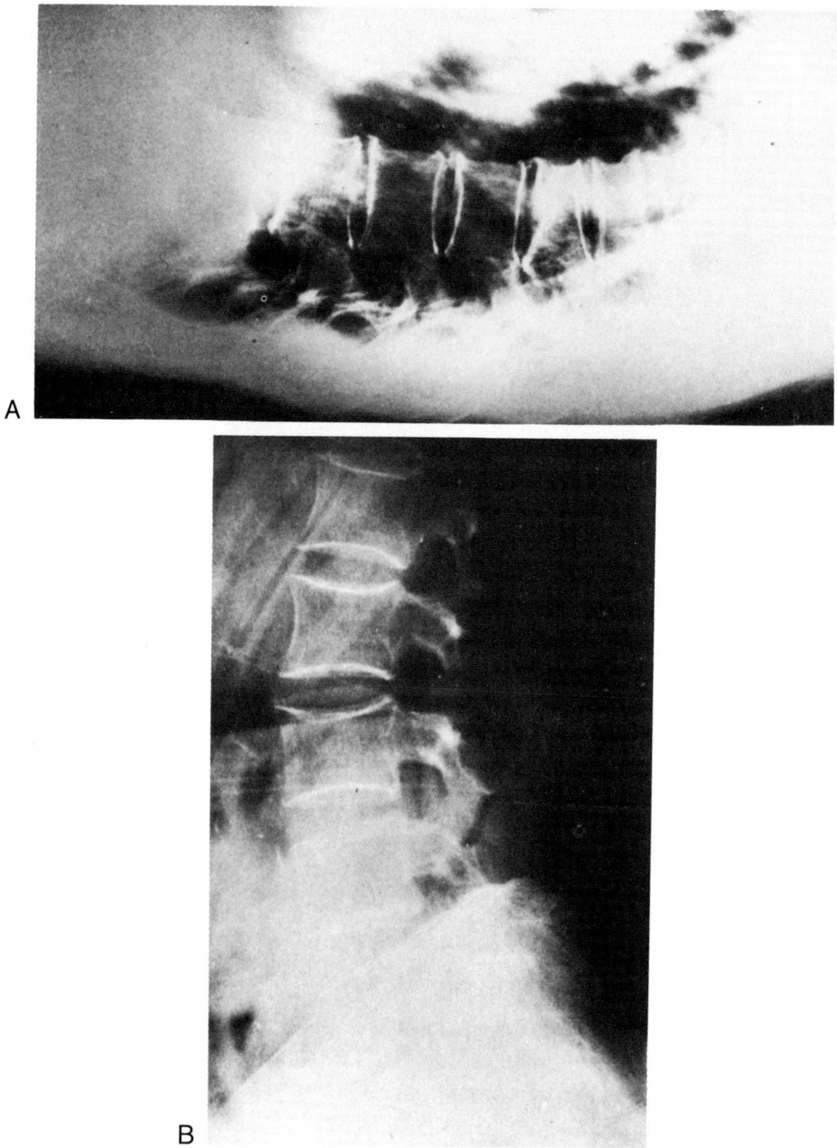

Fig. 7-3 Lateral thoracic (**A**) and lumbar (**B**) spine in a case of early osteoporosis. Note one wedged vertebra, vertebral translucency, and mild biconcavity. (From Nordin,[94] with permission.)

Vertebral compression is present when there is a decrease in the anterior, central, and posterior height of a vertebra (Fig. 7-4). While the significance of a single wedged or compressed vertebra is unclear and may merely represent previous trauma, the presence of two or more deformities almost invariably indicates osteoporosis. The frequency of vertebral fractures is maximal between T8 and L3 vertebral bodies. Fractures above T6 should suggest a cause other than primary osteoporosis and should prompt a search for malignant disease.

In radiographs of the appendicular skeleton, the Singh index has been used as a semiquantitative measure of assessing the status of trabecular bone in the proximal femur (Fig. 7-5). Values of 3 or less are associated with an increased risk of femoral neck fracture. Cortical thinning may also be prominent in the femoral neck (Fig. 7-6).

Newer methods of assessing bone mass in the lumbar spine, wrist, and femoral neck, such as single and dual photon absorptiometry and quantitative computed tomography have surpassed these older radiographic techniques. These more sensitive noninvasive methods are discussed separately in Chapter 3.

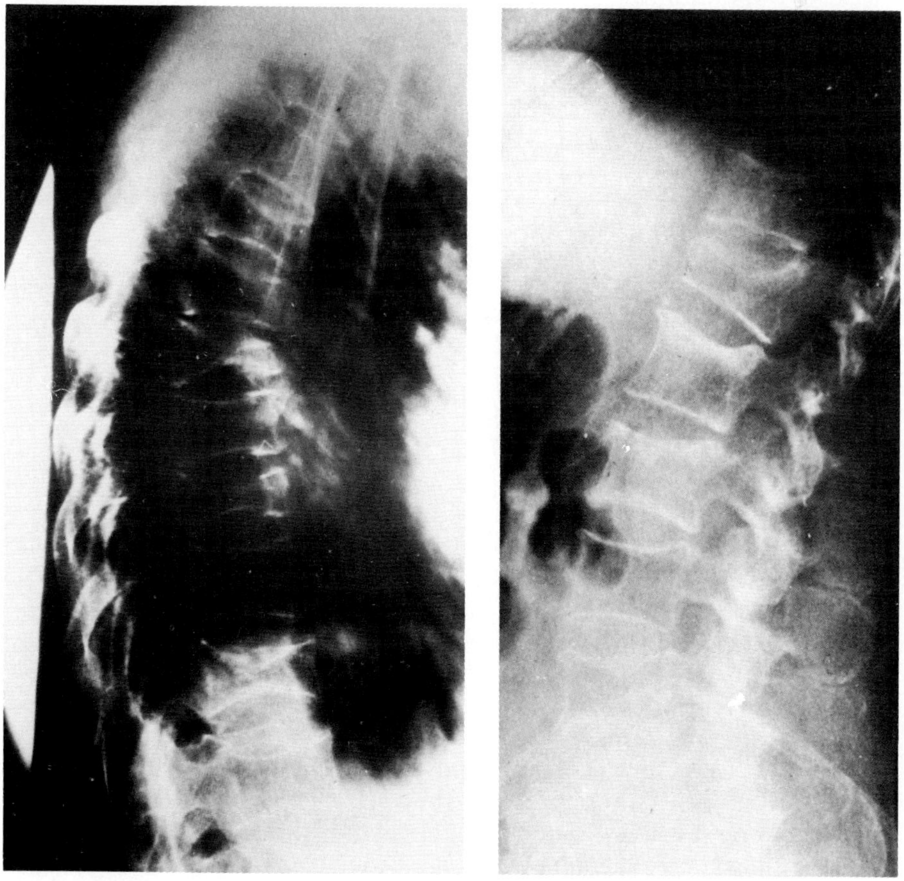

A B

Fig. 7-4 Lateral thoracic (**A**) and lumbar (**B**) spine in a case of severe osteoporosis. Note multiple wedged and compressed vertebrae and irregular deformation of others. (From Nordin,[94] with permission.)

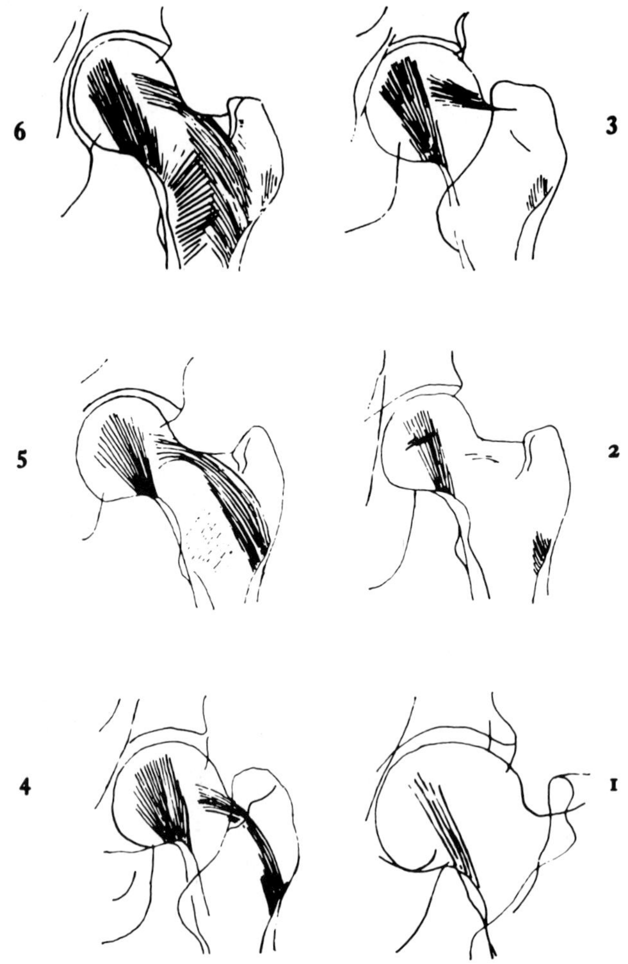

Fig. 7-5 Diagrmmatic representation of the Singh index. Note the progressive radiologic disappearance of trabecular groups at the lower index values. (From Nordin,[94] with permission.)

Histomorphometric Features of Osteoporosis

In recent years several technical advances have established the iliac crest bone biopsy as a useful tool for the study of osteoporosis as well as other metabolic bone diseases. Histomorphometric analyses of undecalcified biopsies have shown a reduction in trabecular bone volume in 70 to 80 percent of patients with vertebral crush fracture. This decrease in trabecular bone volume has been demonstrated to be due to progressive loss of entire trabeculae. Other studies have demonstrated a wide spectrum of bone remodeling activity.[95] Approximately one-third of patients have low-turnover or "inactive" os-

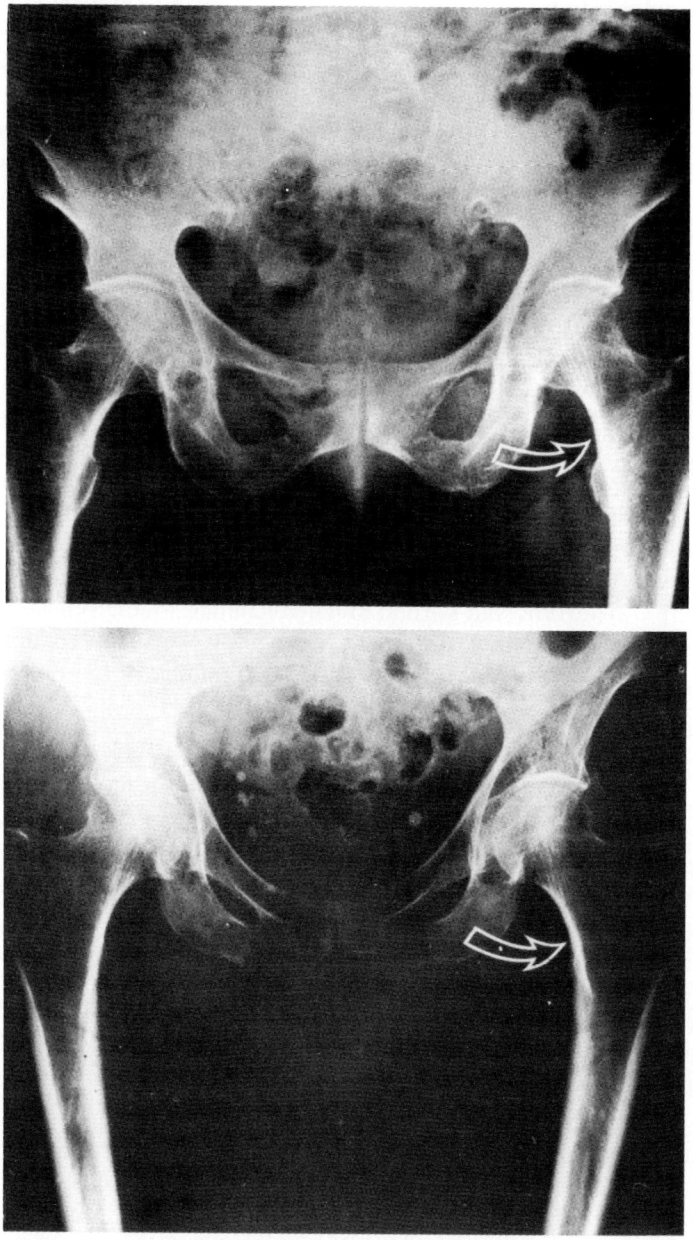

Fig. 7-6 Radiographs of the pelvis in cases of mild (**A**) and severe (**B**) osteoporosis. The diminished thickness of the calcar femorale in (**B**) (the condensation of cortical bone immediately above the lesser trochanter, indicated by the arrow) is readily apparent in comparison to the milder loss in (**A**). The Singh index is about 4 in **A** and 2 in **B**. (From Nordin,[94] with permission.)

teoporosis with a slow rate of remodeling, few osteoclasts and osteoblasts, and diminished bone-forming surfaces as measured by tetracycline fluorescent labeling. Another one-third have accelerated bone turnover with abundant osteoclasts, osteoblasts, osteoid and bone-forming surfaces. Another one-third demonstrate skeletal turnover that is within the normal range. Biochemical indices of bone turnover (alkaline phosphatase, osteocalcin, and urinary hydroxyproline excretion) are not predictive of the histologic picture. It is not currently known whether the histomorphometric heterogeneity of osteoporosis reflects differences in pathogenesis or represents temporal variability within the same disease process. Moreover, there are no data that yet link the histomorphometric appearance of a patient's biopsy to responsiveness to a specific form of therapy.

The indications for bone biopsy in postmenopausal or senile osteoporosis are somewhat controversial. Bone biopsy should not be used to quantitate trabecular bone volume to confirm the diagnosis of osteoporosis, since the overlap between clinically osteoporotic patients and normals is too great to make this useful in the individual case. Bone biopsy does help to exclude subclinical osteomalacia in osteopenic patients. Although osteomalacia is unusual in North America, one study found that 5 percent of patients with typical crush fracture syndrome and normal biochemical and radiographic parameters had osteomalacia. In general, unless there are unusual aspects to an individual case, biopsy of the osteoporotic patient should remain a research tool.

Differential Diagnosis

Primary (postmenopausal and senile) osteoporosis is a diagnosis of exclusion. A major goal of the evaluation is to exclude secondary causes of bone loss (Table 7-1). Secondary osteoporosis should be suspected particularly in those individuals who belong to groups with a low prevalence of the disorder, such as white men, young white women, and blacks.

The history should seek information about renal stone disease, thyroid disease, Cushing's syndrome, diabetes, hypogonadism (primary and secondary), liver disease, gastric or intestinal surgery, intestinal illness, systemic malignancy, alcohol and caffeine consumption, and cigarette smoking. A complete drug history, including use of vitamins, diuretics, glucocorticoids, and anticonvulsant drugs, is essential. A family history of osteoporosis or other metabolic bone disease should be sought. An estimate of calcium intake via food sources or supplements is important (Table 7-4). In women, the time of menopause, surgical or natural, should be ascertained.

The physical examination should note height, weight, and measurement of arm span (which gives an estimate of original height) and include a general physical examination. The laboratory evaluation includes measurement of serum calcium, phosphorus, and alkaline phosphatase levels, thyroid function tests, complete blood count, and serum protein electrophoresis. The 24 hour urinary excretion of calcium and, if clinically indicated, cortisol should be

Table 7-4. Nutritional Sources of Calcium

Nutritional Source	Serving	Calcium (mg)
Dairy		
Cheese (hard)	1 oz	140–275
Cottage cheese (low fat, 1%)	1 cup	155
Milk (skim)	1 cup	302
Yogurt	1 cup	275–415
Ice cream	1 cup	175–240
Seafood		
Salmon, canned (with bones)	3 oz	167
Sardines (with bones)	3 oz	371
Shrimp	3 oz	100
Vegetables		
Broccoli	1 cup	177
Collards	1 cup	357
Kale	1 cup	179
Turnip greens	1 cup	249
Beens		
Navy, pinto, kidney (cooked, drained)	1 cup	90
Soybeans (cooked, drained)	1 cup	131
Miscellaneous		
Molasses	2 tbsp	274
Tofu	4 oz	100–150
Orange	1 med	50
Bread	2 slices	50
Almonds	10 nuts	25

measured. Serum vitamin D metabolite and parathyroid hormone levels are useful in the diagnosis of hyperparathyroidism or osteomalacia.

Evaluation of the Asymptomatic Woman

Although significant loss of both cortical and trabecular bone occurs prior to menopause, the rate of bone loss accelerates after menopause. It is clear that prevention of osteoporosis may be more successful than therapy of established osteoporosis. The time of menopause (or oophorectomy) constitutes a natural point at which to assess a woman's risk for developing osteoporosis. This may be accomplished by determining the woman's risk factors and by obtaining bone mass measurements in those considered to be at increased risk.

The currently recognized risk factors thought to increase bone loss or known to occur frequently in association with clinical osteoporosis are listed in Table 7-2. Most of them have been discussed in preceding sections of this chapter. In a general way, these risk factors may be regarded as additive or cumulative.[2] It is our practice to screen most carefully those women who are caucasian, or Oriental and who are thin, have poor dietary calcium intake, a sedentary lifestyle, early menopause, or a positive family history of osteoporosis. Those women who, on the basis of historical risk factors, may be at increased risk of developing type I osteoporosis may be referred for a measurement of bone density. The available methods to accomplish this are discussed separately (Chap. 3).

The routine use of bone measurements in the perimenopausal population is still controversial. These controversies relate primarily to difficulties with reproducibility and accuracy of the measurements, especially in longitudinal measurements in the individual patient. Since bone mass may be lost at different rates a single measurement of bone mineral density will not differentiate those women who are losing bone rapidly from those who are not. While longitudinal measurements provide a better estimate of fracture risk, twice yearly measurements over a 2 to 3 year period are necessary to estimate individual rates of bone loss.[2] An additional difficulty relates to the fact that measurements at sites in the appendicular skeleton such as the radius or os calcis,[2] which are less expensive and more easily performed, do not correlate well enough with density in the lumbar spine to be predictive for the individual patient. For these reasons, we recommend measurement of bone density at the site of interest (i.e., the vertebral body) only for those women considered to be at increased risk for postmenopausal osteoporosis.

Therapy

Prevention of osteoporosis and therapy of established osteoporosis are best considered separately. Although some therapies overlap, the populations that form these groups are different with regard to demographic composition and the pathophysiologic status of the skeleton.

Prevention

Given the already staggering incidence of osteoporotic fractures in the United States, the increasing size of the elderly population, and the fact that no generally efficacious treatment for osteoporosis exists, prevention of osteoporosis is the most cost-effective approach.

Calcium. While the evidence that increasing calcium intake can enhance peak bone mass, reduce bone loss, or prevent fracture is currently a matter of heated debate, it is reasonable for individuals to ensure that their dietary calcium intake is sufficient to remain in calcium balance. We therefore recommend a daily calcium intake of 1000 mg for adults and 1500 mg for adolescents and postmenopausal women. Although this can be achieved by increasing intake of calcium-containing foods (Table 7-4), concerns about calories and fat (both features of many foods rich in calcium) limits this obvious solution. Thus, calcium supplementation is frequently necessary. Calcium carbonate is most popular since 40 percent of the compound is elemental calcium and fewer tablets are necessary than with preparations of calcium salts that are poorer in their percentage of calcium, such as the lactate (13 percent) or gluconate (9 percent) forms[96] (Table 7-5). Complicance may be better with preparations that contain 500 mg of elemental calcium per tablet, again because fewer tablets are necessary. Calcium carbonate should be taken with meals because absorption is reduced in the presence of achlorhydria. In this regard, some experts recommend calcium citrate because it is more soluble and its absorbability depends less upon gastric acidity. Calcium citrate may be particularly useful in the elderly population in whom achlorhydria is more frequent. In patients without a history of nephrolithiasis and/or hypercalciuria, calcium supplementation appears to be safe.

Exercise. In addition to adequate dietary calcium, all individuals should incorporate regular exercise into their daily routine if possible. For the prevention of osteoporosis, repetitive, gravity-resistant, weight-bearing activities such as walking, jogging, and various forms of aerobic exercise may have a beneficial effect upon the skeleton. Swimming and bicycling, which are not weight-bearing exercises, may not be as useful in this regard. Competitive sports such as racket sports and golf (without the cart) may also be useful. The prescription of an exercise program must be made with consideration of the patient's general state of health. The exercise regimen should not be so intensive to induce amenorrhea, thereby introducing another risk factor for the patient.

Estrogens. While the efficacy of increased dietary calcium and physical activity to prevent bone loss in the postmenopausal woman continues to be debated, prophylactic therapy with estrogens clearly prevents skeletal loss and fracture in this group (Fig. 7-7).[16,50–53] However, the potential risks of estrogen therapy[2] are significant. The issue of who should receive estrogen therapy is therefore a matter of balancing the risks of such intervention in the individual patient with the potential benefits, also a matter of individual assessment. In general those at risk for osteoporosis (small or thin, caucasian or Oriental women, women with a history of early menopause, prolonged amenorrhea, or oligomenorrhea from any cause during young adulthood, a strong family history of osteoporosis, or a low bone mineral density at the lumbar spine) are

Table 7-5. Calcium Supplements

	Common Formulation	% Elemental Calcium	Elemental Calcium per Dose (mg)	Dose for 2000 mg
Calcium carbonate	650 mg tablet	40	250	8 tab
	1300 mg tablet		500	4 tab
	2 g/tsp powder		800	2.5 tsp
Calcium citrate	950 mg tablet	20	200	10 tab[a]
Calcium lactate	650 mg tablet	13	84	24 tab
Calcium gluconate	1000 mg tablet	9	93	22 tab
Calcium glubionate	1.8 g/tsp liquid	6.6	115	18 tsp

[a] There is evidence that calcium citrate may be better absorbed than calcium carbonate, so a dose lower than 2000 mg/day may be acceptable.
(From Downs, et al,[96] with permission.)

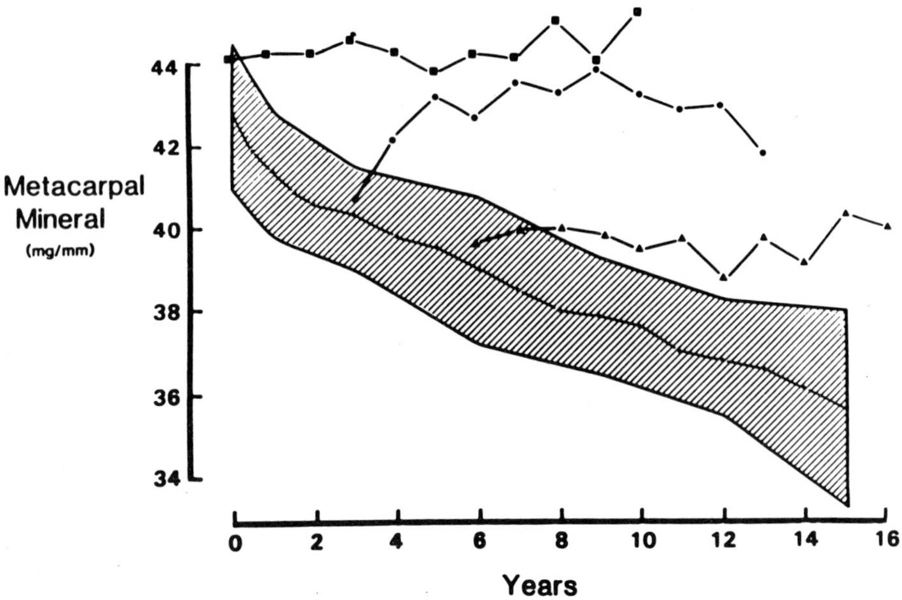

Fig. 7-7 The effect of estrogen treatment on metacarpal bone mass after menopause. Although better protection against bone loss is achieved when estrogens are started in closer proximity to menopause, some degree of protection is obtained even when treatment is not started for many years after menopause. (From Tohme, et al,[76] with permission.)

candidates for estrogen replacement therapy if the risks of such therapy can be justified.

All estrogen compounds appear to be effective in preventing the acceleration in bone loss at menopause. While the efficacy appears to be independent of the route of administration, with both oral and transdermal forms being effective, there is much less experience with transdermal estrogen. The minimum effective dose is 0.625 mg/day of conjugated equine estrogen.[76] One study suggests that when 1.5 g of calcium is provided the minimal effective dose of estrogen may be reduced to 0.3 mg daily.[53] The effectiveness of estrogen therapy is maximal when it is begun soon after menopause and decreases progressively as the time past menopause lengthens. Discontinuation of estrogen therapy results in rates of bone loss comparable to the immediate postmenopausal period.[76]

A major risk of estrogen therapy is an increased incidence of endometrial carcinoma (approximately 1 percent per year). This is largely prevented by the addition, in women with an intact uterus, of a progestagen such as medroxyprogesterone acetate (Provera) 10 mg/day for 10 days every 1 to 3 months. Whether the progestagen itself may enhance the effect of estrogen upon prevention of bone loss is currently not known. Although some studies suggest that estrogen may increase the risk of breast cancer, others have indicated that there may a protective effect when an estrogen–progestin combination is used. For these reasons gynecologic consultation, mammography, and close gynecologic follow-up constitute a mandatory component of estrogen replacement therapy.

Other risks of estrogen therapy are venous thrombosis, hypertension, and gallstones. These side effects are thought to be due to enhanced production of blood coagulation factors, renin substrate, and bile acids induced by the hepatic actions of estogen. The use of transdermal estogen delivery patches that bypass the hepatic circulation may reduce or eliminate these potential difficulties. The effect of estrogens with or without progestins on the incidence of coronary artery disease and cerebrovascular accident in women is currently being debated. Salutary or deleterious effects of estrogen therapy upon the incidence of myocardial infarction and stroke would have an enormous effect upon the practice of prescribing estrogens for the prevention of osteoporosis and other menopause related symptoms. A decision to embark upon estrogen replacement therapy thus requires a careful consideration of the risks and benefits by the patient and her physician.

Calcitonin. Calcitonin, a hormone that specifically inhibits osteoclast-mediated bone resorption, may prove to be an alternative drug for prevention of postmenopausal bone loss when estrogens are contraindicated. However, while small increases in total body calcium have been observed and there is preliminary evidence for retardation of postmenopausal bone resorption,[97] no data are available on the effect of this drug upon fracture rates. The minimal effective dose of calcitonin has not yet been established. Investigators are using dosage schedules that range from 25 MRC units three times weekly to 100 to 200 MRC units daily. Obvious disadvantages of calcitonin therapy include its expense and the necessity for parenteral administration. Lower doses, should they prove to be effective, and newer preparations that can be administered intranasally may obviate these problems, perhaps as well as other side effects such as nausea, headache, and flushing that have been frequently observed.

General Measures. Avoidance of bone toxins such as alcohol and cigarette smoking should be stressed. Individuals at risk should also minimize the use of caffeine, aluminum-containing antacids, excessive dietary fiber, and protein.

Treatment

General Measures. The goals of therapy in the patient with vertebral crush fracture are relief of pain, early mobilization, and prevention of future fractures. The back pain of a vertebral crush fracture may be of such magnitude that narcotic analgesics are necessary. Nonsteroidal anti-inflammatory drugs may also be useful in these patients. Supportive measures such as heat packs and whirlpool therapy may reduce discomfort. Muscle relaxants may alleviate painful paraspinal muscle spasm. Dorsolumbar supports may also be useful initially to permit early mobility. Relief of pain is of great importance since it facilitates mobilization of the osteoporotic patients, which is an essential part of any treatment program. Femoral neck fractures generally require surgical intervention and prolonged periods of rehabilitation.

Pharmacologic Therapy. In general, drugs useful in the therapy of osteoporosis are classified into two categories: those that inhibit bone resorption and those that stimulate new bone formation (Table 7-6).

Antiresorptive Agents. Calcium, estrogen, and calcitonin are the three agents currently approved by the Food and Drug Administration for the treatment of osteoporosis. The primary action of each is to decrease bone resorption, albeit by different mechanisms. In general, the effect of these antiresorptive agents is to stabilize mass or to decrease the rate of bone loss. While there may be a small increase in bone mass during the initial phase of therapy, when bone resorption is suppressed and formation is completed in those bone-remodeling units whose presence antedated the initiation of therapy, a major gain in bone mass cannot be expected.

Calcium therapy decreases the activation of new bone-modeling units indirectly via suppression of parathyroid hormone secretion.[2] Calcium, in doses of 1.5 to 2.0 g/day, should be prescribed in patients with established osteoporosis for the same reasons adequate minimum intake should be encouraged in other populations: it is innocuous and it probably has "skeleton-sparing" effect in the fight to maintain calcium balance. It is reasonable to obtain a measurement of 24 hour urinary calcium excretion during supplementation.

While the effects of estrogen to reduce perimenopausal bone loss are clear, the use of estrogen in the woman more than 15 years postmenopause is more controversial. Recent evidence has suggested that estrogen may slow bone loss even when begun 20 to 25 years after menopause.[98] More information is clearly needed on this point. The effect of estrogen to enhance absorption of dietary calcium may constitute another reason for its use in this age group.[33,39] Estrogens should be prescribed following the guidelines described above. They must be prescribed with greater caution, however, because of the greater prevalence of vascular disease in older women. Calcitonin may be beneficial in that group of patients with established osteoporosis who have high bone turnover. It may prove to be useful in those patients with type I osteoporosis in whom estrogen therapy is not an option.

There is very little evidence that calcitonin or estrogen therapy is of much

Table 7-6. Therapy of Osteoporosis

Agents that inhibit bone resorption
Calcium
Estrogen
Calcitonin
Diphosphonates
Agents that stimulate bone formation
Sodium fluoride
Anabolic steroids
Human PTH 1-34

benefit to patients over the age of 70 with type II osteoporosis who are characterized as a group by low-turnover osteoporosis and are no longer thought to be in a phase of rapid bone loss. It has been recommended that these patients be managed with calcium supplementation and vitamin D (400 to 1000 U daily) to improve calcium absorption as well as instruction in measures designed to avoid trauma and falls.[2]

Agents That Stimulate New Bone Formation. Sodium fluoride,[99] unlike the aforementioned agents, stimulates osteoblast division, causes new bone formation, and increases bone mineral density. It has been reported to reduce vertebral fracture risk in treated patients. Response is indicated by coarsening of vertebral trabeculation and thickening of end-plates, a substantial increase in bone mineral density, or histologic evidence of fluorosis. Regimens of 25 to 100 mg daily have been used, the higher doses being associated with more side effects as well as probably a greater therapeutic effect. There are, however, difficulties with fluoride therapy. The new bone may not mineralize well and supplemental calcium and vitamin D are required to prevent osteomalacia (1 to 2 g/day elemental calcium and 50,000 U vitamin D once or twice weekly). Histologic data suggest that the tensile strength of the new bone may not be as great as normal bone. Despite this however, fracture risk does decrease after the first year of therapy. While fluoride therapy does improve trabecular bone mineral density, cortical bone density does not increase. This fact, together with the observation that calcium balance is not improved with fluoride treatment, has led to the theory that cortical bone mineral may be the source of the trabecular bone mineral and has raised fears that risk of other fractures may increase in fluoride-treated patients. However, a recent multicenter evaluation did not find increased frequency of femoral neck fractures in fluoride-treated patients.[100] Fluoride has been associated with disabling and potentially dangerous side effects such as gastric irritation, ulceration, and gastrointestinal bleeding. In addition, osteophyte formation, ligamental calcification, and a painful arthropathy of weight-bearing joints, thought to be due to metaphyseal microfractures of the long bones, has been described.

A substantial proportion of patients (50 percent) have an incomplete response or no response to fluoride. There is currently no way of predicting whether a given patient will be responsive or unresponsive. Protection from fracture is probably limited to the responders. Fluoride is an experimental drug, and is currently not approved by the Food and Drug Administration for use in osteoporosis. Its use should probably be limited to the clinical research setting.

Other bone-forming regimens have been less widely evaluated than sodium fluoride. Anabolic steroids may stimulate the osteoblast in vitro and have been shown to increase total body calcium.[101] However, because of masculinizing side effects they are poorly tolerated in women. Intermittent infusions of synthetic PTH (1-34) stimulate new bone formation in women and men with osteoporosis.[102,103] The use of this agent remains investigational. Cyclic therapy with different agents targeted to affect different segments of the remodeling cycle (''ADFR'' therapy) is also currently under investigation.[104]

Miscellaneous Agents. Vitamin D may be useful in populations thought to be at risk for deficiency of this hormone, such as elderly individuals with a poor diet, institutionalized people, or those on corticosteroids. Doses of 400 to 1000 units daily are appropriate. Pharmacologic doses place patients at risk for hypercalciuria, hypercalcemia, and possibly enhanced bone resorption. Similarly, while administration of calcitriol, the active metabolite of vitamin D, may circumvent the putative defect in 1-alpha hydroxylase activity in the elderly and has been associated with a decrease in fracture incidence in one study, there is a narrow therapeutic window and careful monitoring is necessary.[105]

Thiazide diuretics have been used in osteoporosis therapy in the expectation that their hypocalciuric actions might improve calcium balance and decrease rates of bone loss or increase bone mineral density. The two available studies have had discrepant results and the presence of any beneficial effect of thiazides on the skeleton is not known.[91,106]

Diphosphonates are stable analog of pyrophosphate that can block osteoclastic bone resorption[107] and may therefore be useful in the treatment of conditions characterized by high rates of bone resorption, such as immobilization. Recent data also suggest a beneficial effect in postmenopausal osteoporosis,[108] but these results are preliminary and the use of these drugs outside the investigational setting is not justified.

In summary, the goal of therapy in the patient with established osteoporosis is prevention of recurrent fracture. General measures including proper diet, a carefully constructed exercise program, and instruction aimed at decreasing the risk of falling are important. In the younger patient with type I osteoporosis who may still be losing bone rapidly, calcium, estrogen, and calcitonin may be beneficial. Older individuals (over 70) with type II osteoporosis may not derive much benefit from these agents, and assessment of the relative risk-to-benefit ratio is particularly important in this age group. Attempts to stimulate new bone formation are reasonable if tolerated. In the near future more data will become available on some of these agents and the outlook for the patient with osteoporosis may improve.

OTHER FORMS OF PRIMARY OSTEOPOROSIS

Juvenile Osteoporosis

This rare disease occurs in prepubertal or adolescent children between the ages of 8 and 15 years.[109] It most commonly presents with acute back pain due to vertebral crush fractures. Significant loss of height and permanent spinal deformity can occur. Although the temporal relationship of the disorder to puberty suggests an endocrine cause, the cause of the disease is completely unknown. Spontaneous remission after 2 to 6 years is the rule.

As with other unusual presentations of osteoporosis, it is important to eliminate other causes such as hematologic neoplasms, Cushing's syndrome, or osteogenesis imperfecta. In general, this can be readily accomplished although transiliac crest bone biopsy may be necessary to exclude osteogenesis imperfecta. In contrast to osteogenesis imperfecta,[110] in juvenile osteoporosis the family history is negative, its onset is later, the axial skeleton is affected more severely than the appendicular skeleton, and other clinical findings of osteogenesis imperfecta such as blue sclera, dental loss, and ligamentous laxity are not present. Histologically, low bone turnover is seen in osteogenesis imperfecta while high turnover with relatively uncontrolled activity of metaphyseal osteoclasts is seen in juvenile osteoporosis. Mild elevations of urinary hydroxyproline levels have been measured and alkaline phosphatase levels are increased during fracture healing.

Therapy consists of pain relief, mobilization, and physical therapy. Therapy with sex steroids is not effective. Diphosphonates may be of some benefit but very few data are available.[111]

Idiopathic Osteoporosis of Young Adults

This uncommon type of osteoporosis occurs in patients between the ages of 20 and 50 and is more frequently seen among men.[112,113] The clinical features, except for the age of onset, are similar to those of postmenopausal or senile osteoporosis, although hypercalciuria and nephrolithiasis occur more often. While these patients may have a history of alcohol abuse, histologic parameters show excessive osteoclastic bone resorption and active remodeling whereas alcohol-induced osteoporosis is associated with depressed parameters of bone turnover. Late-onset osteogenesis imperfecta may also be confused with this entity. The condition may follow a course similar to involutional osteoporosis but can be rapidly progressive. The cause is unknown. Therapy is the same as for other forms of osteoporosis.

Osteoporosis in Men

Osteoporosis occurs much less frequently in males than in females. The incidence of vertebral crush fractures is 10 times greater and femoral neck fractures are twice as common in women than in men.[3–5] Because of its relative rarity, an intensive search should be made for secondary causes in a man who presents with osteoporosis. Common causative factors include alcohol abuse[86,88] and hypogonadism.[86,114,115] Histomorphometric data indicate that a low-turnover type of osteoporosis is characteristic of alcohol-related osteopenia whereas both elevated and depressed states of turnover have been observed in association with hypogonadism. In addition, a form of osteoporosis associated with hypercalciuria and accelerated bone turnover has been described in young men in whom other causes have been excluded.[112]

Regional Osteoporoses

Reflex sympathetic dystrophy (Sudeck's atrophy or shoulder–hand syndrome) is associated with radiographically apparent localized osteoporosis.[114] Histologically, there is accelerated bone resorption secondary to excessive osteoclast activity. The mechanism for these changes is unclear but may involve disuse of the painful limb or neurovascular changes. Treatment is supportive. Corticosteroids and calcitonin have been used.

Transient osteoporosis of the hip[117] is a rare disorder of unknown cause that most commonly presents in the third trimester of pregnancy although it has also been reported in men and nonpregnant young or middle aged women. It is characterized by spontaneous hip pain, limitation of motion, antalgic limp, and osteopenia of the periarticular bones of the hip joint, particularly the femoral head. The symptoms generally resolve spontaneously within a year.

Regional migratory osteoporosis[118] is a syndrome characterized by painful localized bone loss particularly in the lower extremities. Recovery usually occurs spontaneously but the course may be marked by recurrences at other sites. The cause is unknown. Differentiation from various arthritides is based upon the lack of joint involvement. The condition may persist for several years. Treatment is supportive. Nonsteroidal anti-inflammatory drugs and glucocorticoids are beneficial and use of calcitonin may result in dramatic clinical improvement.

SECONDARY OSTEOPOROSIS

Congenital or Inherited Forms

Osteogenesis Imperfecta

Osteogenesis imperfecta, the brittle bone syndrome, is a common inheritable disorder of bone, occurring approximately once per 20,000 live births.[110] It is characterized by defective bone formation that leads to increased bone fragility, fracture, and skeletal deformities. In addition there is a variable incidence of certain extraskeletal manifestations. Most forms of the disease are thought to be caused by abnormalities in collagen biosynthesis or structure. The structural complexity of the collagen molecule probably accounts for the wide range of severity and variable clinical presentation of this heterogeneous disorder. Current research is directed toward identification of these abnormalities of collagen synthesis at the molecular level. Women with this disorder may present with a marked rise in fracture incidence at menopause, when the protective effect of estrogen is lost. Such women would benefit from estrogen replacement therapy.

Osteopenia is a feature of a number of chromosomal disorders including children with XO (Turner's syndrome) gonadal dysgenesis, Klinefelter's (XXY) syndrome, and with XXXY as well as Down's syndrome (trisomy 21).[48,128] It is not clear whether the hypogonadism concomitant with some of these syndromes is the only factor in the development of osteopenia. The osteopenia associated with trisomy 21 appears to reverse at puberty, suggesting that other factors may play a role.[119]

Other genetic disorders leading to defective collagen synthesis or crosslinking, such as the Ehlers-Danlos syndrome, Marfan's syndrome, Menke's syndrome, and homocystinuria, may also be associated with osteopenia. Thalassemia and sickle cell disease, which are anemias characterized by bone marrow hyperplasia, are also accompanied by osteoporosis. Glycogen storage diseases, hypophosphatasia, and familial dysautonomia (Riley–Day syndrome) are also associated with osteoporosis.

Endocrine Causes of Osteopenia

Glucocorticoid Excess

Steroid-induced osteoporosis[76,120,121] is the most common form of secondary osteoporosis. Osteoporosis may accompany or be the presenting sign of Cushing's syndrome due to adrenal tumors or to ACTH-secreting tumors of the anterior pituitary or other nonendocrine tissues (such as carcinoma of the bronchus). However, therapy with glucocorticoids or ACTH and their synthetic analogs constitutes the most frequent source of glucocorticoid excess today. Osteoporosis can complicate any disorder (chronic asthma, various rheumatic diseases, organ transplantation) that requires long-term steroid therapy. Children and the elderly, especially postmenopausal women whose skeletons are already compromised, are at greatest risk. Areas with large proportions of trabecular bone, that is, ribs and vertebrae, are disproportionately affected. Adults may present with rib, long bone, or vertebral crush fractures; children may be severely affected and there may be concomitant growth retardation. There is a positive correlation between the duration of steroid therapy and the degree of bone loss. Doses of prednisone as low as 8 to 10 mg per day have been associated with vertebral bone loss. While there is disagreement regarding the reversibility of demineralization, it may be reversible, in part, in children and young adults.[122]

The pathogenesis of steroid-induced osteoporosis is not well understood. Glucocorticoids inhibit bone formation, through a direct effect to inhibit osteoblast recruitment and activity. Steroids also reduce the efficiency of dietary calcium absorption. The mechanism of this effect is in question but might relate to direct actions on the intestinal epithelial cell to reduce cell division, stabilize cell membranes or decrease synthesis of calcium-binding protein. Antagonism of vitamin D metabolism has also been implicated. These effects are thought to contribute to a state of secondary hyperparathyroidism with increased osteoclastic bone resorption. The combination of increased bone resorption and decreased bone formation leads to particularly rapid and severe demineralization. Histomorphometric analyses of bone in situations of glucocorticoid excess have demonstrated either increased bone resorption or decreased turnover.[95] These discrepancies may be due to sampling at various times during the development of steroid-induced osteoporosis. Glucocorticoids may also increase urinary calcium excretion, due either to a direct effect upon renal handling of calcium or to increased bone resorption. Nephrolithiasis may occur occasionally.

Discontinuation of steroid therapy or successful treatment of Cushing's syndrome is the only effective approach. Particularly in individuals at high risk, attempts to prevent clinical osteoporosis should be instituted. If possible, the duration of glucocorticoid therapy should be minimized and the smallest effective dose should be prescribed. Alternate day therapy, if tolerated, may be useful, particularly in children. One approach might be to monitor patients with serial measurements of trabecular bone density (distal radius or vertebrae) at 3 to 6 month intervals and to institute therapy if significant bone loss occurs. Even if this approach is not possible, the use of calcium supplementation and vitamin D is reasonable in all such patients. Total calcium intake from dietary sources and supplements should be 1.5 g/day. Vitamin D should be prescribed in doses ranging from 1000 units/day to 50,000 units per week. While there is a theoretical basis for prescribing calcitriol, no data exist regarding its efficacy. However in a controlled study, 1 alpha-hydroxyvitamin D (2 μg/day), reduced serum PTH and urinary hydroxyproline excretion and increased calcium absorption and bone mass in patients receiving glucocorticoids.[123] The inhibitory effects of glucocorticoids may be counteracted by fluoride therapy. Since bone loss from glucocorticoids is additive with bone loss from other causes, other risk factors for osteoporosis should be sought and corrected. For example, excessive ingestion of ethanol should be discontinued. Estrogen therapy in the postmenopausal woman should be prescribed if no contraindications are present.

Thyroid Disease

Rarely, thyrotoxicosis may be associated with osteopenia that is indistinguishable from other forms of osteoporosis.[76] Bone loss is thought to be due to a direct effect of thyroid hormone to stimulate osteoclastic bone resorption. Since the coupling mechanism is presumably intact, bone formation has also been observed to be increased. However, the increased bone formation is insufficient to compensate for the loss.[124,125] Biochemically, hyperthyroidism may be characterized by mild hypercalcemia in approximately 10 percent of cases, hypercalciuria, increased urinary hydroxyproline excretion, and elevated levels of bone-derived plasma alkaline phosphatase. The skeletal changes in thyrotoxicosis rarely result in bone pain and fractures and, in general, should be regarded as a contributing factor to osteoporosis from other causes. Thus, older patients, particularly postmenopausal women, may be more severely affected. The bone loss may be reversible in younger patients but not in older ones.

In the elderly population with hypothyroidism, thyroid hormone replacement may have the undesirable effect of increasing bone loss.[76] The requirements for thyroid hormone replacement may decrease with advancing age;

excessive doses may further exacerbate the tendency to osteoporosis in the elderly.

Primary Hyperparathyroidism

The classic bone lesion of primary hyperparathyroidism is osteitis fibrosa cystica, observed today in less than 10 percent of affected patients. Evidence of increased bone turnover however is apparent histologically in up to 90 percent of patients with this disease (Chap. 4). Generalized skeletal demineralization, which has been reported in association with primary hyperparathyroidism, is thought to result when osteoclasic bone resorption exceeds formation of new bone. While this is most likely to occur in postmenopausal women, our experience has suggested that clinical osteoporosis with bone pain and fracture is uncommon in patients with primary hyperparathyroidism. Consistent with the view of this disorder as affecting cortical rather than trabecular bone, we have observed relative densitometric sparing of vertebral bone mineral density and marked decreases in single photon absorptiometry at the distal radius, a site with a much higher proportion of cortical bone than the vertebral column.

Acromegaly

Osteoporosis has been reported to occur in association with acromegaly.[127] However, it is unusual in the absence of concomitant hypogonadism. Fractures are rare. Biochemical changes include hyperphosphatemia, probably due to growth-hormone-mediated increased renal tubular absorption of phosphate, and hypercalciuria secondary to growth-hormone-induced increases in $1,25(OH)_2D$ production and intestinal calcium absorption. Radiographically, acromegaly is characterized by new periosteal bone formation and a characteristic increased concavity of the posterior surfaces of the vertebral bodies. Apparent cortical thinning in the long bones is due to enlargement of the marrow cavity. Histologic data obtained from eugonadal acromegalic patients suggest a high turnover state primarily involving cortical bone.

Hypogonadism

Both primary and secondary hypogonadism are associated with osteoporosis. In addition to the well-known skeletal effects of natural or surgical menopause, both Turner's syndrome and Klinefelter's syndrome are associated with a high incidence of osteoporosis.[44,128] Hypogonadotrophic hypogonadism, such as occurs with pituitary tumors or hypothalmic–pituitary dysfunction (exercise-induced amenorrhea, anorexia nervosa), also is associated with osteoporosis.[47–49] Where there are no contraindications, sex hormone replacement is recommended to prevent osteoporosis.

Hyperprolactinemia

Hyperprolactinemia can be associated with decreased bone mineral density at the distal radius and lumbar spine.[45,46] While some studies have suggested that this is due to the associated hypogonadism, others have implicated a direct effect of prolactin on bone.[129,130] It is not clear whether the osteopenia is reversible when the prolactin levels are lowered.[131,132]

Diabetes Mellitus

Reduced skeletal mass has been observed in patients with type I insulin-dependent diabetes mellitus. In patients with type II diabetes, increased bone mineral density independent of obesity has been reported.[92,133] Biochemical changes associated with diabetes include hypercalciuria that is related to glucose control. Plasma levels of calciotropic hormones are generally normal although a subtle deficiency in renal 1-alpha hydroxylation has been suggested by some studies. The clinical significance of these changes is unclear since there is no evidence of increased fracture risk in diabetic patients.[76]

Pregnancy and Lactation

Rarely, a rapidly progressive syndrome of osteoporosis, particularly involving the spine, may occur during pregnancy or lactation. The cause is unknown.[135] Despite average daily transfers of 200 mg of calcium to the fetus, compensation by the normal regulatory mechanisms to increase 1,25 $(OH)_2D$ synthesis, intestinal calcium absorption, and possibly calcitonin secretion occurs in normal pregnant women. The responses to the demands of lactation are not known but the maternal skeletal mass may increase during pregnancy to compensate. Thus patients who present with vertebral crush fracture during pregnancy or lactation are distinctly unusual. It has been postulated that they may have an underlying defect in mineral metabolism that is unmasked by the physiologic stress of pregnancy. However, since the syndrome is self-limiting and subsequent pregnancies may not be associated with fracture, other mechanisms must be operative.

Neoplastic Disease

Several malignant tumors, primarily of myeloid or lymphocytic cell lines, may be associated with bony involvement that can mimic the clinical and radiographic features of primary osteoporosis. Multiple myeloma is the most common. Vertebral crush fractures and, less frequently, fractures of the long bones may occur. Laboratory evaluation reveals anemia and abnormal serum or urine protein electrophoresis. On histomorphometry, markedly increased osteoclastic bone resorption and absent bone formation are seen. Production of osteoclast-activating factors (OAFs) by myeloma cells is thought to be responsible for the demineralization. Lymphotoxin, interleukin-1, tumor necrosis factor alpha, and prostaglandin E_2 have all been implicated as bone-resorbing principles.[135]

Patients with monocytic leukemia may develop osteoporosis. While a direct effect of the neoplasm upon bone is possible, these patients also demonstrate hypokalemia and elevated excretion of lysozyme. Lysozyme is thought to play a role in bone mineralization and hypokalemia may interfere with skeletal metabolism by lowering bone extracellular fluid potassium.[136] Diffuse bone carcinomatosis may also be associated with demineralization.

Systemic mastocytosis, in which there is diffuse infiltration of mast cells into the liver, spleen, gastrointestinal system, and bones, has also been associated with generalized demineralization. It is postulated that the heparin contained in mast cells may play a role in the development of osteoporosis, although a role for other mediators or cellular infiltration itself has not been excluded.[136]

Gastrointestinal Disease

Malabsorption syndromes, such as gluten-sensitive enteropathy, while perhaps better recognized as causes of osteomalacia (Chap. 5), are associated with osteoporosis in patients who are vitamin D replete from other sources (e.g., sunlight). Such individuals lack intestinal villi, the target organ for vitamin D, and severe calcium malabsorption may develop.

Subtotal gastrectomy, particularly the Billroth II operation, is associated with the development of osteomalacia in 5 to 10 percent of cases many years after the surgery.[137] A larger number of patients, particularly postmenopausal women and elderly men, develop accelerated bone loss. The mechanism may be due to calcium malabsorption, similar to that which may be associated with achlorhydria.

Lactase deficiency[138] is seen in older age persons. The resultant milk intolerance and calcium malabsorption may contribute to the development of osteoporosis in postmenopausal women and elderly men. Patients with lactase deficiency should receive calcium supplements.

Liver Disease

Chronic obstructive liver disease and parenchymal liver disease, probably because of derangements in vitamin D metabolism, lead to osteomalacia. However, some patients, particularly those with primary biliary cirrhosis, develop osteopenia and fractures due to osteoporosis.[139] Histomorphometric studies have demonstrated a low turnover state. The pathogenesis is not understood; the osteoporosis does not respond to treatment with vitamin D.

Drugs Causing Osteopenia

Corticosteroids

The effects of corticosteroids upon the skeleton have been discussed. Osteoporosis has been documented in patients receiving exogenous corticosteroids for a variety of chronic illnesses including asthma, skin conditions such as psoriasis, rheumatoid arthritis, ulcerative colitis, and Crohn's disease. It should be noted that the underlying medical condition may also play a role in the development of osteoporosis.

Chemotherapeutic Agents

Methotrexate and other antimetabolites may be associated with negative calcium balance and osteopenia.

Heparin

Long-term heparin administration (15,000 units or more daily for 6 months or longer) has been reported to cause rapidly progressive demineralization and an increase in fracture incidence.[141] The changes may be reversible with cessation of therapy. Heparin is a potent inhibitor of crystal aggregation and is also an activator of bone collagenase. Heparin-induced activation of lysosomal bone resorption or potentiation of PTH-mediated bone resorption could also account for the demineralization.

Ethanol

Chronic ingestion of ethanol has been associated with osteopenia and increased fracture incidence.[86] The cause of the osteopenia is probably multifactorial. Alcoholism is associated with poor nutritional habits, low dietary calcium intake, and altered hepatic metabolism of vitamin D. Ethanol-induced hypermagnesuria and concomitant hypomagnesemia could alter parathyroid hormone secretion. Moreover, hypogonadism is prevalent in alcoholic men. While all of these factors may have a negative impact upon the skeleton, there is also in vitro evidence for a direct toxic effect of alcohol on osteoblast function.[89] Moreover, well-nourished alcoholics without clinical or biochemical evidence of hepatic dysfunction or hypogonadism are at risk for osteoporosis. Histomorphometric studies in such men have shown a low turnover state.[88]

Miscellaneous Causes

Immobilization

Generalized immobilization results in rapid and diffuse bone loss.[80,81,136] For reasons that are unclear, there is a rapid increase in the rate of bone resorption and only a slight increase in bone formation. Biochemically, this form of high-turnover osteoporosis is characterized by increased urinary excretion of calcium and phosphorus, and, early in the course, mild hypercalcemia and hyperphosphatemia may develop. Levels of parathyroid hormone are decreased.[142] As much as 50 percent of the skeletal mass may be lost in a matter of months. The process is self-limited and may be partially reversible if weight bearing is resumed, although more time is required to restore bone than to lose it. In addition to lack of weight bearing, alterations in vascular, neurogenic, or humoral factors controlling blood flow are thought to be involved. Weight-bearing bones and those characterized by a large proportion of trabecular bone, such as vertebrae, are most severely affected. Paraplegic patients and children with spina bifida may be affected by associated ectopic calcification, particularly around the hips. Nephrolithiasis is also common. Exercises designed to encourage muscle use may retard the process of bone loss. Diphosphonates have been suggested as possible agents to inhibit bone resorption in these patients, but there are no long-term studies of their efficacy.

Rheumatoid Arthritis

Patients with rheumatoid arthritis may develop generalized osteopenia and fractures, even though they have never been treated with corticosteroids.[136] Periarticular trabecular bone is most severely affected, leading to the hypothesis that local inflammatory factors may stimulate bone resorption. Prolonged immobilization and corticosteroid therapy exacerbate this process.

Smoking

The role of cigarette smoking in osteoporosis has been discussed in the section on pathogenesis.[85,87] Smoking is associated with a higher relative risk of vertebral crush fracture in men.[86] Given the prevalence of smoking in the population, it may play a greater role than previously appreciated.[143]

REFERENCES

1. Dempster DW, Shane, E, Horbert, W, Lindsay, R: A simple method for correlative light and scanning electron microscopy of human iliac crest bone biopsies: qualitative observations in normal and osteoporotic subjects. J Bone Mineral Res 1:15, 1986
2. Riggs BL, Melton, LJ: Involutional osteoporosis. N Engl J Med 314:1676, 1986
3. Melton LJ, Riggs BL: Epidemiology of age-related fractures. p.45.In Avioli LV (ed): The Osteoporotic Syndrome. Grune & Stratton, Orlando, 1983
4. Cummings SR, Kelsey JL, Nevitt MC, O'Dowd KJ: Epidemiology of osteoporosis and osteoporotic fractures. Epidemiol Rev 7:178, 1985
5. Holbrook TL, Grazier K, Kelsey JL, et al: The Frequency of Occurrence, Impact, and Cost of Musculoskeletal Conditions in the United States. American Academy of Orthopedic Surgeons, Chicago, 1985

6. America in transition: an aging society. p.23. In: Current Population Reports. US Department of Commerce, Bureau of the Census. Series 128:3, 1983
7. Smith DM, Nance WE, Kang KW, et al: Genetic factors in determining bone mass. J Clin Invest 52:2800, 1973
8. Mazess RB: On aging bone loss. Clin Orthop 165:239, 1982
9. Cohn SH, Abesamis C, Yasumura S, et al: Comparative skeletal mass and radial bone mineral content in black and white women. Metabolism 26:171, 1977
10. Matkovic V, Kostial K, Simonovic I, et al: Bone status and fracture rates in two regions of Yugoslavia. Am J Clin Nutr 32:540, 1979
11. Nilsson BE, Westlin NE: Bone density in athletes. Clin Orthop 77:179, 1971
12. Dalen N, Olsson KE: Bone mineral content and physical activity. Acta Orthop Scand 45:170, 1974
13. Aloia JF, Cohn SH, Babu T, et al: Skeletal mass and body composition in marathon runners. Metabolism 27:1793, 1978
14. Consensus Conference: Osteoporosis. JAMA 232:799, 1984
15. Smith DM, Khairi MRA, Johnston CC, Jr: The loss of bone mineral with aging and its relationship to risk of fracture. J Clin Invest 56:311, 1975
16. Lindsay R, Hart DM, Forrest C, Baird C: Prevention of spinal osteoporosis in oophorectomized women. Lancet 2:1151, 1980
17. Riggs BL, Wahner HW, Dunn WL, et al: Differential changes in bone mineral density of the appendicular and axial skeleton with aging: relationship to spinal osteoporosis. J Clin Invest 67:328, 1981
18. Marcus R, Kosek J Pfefferbaum A, Horning S: Age-related loss of trabecular bone in premenopausal women: a biopsy study. Calcif Tissue Int 35:406, 1983
19. Cann CE, Genant HK, Kolb FO, Ettinger B: Quantitative computed tomography for prediction of vertebral fracture risk. Bone 6:1, 1985
20. Krolner B, Pors Nielsen S: Bone mineral content of the lumbar spine in normal and osteoporotic women: cross-sectional and longitudinal studies. Clin Sci 62:327, 1982
21. Genant HK, Cann CE, Ettinger B, Gordon GS: Quantitative computed tomography of vertebral spongiosa: a sensitive method for detecting early bone loss after oophorectomy. Ann Intern Med 97:699, 1982
22. Frost HM: Bone Remodeling and Its Relationship to Metabolic Bone Diseases. Charles C Thomas, Springfield, IL, 1973
23. Parfitt AM: Quantum concept of bone remodeling and turnover: implications for the pathogenesis of osteoporosis. Calcif Tissue Int 28:1, 1979
24. Parfitt AM: The coupling of bone formation to bone resorption: a critical analysis of the concept and of its relevance to the pathogenesis of osteoporosis. Metab Bone Dis Rel Res 4:1, 1982
25. Bullamore JR, Gallagher JC, Wilkinson R, et al: Effect of age on calcium absorption. Lancet 2:535, 1970
26. Alevizaki CC, Ikkos DG, Singhelakis P: Progressive decrease of true intestinal calcium absorption with age in normal man. J Nucl Med 14:760, 1973
27. Gallagher JC, Riggs BL, Eisman J, et al: Intestinal calcium absorption and serum vitamin D metabolites in normal subjects and osteoporotic patients: effect of age and dietary calcium. J Clin Invest 64:729, 1979
28. Manolagas SC, Culler FL, Howard JE, et al. The cytoreceptor assay for 1,25-dihydroxyvitamin D and its application to clinical studies. J Clin Endocrinol Metab 56:751, 1983
29. Tsai K-S, Heath H III, Kumar R, Riggs BL: Impaired vitamin D metabolism with

aging in women: possible role in pathogenesis of senile osteoporosis. J Clin Invest 73:1668, 1984
30. Slovik DM, Adams JS, Neer RM, et al: Deficient production of 1,25-dihydroxyvitamin D in elderly osteoporotic patients. N Engl J Med 305:372, 1981
31. Riggs BL, Hamstra A, DeLuca HF: Assessment of 25-hydroxyvitamin D alpha-hydroxylase reserve in postmenopausal osteoporosis by administration of parathyroid extract. J Clin Endocrinol Metab 53:833, 1981
32. Sorenson OH, Lumholtz B, Lund B, et al: Acute effects of parathyroid hormone on vitamin D metabolites in patients with the bone loss of aging. J Clin Endocrinol Metab 54:1258, 1982
33. Heaney RP, Gallagher JC, Johnston CC, Jr., et al: Calcium nutrition and bone health in the elderly. Am J Clin Nutr 36:986, 1982
34. Gallagher JC, Riggs BL, Jerpbak CM, Arnaud CD: The effect of age on serum immunoreactive parathyroid hormone in normal and osteoporotic women. J Lab Clin Med 95:373, 1980
35. Wiske PS, Epstein S, Bell NH, et al: Increases in immunoreactive parathyroid hormone with age. N Engl J Med 300:1419, 1979
36. Marcus R, Madvig P, Young G: Age-related changes in parathyroid hormone and parathyroid hormone action in normal humans. J Clin Endocrinol Metab 58:223, 1984
37. Insogna KL, Lewis AM, Lipinski BA, et al: Effect of age on serum immunoreactive parathyroid hormone and its biological effects. J Clin Endocrinol Metab 63:1072, 1981
38. Silverberg SJ, Shane E, Clemens TL, et al: The effect of phosphate on major indices of skeletal metabolism in normal subjects. J Bone Mineral Res 4:383, 1986
39. Heaney RP, Recker RR, Saville PD: Menopausal changes in calcium balance. J Lab Clin Med 92:953, 1978
40. Parfitt AM, Matthews C, Rao D, et al: Impaired osteoblast function in metabolic bone disease. p.321. In DeLuca HF, Frost H, Jee W, et al (eds): Osteoporosis: Recent Advances in Pathogenesis and Treatment. University Park Press, Baltimore, 1981
41. Lips P, Coupron P, Meunier PJ: Mean wall thickness of trabecular bone packets in human iliac crest: changes with age. Calcif Tissue Res 26:13, 1978
42. Richelson LS, Wahner HW, Melton LJ, et al: Relative contributions of aging and estrogen deficiency to postmenopausal bone loss. N Engl J Med 311:1273, 1984
43. Albright F, Bloomberg F, Smith PH: Postmenopausal osteoporosis. Trans Assoc Am Physicians 55:298, 1940
44. Shore RM, Chesney RW, Mazess RB, et al: Skeletal demineralization in Turner's syndrome. Calcif Tissue Int 34:519, 1982
45. Klibanski A, Neer RM, Bettins IZ, et al: Decreased bone density in hyperprolactinemic women. N Engl J Med 303:1511, 1980
46. Koppelman MCS, Kurtz DW, Morrish KA, et al: Vertebral body bone mineral content in hyperprolactinemic women. J Clin Endocrinol Metab 59:1050, 1984
47. Rigotti NA, Nussbaum SR, Herzog DB, et al: Osteoporosis in women with anorexia nervosa. N Engl J Med 311:1601, 1984
48. Drinkwater BL, Nilson K, Chestnut CH III, et al: Bone mineral content of amenorrheic and eumenorrheic athletes. N Engl J Med 311:277, 1984
49. Marcus R, Cann C, Madvig P, et al: Menstrual function and bone mass in elite woman distance runners. Ann Intern Med 102:158, 1985

50. Weiss NS, Ure CL, Ballard JH, et al: Decreased risk of fractures of the hip and lower forearm with postmenopausal use of estrogen. N Engl J Med 303:1195, 1980
51. Hutchinson TA, Polansky JM, Feinstein AR: Postmenopausal oestrogens protect against fracture of the hip and distal radius. Lancet 2:705, 1979
52. Krieger M, Kelsey JL, Holford TR: An epidemiological study of hip fracture in postmenopausal women. Am J Epidemiol 116:141, 1982
53. Ettinger B, Genant HK, Cann CE: Long-term estrogen replacement therapy prevents bone loss and fractures. Ann Intern Med 102:319, 1985
54. Davidson BJ, Ross RK, Perganini-Hill A, et al: Total and free estrogens and androgens in postmenopausal women with hip fracture. J Clin Endocrinol Metab 54:115, 1982
55. Riis BJ, Christiansen C, Deftos LJ, Catherwood BD: The role of serum concentrations of estrogens on postmenopausal osteoporosis and bone turnover. p.333. In Christiansen C, Arnaud CD, Nordin BEC, et al (eds): Osteoporosis. Aalborg Stifsbogtrykkeri, Denmark, 1984.
56. Johnston CC, Jr., Hui SL, Witt R, et al: Early menopausal changes in bone mass and sex steroids. J Clin Endocrinol Metab 61:905, 1985
57. Nisker JA, Hammond GL, Davidson BJ: Serum sex-hormone-binding capacity and the percentage of free estradiol in postmenopausal women with and without endometrial carcinoma: a new biochemical basis for the association between obesity and endometrial carcinoma. Am J Obstet Gynecol 138:637, 1980
58. Siiteri PK, Macdonald PC: Role of extraglandular estrogen in human endocrinology. p.615. Handbook of Physiology. Section 7, Volume II (Part I). American Physiology Society, Washington, DC, 1973
59. Nutick G, Cruess RL: Estrogen receptors in bone. Proc R Soc Exp Biol Med 146:265, 1974
60. Chen TL, Feldman D: Distinction between alpha-feta protein and intracellular estrogen receptors Endocrinology 102:236, 1978
61. Komm BS, Sheetz, L, Baker M, et al: Bone related cells in culture express putative estrogen receptor mRNA and ^{125}I-17beta-estradiol binding. J Bone Mineral Res 2:suppl 237A, 1987
62. Eriksen EF, Berg NJ, Graham ML, et al: Evidence of estrogen receptors in human bone cells. J. Bone Mineral Res 2:suppl 238A, 1987
63. Stern PH: Inhibition by steroids of parathyroid hormone-induced Ca^{45} release from embryonic rat bone in vitro. J Pharmacol Exp Ther 168:211, 1969
64. Canalis E, Raisz LG: Effect of sex steroids on bone collagen synthesis in vitro. Calcif Tiss Res 25:105, 1978
65. Heath H III, Sizemore GW; Plasma calcitonin in normal man: differences between men and women. J Clin Invest 60:1135, 1977
66. Deftos LJ, Weisman MH, Williams GW, et al: Influence of age and sex on plasma calcitonin in human beings. N Engl J Med 302:1351, 1980
67. Body J-J, Heath H III: Estimates of circulating monomeric calcitonin: physiological studies in normal and thyroidectomized man. J Clin Endocrinol Metab 57:897, 1983
68. Hurley DL, Tiegs RD, Wahner HW, Heath H III: Axial and appendicular bone mineral density in patients with long-term deficiency or excess of calcitonin. N Engl J Med 317:537, 1987
69. Heaney RP, Recker RR: Distribution of calcium absorption in middle-aged women. Am J Clin Nutr 43:299, 1986
70. Malm OJ: Calcium requirement and adaptation in adult men. Scand J Clin Lab Invest 10 (suppl 36):1, 1958

71. Neer RM: Calcium and inorganic phosphate homeostasis. p.699. In DeGroot LJ et al (eds): Endocrinology. Vol 2. Grune & Stratton, Orlando, 1979
72. Omdahl JL, Garry PJ, Hunsaker LA, et al: Nutritional status in a healthy elderly population: vitamin D. Am J Clin Nutr 36:1225, 1982
73. Nilas L, Christiansen C, Rodbro P: Calcium supplementation and postmenopausal bone loss. Br Med J 289:1103, 1984
74. Christiansen C, Riis BJ, Thomsen K: Does calcium treatment prevent postmenopausal bone loss? A double-blind controlled clinical trial. J Bone Mineral Res 1 (suppl 1):166, 1986
75. Heaney RP, Recker RR: Effects of nitrogen, phosphorus and caffeine on calcium balance in women. J Lab Clin Med 99:46, 1982
76. Tohme JT, Lindsay R: Osteoporosis. In Becker KL (ed): Principles and Practice of Endocrinology and Metabolism. JB Lippincott, Philadelphia, 1987
77. Moller M, Horsman A, Harrald B, et al: Metacarpal morphometry in monozygotic and dizygotic elderly twins. Calcif Tissue Res 26:197, 1978
78. Cave W, Nordin BEC: p.357. In Nordin BEC (ed): Calcium, Phosphate and Magnesium Metabolism. Churchill Livingstone, New York, 1976
79. Bell NH, Greene A, Epstein S, et al: Evidence for alteration of the vitamin D-endocrine system in blacks. J Clin Invest 76:470, 1985
80. Krolner B, Toft B: Vertebral bone loss: an unheeded side-effect of therapeutic bed rest. Clin Sci 64:537, 1983
81. Mazess RB, Whedon JD: Immobilization and bone. Calcif Tissue Int 35:265, 1983
82. Whedon GD, Lutwak L, Reid J, et al: Mineral and nitrogen metabolic studies on Skylab orbital space flights. Trans Assoc Am Physicians 87:95, 1974
83. Aloia JF, Cohn SH, Ostuni JA, et al: Prevention of involutional bone loss by exercise. Ann Intern Med 89:356, 1978
84. Smith EL, Reddan W, Smith PE: Physical activity and calcium modalities for bone mineral increase in aged women. Med Sci Sports Exercise 13:60, 1981
85. Daniell HW: Osteoporosis of the slender smoker: vertebral compression fractures and loss of metacarpal cortex in relation to postmenopausal smoking and lack of obesity. Arch Intern Med 13:298, 1976
86. Seaman E, Melton LJ III, O'Fallon WM, Riggs BL: Risk factors for spinal osteoporosis in men. Am J Med 75:977, 1983
87. Williams AR, Weiss NS, Ure Cl. et al: Effect of weight, smoking and estrogen use on the risk of hip and forearm fractures in postmenopausal women. Obstet Gynecol 60:695, 1982
88. Bikle DD, Genant HK, Cann C, et al: Bone disease in alcohol abuse. Ann Intern Med 103:42, 1985
89. Farley JR, Fitzsimmons R, Taylor AK, et al: Direct effects of ethanol on bone resorption and formation in vitro. Arch Biochem Biophys 238:305, 1985
90. Baran DT, Teitelbaum SL, Bergfeld MA, et al: Effect of alcohol ingestion on bone and mineral metabolism in rats. Am J Physiol 238:E507, 1980
91. Wasnich RD, Benfante RJ, Yano K, et al: Thiazide effect on the mineral content of bone. N Engl J Med 309:344, 1983
92. Weinstock RS, Goland RS, Shane E, et al: Increased bone mineral density in women with non-insulin dependent diabetes mellitus. J Bone Mineral Res Suppl I, 227A, 1986
93. Riggs BL, Melton LJ III: Evidence for two distinct syndromes of involutional osteoporosis. Am J Med 75:899, 1983
94. Nordin BEC: Osteoporosis with particular reference to the menopause. p.13. In

Avioli LV(ed): The Osteoporotic Syndrome. Detection, Prevention and Treatment. Grune & Stratton, Orlando, 1983

95. Dempster DW, Shane E: Bone quantification and dynamics of bone turnover by histomorphometric analysis. In Becker KL (ed): Principles and Practice of Endocrinology and Metabolism. JB Lippincott, Philadelphia, 1987
96. Downs RW, Jr., Levine MA: Hypoparathyroidism and other causes of hypocalcemia. In Becker KL (ed): Principles and Practice of Endocrinology and Metabolism. JB Lippincott, Philadelphia, 1987
97. Chestnut CH: Synthetic salmon calcitonin, diphosphonates and anabolic steroids in the treatment of postmenopausal osteoporosis. p. 549. In Christiansen C, et al (eds): Osteoporosis. Aalborg Stiftsbogtrykkeri, Copenhagen, 1984
98. Jensen GF, Meinecke B, Boesen J, et al: Does 1,25 $(OH)_2D_3$ accelerate spinal bone loss? A controlled therapeutic trial in a 70 year old woman. Clin Orthop 192:215, 1985
99. Riggs BL: Treatment of osteoporosis with sodium fluoride: an appraisal. p.366. In Peck WA (ed): Bone and Mineral Research, Annual 2: A Yearly Survey of Developments in the Field of Bone and Mineral. Elsevier Science Publishing, New York, 1984
100. Riggs BL, Baylink DJ, Kleerekoper M, et al: Incidence of hip fractures in osteoporotic women treated with sodium fluoride. J Bone Mineral Res 2:123, 1987
101. Chestnut CH, Ivey J, Gruber HE, et al: Stanozolol in postmenopausal osteoporosis: therapeutic efficacy and possible mechanism of action. Metabolism 32:571, 1983
102. Reeve J, Meunier PJ, Parsons JA, et al: Anabolic effects of human parathyroid hormone fragments on trabecular bone in involutional osteoporosis: a multi-center trial. Br Med J 280:1340, 1980
103. Slovik DM, Neer RM, Potts JT, Jr: Short-term effects of synthetic human parathyroid hormone-(1-34) administration on bone mineral metabolism in osteoporotic patients. J Clin Invest 68:1261, 1981
104. Frost HM: Treatment of osteoporosis by manipulation of coherent bone cell populations. Clin Orthop 142:227, 1979
105. Riggs, BL, Nelson KI: Effect of long-term treatment with calcitriol on calcium absorption and mineral metabolism in postmenopausal osteoporosis. J Clin Endocrinol Metab 61:457, 1985
106. Transbol I, Christenson MS, Jensen GF, et al: Thiazide for the postponement of postmenopauseal bone loss. Metabolism 31:383, 1982
107. Russell RGG, Fleisch H: Pyrophosphate and diphosphonates in skeletal metabolism: physiological, clinical and therapeutic aspects. Clin Orthop 108: 241, 1975
108. Sorenson O, Storm T, Tramsborg G: The effect of Didronel therapy in postmenopausal osteoporotic women. J Bone Mineral Res 2:Suppl 1, 226A, 1987
109. Teotia M, Teotia SPS, Singh RK: Idiopathic juvenile osteoporosis. Am J Dis Child 133:894, 1979
110. Whyte MP: Rare disorders of skeletal homeostasis. In Becker KL (ed): Principles and Practice of Endocrinology and Metabolism. JB Lippincott, Philadelphia, 1987
111. Hoekman J, Papapoulos SE, Peters ACB, Bijvoet OLM: Characteristics and bisphosphonate treatment of a patient with juvenile osteoporosis. J Clin Endocrinol Metab 61:952, 1985
112. Perry HM III, Fallon MD, Birkfeld M: Osteoporosis in young men. Arch Intern Med 142:1295, 1982
113. Jackson WPU: Osteoporosis of unknown cause in young people. J Bone Joint Surg 403:420, 1958

114. Finkelstein JS, Klibanski A, Neer RM, et al: Osteoporosis in men with idiopathic hypogonadotropic hypogonadism. Ann Intern Med 106:354, 1987
115. Francis RM, Peacock M, Aaron JE, et al: Osteoporosis in hypogonadal men: role of decreased plasma 1,25 dihydroxyvitamin D, calcium malabsorption, and low bone formation. Bone 7:261, 1986
116. Kozin F, Genant H, Bekerman C, McCarty DJ: The reflex sympathetic dystrophy syndrome: II. Roentgenographic and scintigraphic evidence of bilaterality and periarticular accentuation. Am J Med 60:332, 1976
117. Valenzuela F, Aris H, Jacobelli S: Transient osteoporosis of the hip.J Rheumatol 4:59, 1977
118. McCord WC, Niesk M, Campion DS, Lowie JS: Regional migratory osteoporosis. Arthritis Rheum 10:363, 1973
119. Garn SM, Poznanski AK: Transient and irreversible bone losses. p.114. In Barzel US (ed): Osteoporosis. Grune & Stratton, Orlando, 1970
120. Baylink DJ: Glucocorticoid-induced osteoporosis. N Engl J Med 309:306, 1983
121. Avioli LV: Effects of chronic corticosteroid therapy on mineral metabolism and calcium absorption. Adv Exp Med Biol 171:81, 1984
122. Pocock NA, Eisman JA, Dunstan CR, et al: Recovery from steroid-induced osteoporosis. Ann Intern Med 107:319, 1987
123. Braun JJ, Birkenhager-Frenkel DH, Rietvald AH: Influence of 1-alpha-hydroxyvitamin D administration on bone and mineral metabolism in patients with chronic glucocorticoid treatment. Clin Endocrinol 18:265, 1980
124. Eriksen EF, Mosekilde L, Melsen F: Trabecular bone remodeling and bone balance in hyperthyroidism. Bone 6:421, 1985
125. Coindre JM, David JP, Riviere L, et al: Bone loss in hypothyroidism with hormone replacement: A histomorphometric study. Arch Intern Med 146:48, 1986
126. Fallon MD, Perry HM, Bergfield M, et al: Exogenous hyperthyroidism with osteoporosis. Arch Intern Med 143:442, 1983
127. Riggs, BL, Randall RV, Wahner HW, et al: The nature of the metabolic bone disorder in acromegaly. J Clin Endocrinol Metab 34:911, 1972
128. Smith DAS, Walker MS: Changes in plasma steroids and bone density in Klinefelter's syndrome. Calcif Tissue Int 22 (Suppl):225, 1977
129. Schlechte JA, Sherman B, Martin R: Bone density in amenorrheic women with and without hyperprolactinemia. J Clin Endocrinol Metab 56:1120, 1983
130. Kumar R, Abboub CF, Riggs BL: The effect of elevated prolactin levels on plasma 1,25 dihydroxyvitamin D and intestinal absorption of calcium. Mayo Clin Proc 55:51, 1980
131. Klibanski A, Greenspan SL: Increase in bone mass after treatment of hyperprolactinemic amenorrhea. N Engl J Med 315:542, 1986
132. Schlechte J, El-Khoury G, Kathol M, Walkner L: Forearm and vertebral bone mineral in treated and untreated hyperprolactinemic amenorrhea. J Clin Endocrinol Metab 64:1021, 1987
133. Johnston CC Jr, Hui SL, Longcope C: Bone mass and sex steroid concentration in postmenopausal Caucasian diabetics. Metabolism 34:544, 1985
134. Smith R, Stevenson JC, Winearls JC, et al: Osteoporosis of pregnancy. Lancet 1:1178, 1985
135. Mundy GR, Ibbotson KJ, D'Souza SM, et al: The hypercalcemia of malignancy: clinical implications and pathogenic mechanisms. N Engl J Med 310:1718, 1984
136. Russell RGG: Osteoporosis. p.873. In DeGroot, LJ et al (eds): Endocrinology. Vol 2. Grune & Stratton, Orlando, 1979

137. Rao SD, Kleerekoper M, Rogers M, et al: Is gastrectomy a risk factor for osteoporosis. p. 775. In Christiansen C, Arnaud CD, Nordin BEC, et al. (eds): Osteoporosis. Aalborg Stifsbogtrykkeri, Copenhagen, 1984
138. Newcomer AD, Hodgson SF, McGill DB, Thomas BJ: Lactase deficiency: prevalence in osteoporosis. Ann Intern Med 89:218, 1978
139. Hodgson SF, Dickson ER, Wahner HW, et al: Bone loss and reduced osteoblast function in primary biliary cirrhosis. Ann Intern Med 103:855, 1985
140. Weinblatt ME: Toxicity of low-dose methotrexate in rheumatoid arthritis. J Rheumatol 12 (supp 12) 35, 1985
141. Avioli LV: Heparin-induced osteopenia. p. 375. In Bradshaw RA: Wessler S (eds): Heparin: Structure, Function and Clinical Implications. Plenum, New York, 1975
142. Stewart AF, Adler M, Byers CM, et al: Calcium homeostasis in immobilization: an example of resorptive hypercalciuria. N Engl J Med 306:1136, 1982
143. The Health Consequences of Smoking for Women: A Report of the Surgeon General. US Dept of Health and Human Services, Public Health Service, Office on Smoking and Health, DHHS Publication No (PHS) 81-50156, p 17–63, 1981

8 Bone Disease with Renal Insufficiency and During Total Parenteral Nutrition

Isidro B. Salusky
Jack W. Coburn

Over the last two decades certain technical advances in the domains of nephrology and gastroenterology have markedly altered the management and survival of many patients. The widespread use of dialysis for patients with renal failure and the establishment of long-term treatment with total parenteral nutrition (TPN) are also responsible for the appearance of new syndromes in patients whose lives are now prolonged. Indeed, renal osteodystrophy has become prevalent in patients treated for prolonged periods with maintenance dialysis. Also, bone disease has become prevalent in patients treated with long term TPN. This chapter describes the bone diseases that are seen in patients with renal failure and in those receiving long-term treatment with TPN.

RENAL OSTEODYSTROPHY

The term *renal osteodystrophy* is used in a global sense to include all the skeletal syndromes and alterations of mineral metabolism associated with progressive renal failure. The kidneys play a central role in the equilibrium of mineral metabolism. They maintain the external balance of calcium, phosphorus, and magnesium; they synthesize 1,25-dihydroxyvitamin D_3 ($1,25(OH)_2D_3$) and 24-25-dihydroxyvitamin D_3; they act as a major target organ for the action of parathyroid hormone (PTH); and they serve as a major organ for the degradation and clearance of PTH from the circulation. Also, certain elements, such as aluminum, are mainly excreted through the kidneys; with renal failure, these substances accumulate in the body and can be associated with altered mineral homeostasis.[1] Thus, it is not surprising that progressive reduction of nephron function is associated with altered mineral metabolism. In this chapter, the pathogenesis, histologic features, clinical symptoms, radiologic characteristics, prevention, and treatment of renal osteodystrophy are reviewed.

Pathogenesis

The two major hormones that regulate calcium homeostasis are PTH and the active form of vitamin D_3, calcitriol or $1,25(OH)_2D_3$. In addition, aluminum toxicity reduces the release of PTH by the parathyroid gland and causes impaired bone mineralization. Also, phosphate retention and hyperphosphatemia are important both because they can directly lower the serum calcium levels and because hyperphosphatemia directly potentiates the precipitation of extraskeletal calcifications. Thus, PTH, hyperphosphatemia, $1,25(OH)_2D_3$, and aluminum accumulation are major known factors involved in the pathogenesis of the bone diseases that appear in patients with end-stage renal failure. The spectrum of bone disease can range from a high-turnover bone disease, with elevated PTH levels being the major driving force, to low-turnover bone disease, which arises mainly secondary to aluminum accumulation. These pathogenic factors and the interplay between them are considered below.

Secondary Hyperparathyroidism (High-Turnover Bone Disease)

One factor leading to PTH secretion and parathyroid hyperplasia is perfusion of the parathyroid glands with blood containing low levels of ionized calcium; such hypocalcemia has been thought to be responsible for the development of secondary hyperparathyroidism with the appearance of renal failure. The factors that contribute to hypocalcemia include phosphate retention and hyperphosphatemia, diminished synthesis of $1,25(OH)_2D_3$, and skeletal resistance to the calcemic action of parathyroid hormone.[1]

In vitro studies of cells from normal parathyroid glands have shown that the half-maximal inhibition of PTH release by an increase in ionized calcium concentration, or the "set point," occurs at a calcium concentration of 1.03 mM/L. When the same studies were performed using parathyroid cells obtained from uremic patients, the "set point" was higher than 1.03 mM/L.[2,3] The implication is that a higher serum calcium level is needed to suppress PTH secretion in uremic patients. The mechanism involved in the change in the "set point" is not known, but a change in the adenylate cyclase activity in the hyperplastic parathyroid gland of uremic patients could be one factor.[4] Also, the number of receptors for $1,25(OH)_2D_3$ in the parathyroid gland from uremic patients is diminished.[5] These abnormalities may play a role in the development of the abnormal "set point." These studies have been performed in patients treated with maintenance hemodialysis, and further studies are needed to clarify the role of altered numbers of receptors for $1,25(OH)_2D_3$ in the early development of renal failure.

Another factor that affects PTH secretion by the parathyroid glands is hyperplasia with an increased mass of parathyroid glands. Varying degrees of hyperplasia are important in causing clinically overt secondary hyperparathyroidism in chronic renal failure, and the parathyroid glands may be increased up to 100 times the normal size. The study of the pathogenesis of hyperplasia of the parathyroid glands is more difficult to characterize than the evaluation of PTH secretion by individual cells, per se. However, hyperplasia is very important in that it regresses only very slowly if at all after its causes have been reversed, largely due to the longevity of the parathyroid cells. The presence of hyperplasia adds greatly to the hypersecretion of PTH that occurs from individual parathyroid cells due to the change in the "set point." Moreover, some basal PTH secretion by the parathyroid glands persists even in the presence, of hypercalcemia; thus, such hyperplasia can lead to elevation of PTH levels even in the presence of substantial hypercalcemia.

The role of phosphate retention in causing hypocalcemia as a pathogenic factor in secondary hyperparathyroidism in patients with renal failure is well appreciated.[1,6] The important role of dietary phosphate intake in the development of secondary hyperparathyroidism with advanced renal failure has been documented in studies with dogs. When "uremic" dogs are fed a diet reduced in phosphate content in proportion to the decrease in glomerular filtration rate, the secondary hyperparathyroidism is markedly diminished over a 2-year period. On the other hand, severe and progressive secondary hyperparathyroidism develops in animals fed a normal-phosphate diet.[6] The mechanism by which phosphate retention stimulates PTH is not well understood. The original suggestion that hypocalcemia arose directly from the increase of serum phosphorus levels and that this was responsible for the elevation of serum PTH levels has recently been revised. It is now thought that phosphate retention is directly responsible for reduced production of $1,25(OH)_2D_3$, thereby leading to decreased absorption of calcium from the diet with resultant hypocalcemia.

Patients with advanced renal failure usually have low or even undetectable serum calcitriol levels. In adult patients with mild to moderate renal failure, the serum calcitriol levels have been reported to be normal or slightly reduced.[7,8] In children with moderate renal failure, the mean levels of $1,25(OH)_2D_3$ were slightly low compared to age-matched controls[7]; however, the levels of calcitriol increased significantly (and the serum iPTH decreased) when these children were fed a low-phosphate diet.[9] Similar findings have been reported in adult patients with mild renal failure.[10]

Recent experimental studies in dogs with severe renal failure indicate that hypocalcemia, per se, might not be necessarily involved in the genesis of secondary hyperparathyroidism.[11] Instead, low levels of $1,25(OH)_2D_3$, independent of changes in serum calcium level, may contribute to the oversecretion of PTH.[11] Nonetheless, phosphate restriction may prevent the development of secondary hyperparathyroidism without any changes in the serum calcitriol levels of uremic dogs,[12] an observation suggesting that dietary phosphate may have a direct effect on the secretion of PTH.

Skeletal resistance to the calcemic action of PTH contributes to the hypocalcemia and secondary hyperparathyroidism present in renal failure. The calcemic response to a standardized infusion of parathyroid extract is subnormal in patients with moderate and advanced renal failure. Moreover, the recovery from induced hypocalcemia is delayed and blunted despite a greater increment in serum PTH in patients with mild renal insufficiency compared to the response in normal individuals.[13,14] The mechanisms responsible for the reduced calcemic response to PTH are not understood, and different factors, including alterations of vitamin D metabolism, "uremic toxins," disorders of PTH metabolism, and altered PTH receptors, have been postulated.

Low-Turnover Bone Disease (Osteomalacia/Aplastic Bone Disease)

The pathogenesis of osteomalacia in patients with advanced renal failure and those treated with maintenance dialysis has changed substantially since the original description of patients from China and the United Kingdom.[15,16] Low serum levels of 25(OH)-vitamin D were predictive of the presence of osteomalacia in patients with stable renal failure in England. However, more recent studies from the United States have not demonstrated a relationship between serum levels of vitamin D and osteomalacia; this is probably related to greater exposure to sunlight and more supplementation of foods with vitamin D in the United States.

Long-term treatment with phenytoin, phenobarbital, or both has been associated with the development of osteomalacia in nonrenal patients. A higher incidence of symptomatic bone disease has been reported in dialysis patients who were treated with barbiturates and phenytoin compared to dialysis patients who did not receive these drugs.[17]

As recently as 1980, little was known about the biologic consequences of aluminum accumulation in patients with renal failure.[18] Presently, aluminum accumulation is the leading cause of the vitamin-D-resistant osteomalacia or aplastic bone disease occurring in uremic patients. Epidemiologic studies in dialyzed patients showed a strong correlation between the incidence of both osteomalacia and a neurologic syndrome, termed "dialysis encephalopathy," and the aluminum concentrations in the water used to prepare dialysate solutions.[19–21] These syndromes have become much less frequent with the introduction of water purification in dialysis centers.[21] However, both dialysis encephalopathy and aluminum-related bone disease have been described in occasional adult and pediatric patients with renal failure prior to the initiation of dialysis.[22–28] The aluminum content of the aluminum-containing, phosphate-binding agents, which are widely used to control hyperphosphatemia and secondary hyperparathyroidism in dialysis patients, is a major source for aluminum accumulation in such patients. Indeed, a close correlation was found between plasma aluminum levels, which reflect the recent load of aluminum, and the daily dosage of aluminum in the phosphate-binding agents[29] (Fig. 8-1). After aluminum-containing gels have been discontinued and replaced by alternative agents, the plasma aluminum levels have decreased significantly in dialysis patients [30–32] (Fig. 8-2). Such observations suggest that the oral route is a major source of aluminum accumulation in dialysis patients despite proper water purification to prepare dialysate.

There are strong epidemiologic associations between aluminum-contaminated water and the occurrence of low-turnover bone disease. Moreover, the administration of aluminum can produce either osteomalacia or an aplastic lesion experimentally.[33–37] It has been argued that aluminum accumulation may be merely an epiphenomenon in the development of osteomalacia in a model with vitamin D deficiency.[38] However, there are several important differences between the osteomalacia of vitamin D deficiency and that arising from aluminum accumulation; thus, the relevance of these observations to the disease observed in patients with renal failure is not obvious.

The mechanism whereby aluminum acts on bone is not understood. The identification of aluminum along the mineralization front in biopsies of affected

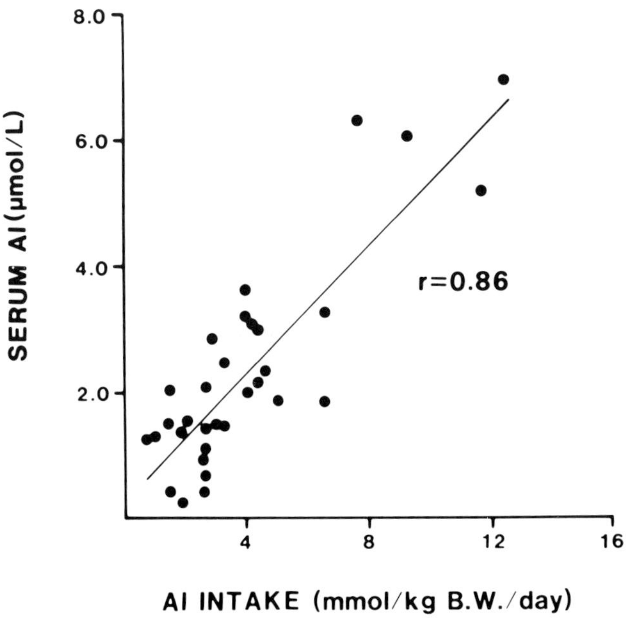

Fig. 8-1 The relation between serum aluminum levels and the oral intake of aluminum hydroxide in children treated with CAPD. (From Salusky, et al.,[29] with permission.)

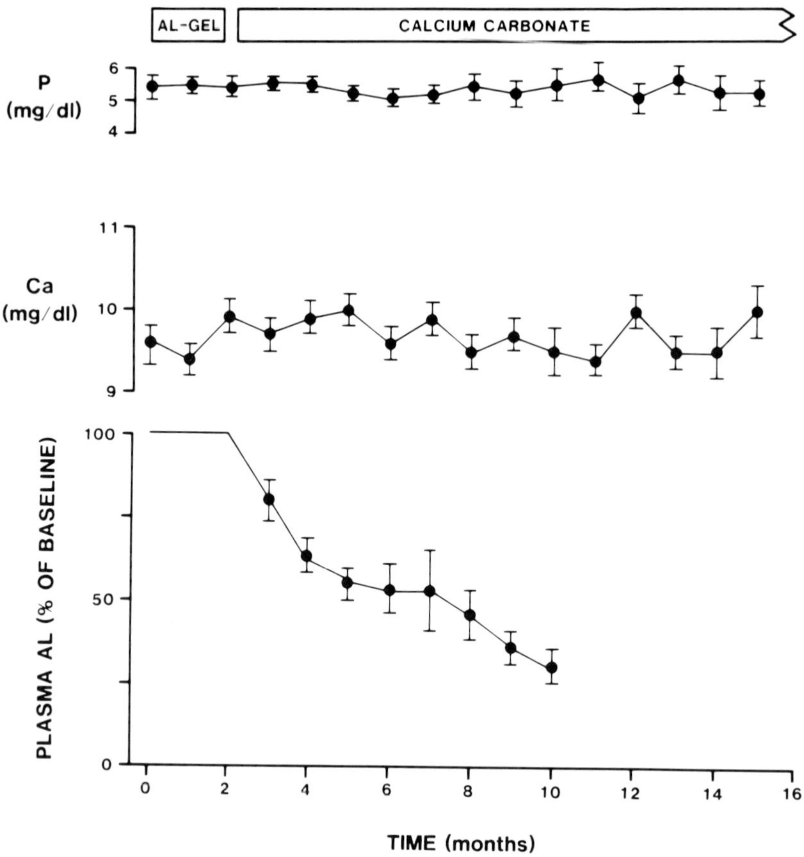

Fig. 8-2 Serial changes in serum phosphorus, calcium, and aluminum levels in patients treated with hemodialysis when aluminum hydroxide gels (AL-GEL) were replaced by calcium carbonate. Data are mean ± SE. (From Hercz, et al.,[32] with permission.)

cases has suggested that aluminum may prevent the mineralization of bone, and data from in vitro studies indicate that aluminum can prevent both the generation and growth of hydroxyapatite crystals.[39] Other studies suggest that aluminum citrate may inhibit crystal formation.[40] Furthermore, aluminum can inhibit the activity of the osteoblast, with decreased alkaline phosphatase activity and lower calcium uptake.[41,42]

Certain risk factors are more prevalent in patients with aluminum-related bone disease than in those with other types of bone disease. These include: previous parathyroidectomy,[43,44] earlier renal transplantation that has failed, bilateral nephrectomy, and the presence of diabetes mellitus.[45] High levels of PTH may "protect" from the development of osteomalacia when there is substantial aluminum loading.[33] After parathyroidectomy, the reduction of PTH levels leads to diminished bone formation rate, thereby predisposing to the surface accumulation of aluminum.[43,44]

Clinical Manifestations

The symptoms and signs of renal osteodystrophy are usually nonspecific, and the laboratory and radiographic abnormalities can sometimes predict the clinical manifestations. Among the symptoms and signs noted are bone pain, muscle weakness, skeletal deformities, and growth retardation.

Bone Pain

Bone pain is a common manifestation of severe bone disease in patients with renal osteodystrophy. Its appearance is insidious and often exacerbated by weight-bearing or a change in posture. The physical examination is often negative. Pain is most common in the lower back, hips, and legs, but it can also occur in the peripheral sites. In some instances, the pain presents as an acute arthritis or periarthritis that is not relieved by massage or local heat. Bone pain tends to be more common in patients with aluminum-related bone disease than in those with osteitis fibrosa, but there is marked variability from one patient to another.

Muscle Weakness

Patients with advanced renal failure may develop proximal myopathy, with symptoms appearing very slowly. The pathogenesis of the myopathy is multifactorial, and several different therapeutic interventions have been associated with substantial clinical improvement. Among the treatments with beneficial effects are treatment with $25(OH)D_3$ or $1,25(OH)_2D_3$, parathyroidectomy, successful renal transplantation, and chelation of aluminum with deferoxamine. Improvement of gait posture has been reported in children with moderate renal failure after treatment with $1,25(OH)_2D_3$, but the mechanism for such a beneficial effect is not clearly understood.

Skeletal Deformities

Deformities of bone can be a manifestation of severe renal osteodystrophy, particularly in children with long-standing renal failure. Deformities occur in children because their bones undergo rapid growth as well as modeling and remodeling. In adults, particularly those with aluminum-related bone disease, bone deformities include lumbar scoliosis, kyphosis, and deformities of the thoracic cage.[1] Pseudoclubbing is a feature indicating the presence of severe osteitis fibrosa.

Growth Retardation

Children with chronic renal failure commonly exhibit growth retardation; the factors implicated include chronic acidosis, malnutrition, renal bone disease, and abnormal somatomedin metabolism. Treatment with calcitriol has been associated with improvement of growth in selected children, but such results have not been confirmed in other patients. It seems likely that calcitriol may improve the growth retardation but only in selected patients with very severe and untreated osteitis fibrosa.

Extraskeletal Manifestations

Several types of soft tissue calcification can be detected by radiographic evaluation of patients with end-stage renal failure. One type of extraskeletal calcification is tumoral calcification or periarticular calcification. The latter is sometimes accompanied by acute periarthritic or periarticular inflamatory symptoms and signs that suggest an acute arthritis. These types of extracellular calcifications are common when serum phosphorus levels in dialysis patients were above 8 to 9 mg/dl related to a very high serum Ca × P product. There is an association between such calcifications and the presence of severe secondary hyperparathyroidism, probably because severe secondary hyperparathyroidism itself increases the serum Ca × P product. Such calcifications can regress substantially following an appropriate reduction of serum phosphorus levels.

Calcifications can involve the media of the arteries; these type of calcifications are diffuse and continuous along the vessel. Their radiographic appearance differs from the irregular, discrete appearance of calcified intimal plaques. Medial calcifications (Monckerberg's sclerosis) usually occur in asymptomatic patients; however, the pulse and blood pressure may be difficult to detect because of the noncompressible vessel. The vascular calcifications can be best detected by lateral radiographs of the ankle or anteroposterior view of the hands or feet (Fig. 8-3) and with the use of magnification techniques.[46] It has been suggested that a high serum Ca × P product is a principal factor in the development of vascular calcifications; however, more recent studies have failed to show such a relationship, but have demonstrated that high serum magnesium levels were associated with less severe vascular calcification in dialysis patients.[46]

Visceral calcifications can occur in the lungs, heart, kidneys, skeletal muscle, and stomach. Pulmonary calcifications can cause restrictive lung disease and they usually persist after successful kidney transplantation or parathyroidectomy. The pathogenesis of visceral calcifications seems to be different from other types of calcifications.[1]

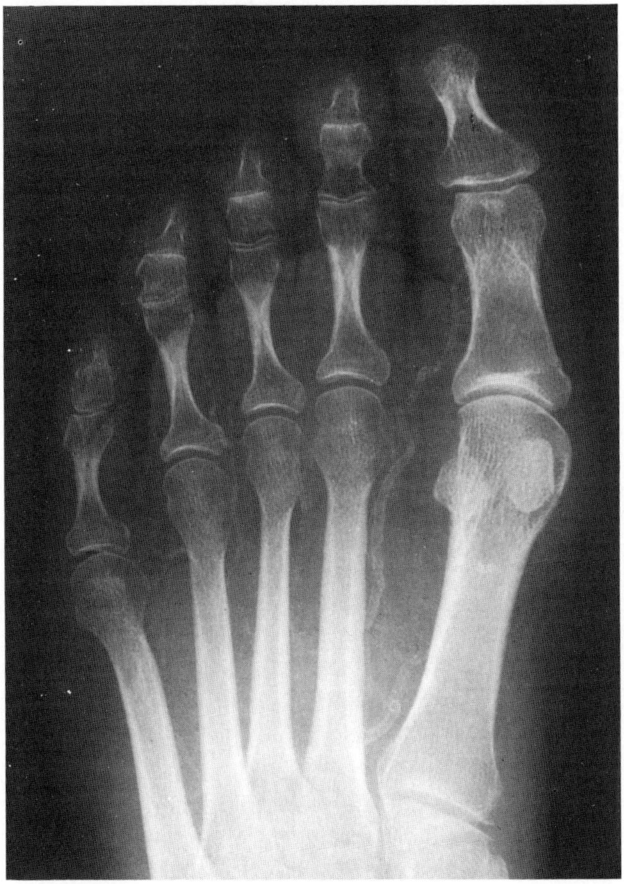

Fig. 8-3 Radiograph shows extensive medial calcifications of the arteries of the foot, resembling an arteriogram.

Biochemical Features

The progressive decline in glomerular filtration rate (GFR) is associated with biochemical changes of parameters of bone and mineral metabolism. Serum calcium levels are often subnormal in patients with advanced renal failure. With the initiation of hemodialysis, serum calcium levels commonly increase into the normal range, and the degree of rise is partially related to the calcium concentration in dialysate. In patients treated with continuous ambulatory peritoneal dialysis (CAPD) and not receiving vitamin D supplements, serum calcium levels remain within the lower limits of normal; secondary hyperparathyroidism can progress in such patients.[47]

Several conditions are associated with hypercalcemia in patients receiving maintenance dialysis; these include aluminum-related bone disease,[1] marked hyperplasia of the parathyroid glands, therapy with calcitriol or another vitamin D sterol, administration of calcium carbonate as a phosphate-binding agent,[30,31] and sarcoidosis or tuberculosis in association with ectopic generation of $1{,}25(OH)_2D_3$.

With advanced renal failure, serum magnesium levels often increase. Upon initiation of regular hemodialysis, the levels are generally at the upper limit of normal provided the dialysate magnesium concentration is 0.5 to 0.8 mEq/liter. The ingestion of magnesium-containing laxatives or antacids can markedly elevate the serum magnesium levels.

The plasma alkaline phosphatase levels are fair markers of the severity of skeletal disease, and changes in alkaline phosphatase can provide a guide to the response to therapy. Plasma alkaline phosphatase levels correlate with the histologic features of osteitis fibrosa, and the response to treatment with a vitamin D sterol. They can also reflect the improvement of osteomalacia that follows treatment of aluminum toxicity with deferoxamine. However, elevated alkaline phosphatase levels will *not* allow one to distinguish between osteitis fibrosa and osteomalacia. It is worth noting that increases of serum alkaline phosphatase levels can reflect underlying liver disease, and hence the measurement of specific isoenzymes would theoretically be advantageous. From a practical standpoint, one can utilize the measurement of certain hepatic enzymes, such as gamma glutamyl-transpeptidase or 5′ nucleotidase, to exclude the presence of hepatic abnormalities as the cause of an elevated alkaline phosphatase activity.[1]

Serum iPTH levels are substantially above normal in most patients with advanced renal failure, but the magnitude of this elevation is determined by the assay method utilized. These assays use an antiserum containing antibodies directed against a specific region or regions of the PTH molecule. Using a mid-C-terminal assay, Hruska et al. found moderately good correlations between serum iPTH levels and several bone parameters, including osteoblastic osteoid surface, osteoclastic osteoid surface, osteoclast count, and trabecular surface in apposition to fibrosis.[48] Andress et al. compared an N-terminal and a C-terminal assay in adult patients treated with hemodialysis. They found that the N-terminal assay gave a good differentiation between patients with osteitis fibrosa and from those with either osteomalacia or a mild lesion. The degree of marow fibrosis correlated somewhat more closely with the N-terminal assay than the C-terminal assay.[49] In patients with aluminum-related bone disease, serum PTH levels are often lower than are usual for dialysis patients. However, the finding of a markedly elevated PTH levels does not exclude the existence of aluminum-related bone disease; therefore, when there is the suspicion of aluminum accumulation in a patient with a markedly elevated PTH level, a bone biopsy is often mandatory. To interpret a serum PTH level properly, one should know the correlation between the PTH levels and the severity of osteitis fibrosa or other features of renal bone disease, as shown in Figure 8-4. Of the commercially available PTH immunoassays, data on the relationship between

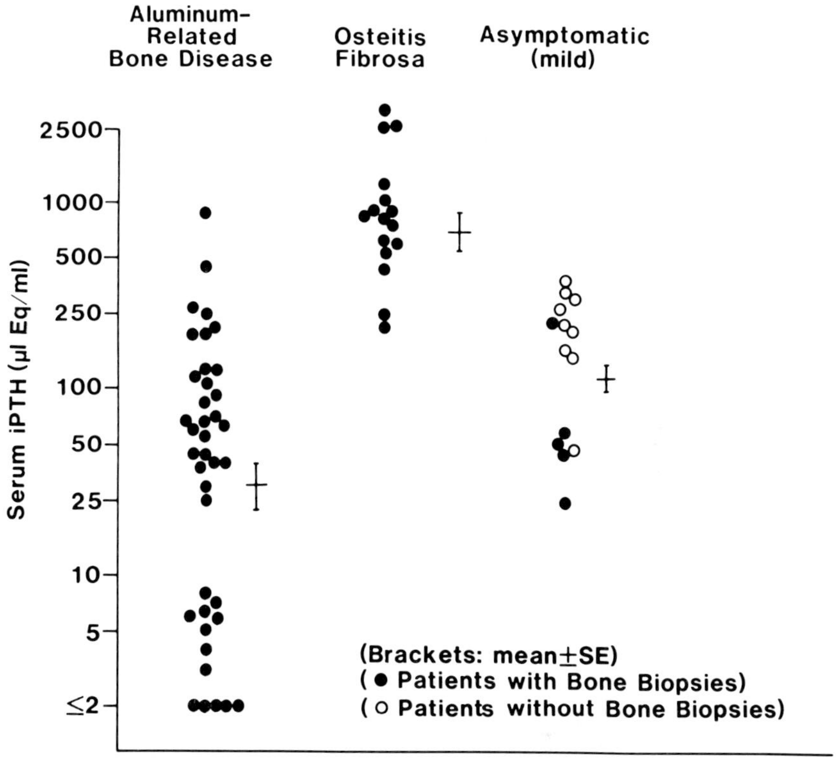

Fig. 8-4 Serum iPTH levels, measured with an antiserum (Ch 9), specific to the midregion of the PTH molecule, and the types of bone diseases determined from iliac crest bone biopsy in patients with end-stage renal disease. The normal iPTH level with this assay is 2 to 6 μlEq/ml. Note the log scale for PTH.

bone histologic features and PTH levels are available in only a few.[1,48,49] We found the results with the mid-C-terminal PTH assay described above[48] were not a good predictor of the type of bone disease in pediatric patients treated with CAPD[50]; bone biopsies were needed to identify the type of bone disease present in such patients.

Plasma aluminum levels are elevated both in patients with chronic renal failure and in those treated with maintenance dialysis.[21–30] Although substantial differences exist among the different reported normal values, the application of electrothermic atomic absorption spectroscopy has provided an accurate method to measure aluminum in both tissues and plasma. Plasma aluminum levels probably reflect the recent load of aluminum, either from contaminated dialysate or from the ingestion of aluminum-containing phosphate binding agents. To detect patients with a high risk of aluminum intoxication, plasma aluminum levels should be monitored every 3 to 4 months in patients treated with maintenance dialysis or in patients with chronic renal failure receiving aluminum-containing gels (Fig. 8-5).

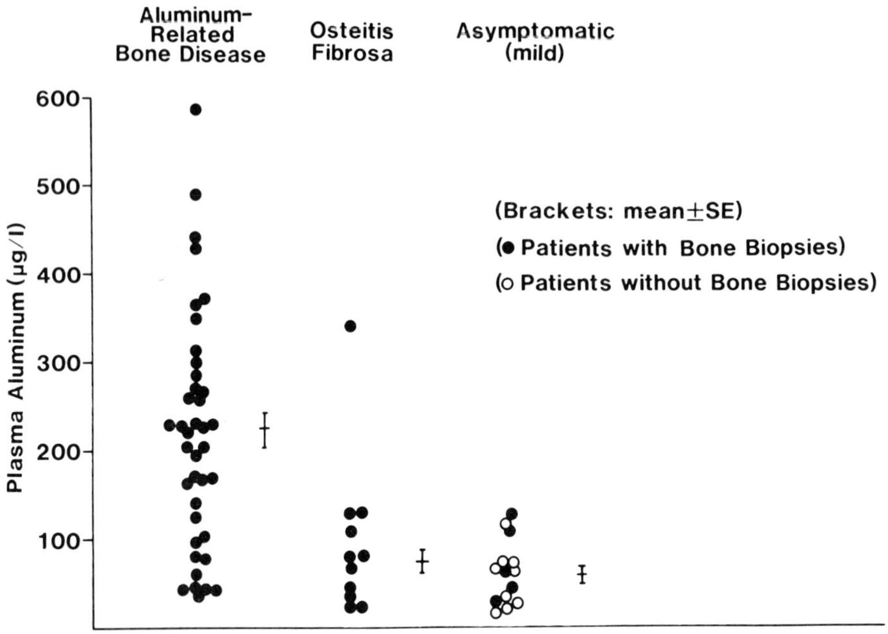

Fig. 8-5 Plasma aluminum levels in groups of patients with end-stage renal failure. Normal plasma Al < 8 μg/L.

Plasma aluminum levels correlate with the oral ingestion of aluminum present in phosphate binding agents,[29] and they reflect less well the tissue stores of aluminum. Deferoxamine, an iron chelating agent, is known to bind aluminum avidly.[51] Since the infusion of deferoxamine will elevate the plasma aluminum levels in patients with aluminum bone disease, a test has been developed to predict the body stores of aluminum. This "deferoxamine infusion test" is performed as follows: patients receive a standardized dose of deferioxamine (40 mg/kg body weight dissolved in 100 ml of 5 percent dextrose) intravenously over 2 hours after a usual hemodialysis procedure. Plasma aluminum levels are measured before and 24 to 48 hours after the infusion.[52] The increment of plasma aluminum after deferoxamine predicts more closely the aluminum content of bone than does the basal plasma aluminum concentration. It was suggested that an increment in plasma aluminum levels might predict the presence of aluminum-related bone disease. However, Malluche et al. found that a deferoxamine infusion test was not specific in all cases[53]; Hodsman et al. demonstrated that dialysis patients with secondary hyperparathyroidism can exhibit a substantial increment in plasma aluminum levels following the infusion of deferoxamine despite low surface stainable aluminum in their bone biopsies.[54] Bone aluminum content was not measured in this study, and the tissue distribution of aluminum is substantially different within the bone of osteitis fibrosa than osteomalacia. Thus, some patients with osteitis fibrosa may have a high tissue content of aluminum and thereby exhibit a "positive" deferoxamine infusion test without showing surface aluminum staining, a major histologic feature of aluminum-related bone disease. However, such patients may be at high risk of developing aluminum-related bone disease after parathyroidectomy.

Radiologic Features

Radiographic Characteristics of Osteitis Fibrosa

The presence of subperiosteal erosions is a common feature of severe secondary hyperparathyroidism; the degree of subperiosteal erosions has been found to correlate with serum iPTH and alkaline phosphatase levels. Skeletal radiographs, however, can be normal in patients with mild to moderate degrees of osteitis fibrosa.[48] Erosions can be present in patients with aluminum-related disease; under such conditions they represent the residual of earlier osteitis fibrosa that failed to mineralize.

Subperiosteal erosions are most readily seen in the hands (Fig. 8-6), the distal ends of the clavicles, the surface of the ischium or pubis (Fig. 8-7), at the sacroiliac joints, and at the junction of the metaphysis and diaphysis of long

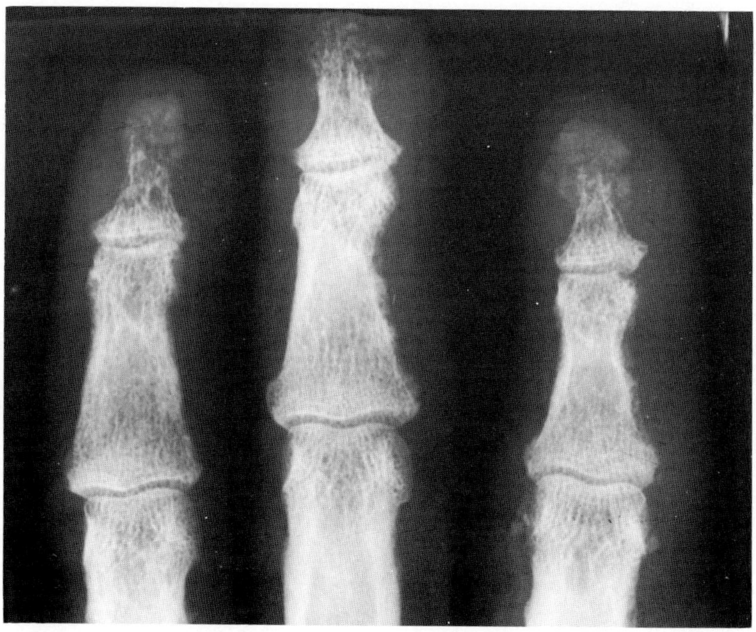

Fig. 8-6 Severe subperiosteal erosions of the phalanges of the left hand of a patient with marked secondary hyperparathyroidism and severe osteitis fibrosa. The abnormalities are much more pronounced on the radial surfaces.

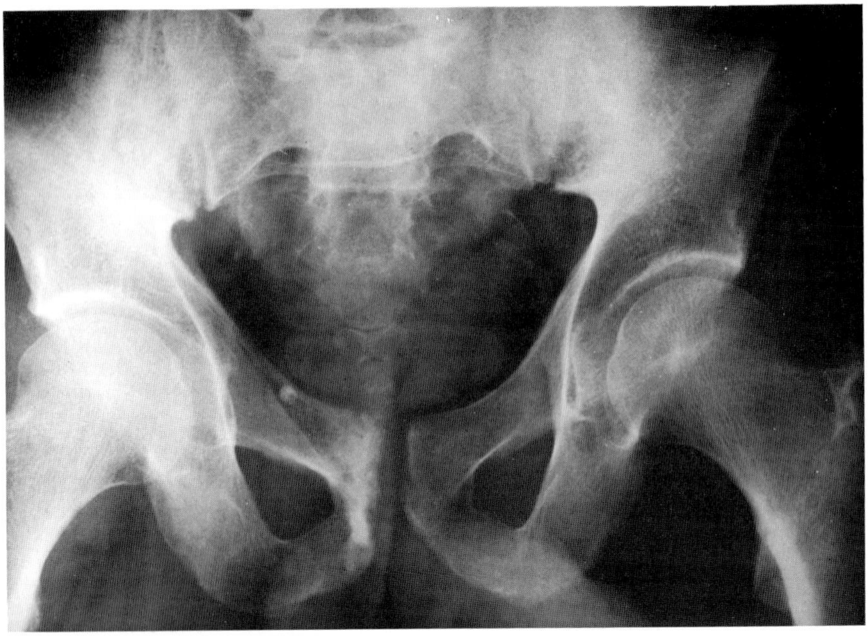

Fig. 8-7 Severe subperiosteal erosion and an area of osteosclerosis of the pubic symphysis in a patient with severe secondary hyperparathyroidism.

bones. Meema et al, use fine-grain films of the hand and magnify them six to sevenfold with a hand lens to increase the sensitivity of such radiographs.[55] In pediatric patients, metaphyseal changes (i.e., growth zone lesions that are also termed *rickets-like lesions* are common. This radiologic feature of secondary hyperparathyroidism is different from the true rachitic changes that arise from vitamin D deficiency.

Radiographic Features of Osteomalacia

The radiographic features of osteomalacia are less specific than those of secondary hyperparathyroidism. Indeed, pseudofractures, which are straight, wide bands of radiolucency that are perpendicular to the long axis of the bone, are the only pathognomonic radiographic feature found in adult patients.[1] True fractures of the ribs, vertebral bodies, and hips also occur, and they are more common in renal patients with osteomalacia than in those with osteitis fibrosa.

Bone Scans

The most frequently used bone-seeking compound for skeletal scintigraphy is the technetium-tagged biphosphonate, 99m-methylene diphosphonate. Bone scans can be used to evaluate the severity of skeletal disease in patients with advanced renal failure, to follow the response to therapy, to detect the presence of pseudofractures, and to identify extraskeletal calcifications.

Osteitis fibrosa is usually manifested by a symmetrical increase of activity over the skull, mandible, sternum, shoulders, vertebrae, and distal aspects of the femur and tibia. In a comparison of bone scan and bone histologic studies by Hodson et al., there was no good correlation between the findings from the two methods, and it was not possible to predict the type of renal osteodystrophy.[56] In contrast, Karsenty et al. demonstrated much greater isotope uptake in patients with osteitis fibrosa than in those with osteomalacia secondary to aluminum accumulation.[57] There was no ability to identify patients with a mixed lesion. At the present time, bone scans provide a noninvasive diagnostic method that may suggest the specific diagnosis of certain bone diseases and can detect the presence of extraskeletal calcifications in patients with end-stage renal failure. However, bone biopsies may still be needed to define specifically the type of renal bone disease.

Histologic Characteristics

Our understanding of the pathophysiology of bone disease has significantly improved with the increased use of iliac crest bone biopsies and wider availability of improved methods for obtaining, preparing, and interpreting thin sections of bone. The bone biopsy procedure can be done safely and with minimal morbidity in an outpatient setting.[58] In addition to the evaluation of static parameters of bone histologic studies, the dynamic characteristics of bone turnover, including the rate of bone formation and mineralization, can be evaluated using the double tetracycline technique. The following schedule for tetracyline has been utilized: demeclocycline 300 mg is taken twice daily for 2 or 3 days; no drug is taken for 11 to 14 days; and then tetracycline, 500 mg twice daily, is ingested for 2 or 3 days with the bone biopsy done 5 to 7 days later. In sections of bone, the areas of uptake of the two tetracyclines are identified by their fluorescent characteristics, and the separation of the two bands and the length of bone surface showing a double label allow calculation of bone formation rate. The aluminum content of bone can be evaluated using a histochemical stain or a chemical method. The histochemical stain can be expressed as the percentage of trabecular surface that stains positive for aluminum, and the total aluminum content, determined chemically in small bone sample obtained with a Jamshidi needle, is measured after EDTA extraction and expressed per weight of bone.[1]

The most common type of bone disease in both adult and pediatric patients with advanced renal failure is osteitis fibrosa arising from excess PTH.[50,58–60] The bone exhibits increased numbers of osteoblasts and osteoclasts and a variable amount of peritrabecular fibrosis; bone formation rate is increased compared to values from nonuremic control subjects.

Another feature of bone in dialysis patients is the presence of osteomalacia or defective mineralization. In this situation, the double tetracycline labeling technique provides the best method to identify defective mineralization. The characteristics of osteomalacia include the presence of wide osteoid seams, increased numbers of osteoid lamellae, an increase in the trabecular surface covered with osteiod, and a diminished rate of mineralization. At the present time, the most frequent cause of osteomalacia in patients with advanced renal failure is the accumulation of aluminum, with aluminum staining more than 25 to 30 percent of trabecular surface. The chemical bone aluminum content is elevated in such patients, but this abnormality is not as specific as the finding of surface staining of aluminum.[60]

Another group of patients with symptomatic bone disease may show normal osteoid volume, the absence of fibrosis, but markedly reduced bone formation rate as indicated by the double tetracycline labeling. This lesion has been classified as "aplastic" or "adynamic" bone disease.[59–60] In the majority of patients with this lesion, substantial aluminum staining is observed on the bone surface. However, the aluminum stain is negative in 10 percent of pediatric patients undergoing maintenance dialysis and identified to have the aplastic bone lesion[50]; the mechanism responsible for low bone turnover in these patients has yet to be established.

Osteitis fibrosa, a finding of secondary hyperparathyroidism, can coexist with osteomalacia in some patients; this pattern is called a "mixed" lesion.[59,60] This lesion sometimes represents a transition from osteitis fibrosa to aluminum-related bone disease or the reverse.

Treatment

The general principles for the management of renal osteodystrophy are to maintain serum calcium and phosphorus levels within the normal limits in order to prevent parathyroid hyperplasia, to avoid the development of extraskeletal calcifications, and to prevent the accumulation of toxic substances such as aluminum. Thus, an optimal dietary regimen, the intake of phosphate binding agents, and vitamin D treatment are needed to manage and treat bone disease in many patients with advanced renal failure.

Dietary Manipulation

The control of serum phosphorus levels in uremic patients is extremely important to minimize the progression of secondary hyperparathyroidism and prevent extracellular calcification. Studies in dogs with chronic uremia have shown that restriction of dietary phosphate intake in proportion to the degree of renal insufficiency can largely prevent the progression of secondary hyperparathyroidism.[6] Moreover, dietary phosphate restriction is associated with reductions of serum PTH levels in patients with mild to moderate renal failure. The principal sources of dietary phosphorus are meat and dairy products, and the phosphorus intake ranges from 1.0 to 1.8 g/day in normal adults.[1] Ideally, phosphorus ingestion should be restricted to 400 to 800 mg/day in patients with advanced renal failure and in those treated with maintenance dialysis. Such diets are effective but are not palatable, and it is difficult to obtain patient compliance over a prolonged period of time; thus, phosphate-binding agents are required in most patients with end-stage renal disease.

Calcium absorption is generally impaired in patients with advanced renal failure, and the calcium content of the diets of these patients is usually suboptimal.[1] Calcium supplements can have two beneficial effects in uremic patients. (1) There is an increased amount of calcium available for absorption and (2) the calcium salt can act as a phosphate-binding agent. Optimal calcium balance can be reached with the intake of calcium as calcium carbonate, calcium citrate, or calcium lactate, and the calcium balance reaches neutral when the diet is supplemented by 1000 to 1200 mg calcium per day.

Phosphate Binding Agents

These agents reduce intestinal phosphate absorption and thereby prevent hyperphosphatemia or an increase of body stores of phosphate. Until very recently, the aluminum-containing gels were the agents most widely used to reduce phosphorus absorption in patients with advanced renal failure and those treated with maintenance dialysis.[1] Now it is known that the long-term ingestion of large doses of such agents is accompanied by an increased accumulation of aluminum in patients with renal failure.[21–29] Plasma aluminum levels correlate with the amount of aluminum ingested in the phosphate-binding agents,[29] and the absorption of aluminum from the gastrointestinal tract is a major source of aluminum loading and toxicity. The optimal safe dose of aluminum hydroxide to avoid such toxicity has not been established; Sedman et al. suggested that uremic children who receive more than 30 to 50 mg/kg/day of aluminum hydroxide are at a high risk of developing aluminum toxicity.[28] Winney et al. reported that plasma aluminum levels are below those associated with aluminum toxicity when the dose is less than six capsules of aluminum hydroxide per day.[61]

Calcium carbonate can also reduce intestinal phosphorus absorption[62]; however, its initial use was associated with multiple episodes of hypercalcemia, diarrhea, and metabolic alkalosis. In subsequent studies in both adult and pediatric patients on maintenance dialysis, calcium carbonate has led to adequate control of serum phosphorus levels; hypercalcemia has been the major side effect.[30,31,63] When calcium carbonate is used as phosphate binding agent, it should be ingested with a meal to increase the phosphate binding efficiency and minimize the intestinal absorption of calcium. The dosages required to obtain an acceptable control of serum phosphorus levels have ranged from 4.5 to 14 g/day.[30–32,62–63] Calcium carbonate should not be initiated until the serum phosphorus levels are below 6.0 mg/dl to avoid a high Ca × P product, which can predispose to extraskeletal calcifications. Fournier et al. have found that calcium carbonate alone could control hyperphosphatemia in only half of adult patients undergoing long-term dialysis,[63] and some patients require the administration of both calcium carbonate and low doses of aluminum hydroxide for control of serum phosphorus levels. Whether long-term treatment with calcium carbonate will lead to extraskeletal calcifications is not known at the present time.

Other phosphate binding agents that have been used in limited numbers of patients and with variable results include magnesium salts and polyuronic acid. Magnesium oxide was reported to be ineffective in one study,[64] while magnesium carbonate was effective when given in conjunction with a magnesium-free dialysate solution.[65] A complex polymer of uronic acid was reported to be an effective phosphate binder in hemodialysis patients.[66] Hypercalcemia was a side effect in one study; but the number of patients included was small and it was used for a relatively short period of time. Further studies are needed to evaluate better the efficacy and safety of this agent.

Vitamin D Sterols

Despite dietary phosphate restriction, the use of phosphate binding agents, an appropriate level of calcium in the dialysate, and an adequate intake of calcium, a significant fraction of renal patients still develop severe secondary hyperparathyroidism. The use of dihydrotachysterol, 25-hydroxyvitamin D_3, 1-alpha-hydroxyvitamin D_3, 1,25 dihydroxyvitamin D_3, or even large doses of vitamin D_3 or D_2 is often followed by improved clinical symptoms and correction of certain biochemical and radiologic features of secondary hyperparathyroidism.[1] There are no carefully controlled studies that compare the effectiveness of these vitamin D sterols.

Calcifediol, $25(OH)D_3$, is often effective in the control of secondary hyperparathyroidism in adults and children treated with maintenance dialysis.[67,68] A six-center study of dialysis patients demonstrated improvement of musculoskeletal symptoms, a fall in the serum alkaline phosphatase activity, and a decrease in the extent of osteitis fibrosa during treatment with this sterol. Hypercalcemia occurred in association with supranormal plasma levels of 25-hydroxyvitamin D_3.

Several clinical trials have documented the efficacy of calcitriol for the treatment of patients with symptomatic renal osteodystrophy.[1] These studies have shown a decrease in bone pain, improvement in muscle strength and gait-posture, and an increase of growth velocity in some uremic children. Bone histologic studies have demonstrated healing or improvement of osteitis fibrosa.[69]

The dosages of oral calcitriol utilized in these trials have ranged from 0.25 to 1.5 μg/day. The major side effect noted was hypercalcemia. The appearance of hypercalcemia during treatment with calcitriol may predict the type of bone disease.[1] Hypercalcemia that occurs after many weeks or months of calcitriol treatment and is associated with a fall in alkaline phosphatase activity to normal is common with healing of osteitis fibrosa. When patients develop hypercalcemia within the first few weeks of calcitriol treatment, either aluminum-related bone disease or marked and autonomous hyperparathyroidism that requires parathyroidectomy may be present. Ideally, the dose of calcitriol should be adjusted to maintain serum calcium levels between 10.5 and 11.0 mg/dl, an approach that led to optimal PTH suppression in most pediatric patients treated with dialysis.[70]

Slatopolsky et al. have shown that the intravenous administration of calcitriol substantially reduces the secretion of PTH in dialysis patients.[71] These studies suggest that the suppression of PTH is significantly greater than that occurring after the serum calcium level is raised with oral calcium carbonate or possibly even after oral calcitriol. Delmez et al. demonstrated that the intraperitoneal administration calcitriol can suppress PTH levels in patients treated with continuous ambulatory peritoneal dialysis.[72] The optimal route and dose schedule of calcitriol administration that is needed to produce appropriate PTH suppression remains to be evaluated; long-term prospective studies are needed to compare the efficicy of different routes of calcitriol administration in dialysis patients.

Parathyroidectomy

Certain features of secondary hyperparathyroidism indicate a need for parathyroid surgery.[1] In all instances, the presence of aluminum-related bone disease must be excluded prior to parathyroid surgery and the presence of severe secondary hyperparathyroidism must be documented by biochemical, radiographic, and bone histologic parameters. The indications include (1) persistent hypercalcemia (serum calcium level between 11.5 and 12.0 mg/dl); (2) intractable pruritus that does not respond to dialysis or other medical treatment; (3) progressive extraskeletal calcifications despite appropriate phosphate restriction; (4) severe skeletal pain or fractures; and (5) the appearance of calciphylaxis. Other causes of hypercalcemia, including sarcoidosis, malignancy-related hypercalcemia, and the intake of calcium supplements, must be excluded. Because of a greater risk of aluminum toxicity after parathyroidectomy, aluminum hydroxide should be avoided after surgery and calcium carbonate should be the phosphate binding agent of choice.

Management of Aluminum Intoxication

Following the initial reports of the use of deferoxamine for aluminum removal, others have documented a significant improvement of symptoms and bone histologic findings after long-term treatment in patients undergoing maintenance dialysis.[51,53] After the administration of deferoxamine, the removal of aluminum is substantially increased by both hemodialysis and CAPD, in contrast to the rather ineffective removal of aluminum during regular dialysis without deferoxamine.[73,74] Lethal infections with mucormycosis have been described in several dialysis patients treated with deferoxamine.[75] Such complications raise a question regarding the appropriate indications for the use of deferoxamine for the treatment of aluminum intoxication. Asymptomatic patients with aluminum accumulation and aplastic bone lesion have shown improvement following the substitution of calcium carbonate for aluminum gels. Thus, deferoxamine should be given only to patients with severe aluminum intoxication, and the dose should be kept at 1.0 to 2.0 g per week or less according to the plasma aluminum levels.

BONE DISEASE ASSOCIATED WITH LONG-TERM TOTAL PARENTERAL NUTRITION

Since 1968, concentrated nutrient solutions have been infused via a central venous catheter to prevent and treat malnutrition in patients who are unable to assimilate oral nutrients. Such treatment is usually given each night, and it has been continued successfully at home in selected patients for periods up to several years.[76,77] Several metabolic abnormalities, which generally arose due to the omission of required nutrients, were encountered during such long-term treatment. A metabolic bone disease was described independently from two separate centers, in Toronto and in Los Angeles, in patients receiving long-term treatment with total parenteral nutrition (TPN).[78,79] Whether this bone disease represents a single disorder or several problems appearing in patients treated for a prolonged periods with parenteral solutions remains uncertain.

Clinical Features

The patients in southern California had received treatment with TPN for periods of several months to 1 to 2 years; initially the patients fared well and gained weight despite minimal oral intake.[78,80] There was then the insidious appearance of pain that was worsened by weight-bearing and involved the feet, ankles, and knees. The pain gradually intensified and involved the axial skeleton; some patients were confined to bed and were unable to walk without severe pain. The patients had not received medications known to have an adverse effect on bone. Examination revealed tenderness at the articular margin and periarticular areas of the affected joints, but there was no swelling or redness. On discontinuing the TPN, substituting an intravenous solution with only dextrose and electrolytes, and encouraging oral intake, the pain gradually improved despite the recurrence of diarrhea and weight loss with deterioration of nutritional status.

Twenty percent of the patients treated with TPN for more than 3 months in Southern California had bone pain involving the lower extremities, back, or ribs.[80] Prior to the initiation of TPN, all these patients had severe malnutrition and most had previously undergone multiple abdominal operations. Two of 16 patients who were receiving TPN for 7 to 89 months in Toronto noted back pain and crush fractures.[79] The TPN solution used in Los Angeles and given over 12 night-time hours contained essential nutrients that included calcium 200 to 300 mg/day, phosphorus 1000 to 1500 mg/day, casein hydrolysate as the protein source, and vitamin D2 1000 IU/day.[80] The composition of the TPN solution in Toronto had a moderately lower phosphorus content, a slightly higher calcium content, and 50 percent less vitamin D_2.[79]

In both groups, the serum levels of calcium and phosphorus were normal or slightly above, while the levels of magnesium, total CO_2, copper, zinc, total protein, and albumin were normal. Serum alkaline phosphatase activity was elevated. In the Los Angeles patients, there were normal or elevated levels of the vitamin D metabolite, $25(OH)D_2$, and low levels of the D_3 sterol, $25(OH)D_3$.[81] Low plasma levels of $1,25(OH)_2D$ were observed in both Toronto and Los Angeles.[81,82] There was marked hypercalciuria, particularly during the night-time hours while the TPN solutions were being infused. Serum iPTH levels were in the low range of normal or undetectable. No clinical or biochemical parameters distinguished the Los Angeles patients with symptoms of bone disease from the other patients without musculoskeletal symptoms but treated with TPN. Skeletal radiographs showed diffuse osteopenia or crush vertebral fractures and photon absorptiometry revealed decreased bone mineral content. Bone biopsies, carried out with double tetracycline labeling in the symptomatic patients in Los Angeles, showed mild or patchy osteomalacia, a reduced number of osteoclasts (which suggested reduced bone resorption), and a low bone formation rate.[80,81] Bone biopsies were carried out on two occasions in Toronto: first during the first 1 to 4 months of TPN treatment and again after 8 to 73 months of treatment.[79] Between the first and second biopsies, the width of unmineralized osteoid rose, the surface covered with osteoid increased, and the fractional surface of bone taking up a single dose of tetracycline decreased; these observations were interpreted as consistent with the development of osteomalacia. The initial biopsies had showed "a hyperkinetic state" in most patients; however, double tetracycline labeling was not performed to permit more precise evaluation of bone formation rate.

Role of Vitamin D

In Toronto, vitamin D_2 was totally withdrawn from the TPN solutions; this was associated with a reduced urinary calcium, a lowering of serum calcium, and a reduced quantity of unmineralized osteoid in bone biopsies obtained 6 or more months later. The serum levels of 25(OH)D were normal, and it was concluded that the parenteral vitamin D_2 500 I U /day, accounted for the abnormalities of bone.[82] Fractures and radiographic features of rickets were noted in several children undergoing TPN in Los Angeles; these abnormalities improved following the administration of increased doses of vitamin D_2.[83] Thus, the clinicians in Los Angeles were unwilling to accept the view that vitamin D was the cause of the bone disease. The role of low levels of $1,25(OH)_2D$ in causing the skeletal disease was uncertain.

Aluminum Loading as a Cause of Bone Disease

In Los Angeles, it was discovered that the casein hydrolysate utilized as the source of protein in the TPN solutions for nearly all the Los Angeles patients[84] and probably for most in Toronto was contaminated with aluminum; this contamination resulted in the long-term intravenous infusion of aluminum, 1000 to 3000 μg/day.[84,85] In Los Angeles, the plasma aluminum levels were markedly elevated, as was the urinary excretion of aluminum. In addition, specific histochemical stains showed aluminum to be localized along the mineralization front. Thus, the histologic and histomorphologic features of bone from patients treated with TPN were very similar to findings in dialysis patients with aluminum accumulation. It was concluded in Los Angeles that aluminum accumulation was the cause of the skeletal disease.[85] Following this observation, casein hydrolysate was withdrawn from the TPN solutions as the protein source. This change from casein hydrolysate to amino acids resulted in a modest reduction in the total quantity of protein administered; also, the quantity of vitamin D_2 in the multivitamin additive was lowered from 1000 to 400 IU/day when the multivitamin additive was changed from MVI-1 to MVI-12. Clinically apparent bone disease has become unusual in Los Angeles since that time.[86]

In a longitudinal evaluation of both biochemical features and histologic parameters of bone of patients who converted from casein hydrolysate to amino acid as a protein source, there was improvement of the bone disease following the change.[86] Bone formation rate was higher and the osteoid surface area was lower in patients receiving amino acids than in those receiving casein hydrolysate. During treatment with the amino acid solutions, the serum levels of both $1,25(OH)_2D$ and PTH were higher and the plasma levels of aluminum and urinary excretion in both aluminum and calcium were substantially lower. The serum levels of $1,25(OH)_2D$ correlated directly with serum iPTH and inversely with both serum phosphorus and the plasma aluminum levels; moreover, the degree of correlation was greatest with the plasma aluminum level. Other studies [87,88] have shown that aluminum loading can reduce PTH secretion and lower the serum levels of $1,25(OH)_2D$. A reduction of serum PTH levels plus any other factor that favors a reduction of bone turnover are known to predispose to the toxic effect of aluminum on bone in renal failure patients.[1,43–45] Thus, one may speculate that the administration of large quantities of calcium and vitamin D in the TPN solution contributed to the mild elevation of serum calcium level; this would suppress PTH levels and contribute to the low turnover of bone, a factor that could enhance the pathologic effect of aluminum on bone. Conversely, a withdrawal of vitamin D or a reduction of the calcium content of the TPN solution would increase PTH secretion, enhance bone turnover, and reduce the toxic effect aluminum on bone. If aluminum loading was or had been a problem in patients in Toronto, this might explain how alterations in vitamin D dosage might affect aluminum toxicity. The positive correlation between urinary aluminum excretion and urinary calcium raises the possibility that aluminum toxicity may contribute to the loss of calcium from bone and thereby contribute to the hypercalciuria.[86] Alternatively, aluminum could affect the renal tubule to decrease calcium reabsorption.

Hypercalciuria During TPN

A striking finding of most studies of patients treated with TPN has been substantial hypercalciuria.[78–81,86] It is probable that the continued urinary losses of calcium could contribute to the loss of bone mineral and the osteopenia or osteoporosis observed in patients undergoing long-term TPN. Several factors probably contribute to the hypercalciuria.[89] A rise in the filtered load of calcium or an increase in serum calcium concentration per se, could depress the tubular reabsorption of calcium. The infusion of large quantities of sodium and consequent extracellular volume expansion[90] and the infusion of dextrose could contribute to the increased urinary calcium.[91] The quantity of amino acids given[89,92] and the administration of the TPN infusion over 12 to 14 hours of the day, rather than over the total 24 hour period, increases the total urinary calcium excretion over the 24 hour period.[93] The acute acid load that arises from the sulfur-containing amino acids also would contribute. The amount of alkali added, (i.e., acetate or other source of bicarbonate) would be expected to affect the urinary calcium excretion. The quantity of phosphate infused can also affect the tubular reabsorption of calcium and modify the quantity of calcium present in the urine.[94] Furthermore, the physiologic hypoparathyroid state that existed in many of the TPN patients[79,81] would contribute to the hypercalciuria. Further studies should characterize the contributions of the loads of protein and alkali on the urinary calcium losses in these patients. It remains uncertain whether an "appropriate" change in the solution to lower urinary calcium would lead to increased bone mineral content.

TPN Bone Disease: A Heterogeneous Problem

Since the reports from Los Angeles and Toronto, there have been additional studies of bone among patients treated with long-term TPN using crystalline amino acids as the protein source. The results have been somewhat variable. de Vernejoul et al. reported results of bone biopsies in seven patients treated with TPN in Paris for a relatively short period of time, averaging near 7 months.[95] There was reduced bone formation and bone apposition and a decrease in osteoid volume. Hypercalciuria was prominent and the plasma levels of $1,25(OH)_2D$ were in the low normal range. These patients had significantly elevated plasma aluminum levels believed to be related to a moderate aluminum content of the phosphate salts added to the solution; however, aluminum staining of the bone biopsies was negative. In a study of 11 patients from New York who had received treatment with TPN for 51 ± 21 months[96] the bone apposition rate, termed "mineralization rate," was subnormal in 3 of 9 patients; however, the bone formation rate, not reported but estimated from the data provided, was below normal in 10 of 12 patients. Osteoid volume was increased in 2 of 11 patients. There were modest elevations of plasma aluminum in 4 of 6 patients; surface staining for aluminum was present in 3 of 12 patients, and 1 additional patient had an elevated aluminum content of bone. Among 12 patients treated with TPN in Seattle for 9 to 90 months,[97] osteoid volume was above normal in 5 of 12 patients, bone apposition rate was normal, but bone formation rate was moderately to severely depressed in 6 of 12 patients. Substantial hypercalciuria was noted by de Vernejoul et al.[95] and urinary calcium was elevated in several New York patients.[96] The phosphate salt added to the TPN solution was identified as a main source of "moderate aluminum" loading in Paris[95]; the aluminum levels in the TPN solution were not measured in Seattle or New York, although the absence of positive aluminum stains argue against the possibility that aluminum was a major factor. Serum PTH levels were normal or even slightly elevated in most of these patients,[95-97] which contrast with the low levels of PTH in earlier studies from Los Angeles and Toronto.[79,81] A substantial number of both the patients from New York and Seattle had back pain, osteopenia, and compression fractures of the lumbar spine on radiographs, while the patients studied in Paris were largely asymptomatic.

The more recent observations point to the heterogeneity of the bone disease observed in patients treated with long-term TPN; whether this is due to minor differences in the solutions administered, the length of time on TPN treatment, or the age and sex of the patients remains to be clarified. There could be the administration of some unknown toxic substance, such as cadmium,[98] or a deficiency of some essential trace substance, such as silicon,[99] which could be pathogenic. Moreover, it is possible that the relatively low amounts of aluminum that continue to occur in the TPN solutions may contribute to the pathogenesis.

The Future

Recent studies suggest that the bone disease appearing during long-term TPN is heterogenous. The continued treatment of larger number of such patients indicate that surveillance for these problems should continue. The lesson learned from aluminum loading indicates that the search for other toxic substances needs to continue. Further studies are needed to determine the optimal quantity of calcium to add to the TPN solution for a patient of specific ages and sex and to identify the optimal quantities of both protein and acetate to reverse or minimize the hypercalciuria and optimize the net balance for calcium. The possible role of menopause and other hormonal factors that will occur with the advancing age of these patients also requires consideration. Thus, TPN bone disease is a "disease of progress" that offers the opportunity to understand how various nutritional factors can affect bone. Further research is required to optimize the effect of long-term TPN treatment on mineral metabolism and bone.

ACKNOWLEDGMENTS

Part of the work reported herein was supported by USPHS Grants DK35423,RR-865 and by research funds from the Veterans Administration. We are indebted to Al Walker for secretarial assistance.

REFERENCES

1. Coburn JW, Slatopolsky E: Vitamin D, parathyroid hormone, and renal osteodystrophy. p.1657. In Brenner BM, Rector FC. (eds): The Kidney. 3rd Ed. WB Saunders, Philadelphia, 1985
2. Brown EM: Set point for calcium: its role in normal and abnormal secretion. p. 35. In Cohn DV, Talmage RV, and Matthews JL (eds): Hormonal Control of Calcium Metabolism. Excerpta Medica, Amsterdam, 1981
3. Brown EM, Wilson RE, Eastman RC, et al: Abnormal regulation of parathyroid hormone release by calcium in secondary hyperparathyroidism due to chronic renal failure. J Clin Endocrinol Metab 54:172, 1982
4. Bellorin-Font EK, Martin JJ, Freitag C, et al: Altered adenylate cyclase kinetics in hyperfunctioning human parathyroid glands. J Clin Endocrinol Metab 52:499, 1981
5. Korkor AB: Reduced binding of [^{3}H]1,25-dihydroxyvitamin D_3 in the parathyroid glands of patients with renal failure. N Engl J Med 316:1573, 1983
6. Slatopolsky E, Caglar S, Gradowska L, et al: On the prevention of secondary hyperparathyroidism in experimental chronic renal disease using "proportional reduction" of dietary phosphorus intake. Kidney Int 2:147, 1972
7. Portale AA, Booth BE, Tsai HC, and Morris RC, Jr: Reduced plasma concentration of 1,25-dihydroxyvitamin D in children with moderate renal insufficiency. Kidney Int 21:267, 1982
8. Cheung AK, Manolagas SC, Catherwood BD, et al: Determinants of serum 1,25$(OH)_2D_3$ levels in renal disease. Kidney Int 24:104, 1983
9. Portale AA, Booth BE, Halloran BP, Morris RC, Jr: Effect of dietary phosphorus on circulating concentrations of 1,25-dihydroxyvitamin D and immunoreactive parathyroid hormone in children with moderate renal insufficiency. J Clin Invest 73:1580, 1984
10. Llach F, Massry SG: On the mechanism of secondary hyperparathyroidism in moderate renal insufficiency. J Clin Endocrinol Metab 61:601, 1985
11. Lopez-Hilker S, Galceran T, Chan YL, et al: Hypocalcemia may not be essential for the development of secondary hyperparathyroidism in chronic renal failure. J Clin Invest 78:1097, 1986
12. Lopez-Hilker S, Rapp N, Martin K, Slatopolsky E: On the mechanisms of the prevention of secondary hyperparathyroidism by phosphate restriction. (abstract) Kidney Int 29:164, 1986
13. Evanson JM: The response to the infusion of parathyroid extract in hypocalcemic states. Clin Sci 31:63, 1966
14. Massry SG, Coburn JW, Lee DBN, et al: Skeletal resistence to parathyroid hormone in renal failure: study in 105 human subjects. Ann Intern Med 78:357, 1973
15. Liu SH, Chu HI: Studies of calcium and phosphorus metabolism with special reference to pathogenesis and effects of dihydistachysterol and iron. Medicine 22:103, 1943
16. Lumb GA, Mawer EB, Stanbury E: The apparent vitamin D resistance of chronic renal failure: a study of the physiology of vitamin D in man. Am J Med 50:421, 1971
17. Pierides AM, Kerr DN, Ellis HA, et al: 1 -Hydroxy-cholecalciferol in hemodialysis renal osteodystrophy: adverse effects of anticonvulsant therapy. Clin Nephrol 5:189, 1976
18. Coburn JW, Nebeker HG, Hercz G, et al: Role of aluminum accumulation in the pathogenesis of renal osteodystrophy. p.1383. In Robinson RR (ed): Nephrology. Vol. II. Springer-Verlag, New York, 1984
19. Ward MK, Feest TG, Willis HA, et al: Osteomalacic dialysis osteodystrophy:

evidence for a waterborne aetiologic agent, probably aluminum. Lancet 1:841, 1978
20. Parkinson IS, Feest TG, Ward MK, et al: Fracturing dialysis osteodystrophy and dialysis encephalopathy: an epidemiological survey. Lancet 1:406, 1979
21. Pierides AM, Edwards WG, Cullum UX, et al: Hemodialysis encephalopathy with osteomalacia fractures and muscle weakness. Kidney Int 18:115, 1980
22. Nathan E, Pedersen SE: Dialysis encephalopathy in a non-dialyzed uremic boy treated with aluminum hydroxide orally. Acta Pediatr Scand 69:793, 1980
23. Felsenfeld AJ, Gutman RA, Llach F, Harrelson JM: Osteomalacia in chronic renal failure: a syndrome previously reported only with maintenance dialysis. Am J Nephrol 2:147, 1982
24. Griswold WR, Reznik KV, Mendoza SA, et al: Accumulation of aluminum in an non-dialyzed uremic child receiving aluminum hydroxide. Pediatrics 71:56, 1983
25. Randall ME: Aluminum toxicity in an infant not on dialysis. Lancet 1:1327, 1983
26. Kaye M: Oral toxicity in a non-dialyzed patient with renal failure. Clin Nephrol 20:208, 1983
27. Andreoli SP, Bergstein JM, Sherrard DJ: Aluminum intoxication from alumium-containing phosphate binders in children with azotemia not undergoing dialysis. N Engl J Med 310:1079, 1984
28. Sedman AB, Miller NL, Warady BA, et al: Aluminum loading in children with chronic renal failure. Kidney Int 26:201, 1984
29. Salusky IB, Coburn JW, Paunier L, et al: Role of aluminum hydroxide in raising serum aluminum levels in children undergoing continuous ambulatory peritoneal dialysis (CAPD). J Pediatr 105:717, 1984
30. Moriniere PH, Roussel A, Tahiri Y, et al: Substitution of aluminum hydroxide by high doses of calcium carbonate in patients on chronic hemodialysis: disappearances of hyperaluminemia and equal control of hyperparathyroidism. Proc Eur Dial Transplant Assoc 19:784, 1982
31. Salusky IB, Coburn JW, Foley J, et al: Effects of oral calcium carbonate on control of serum phosphorus and changes in plasma aluminum levels after discontinuation of aluminum-containing gels in children receiving dialysis. J Pediatr 108:767, 1986
32. Hercz G, Kraut JA, Andress DA, et al: Use of calcium carbonate as a phosphate binder in dialysis patients. Miner Electrolyte Metab 12:314, 1986
33. Ellis HA, McCarthy JH, Herrington J: Bone aluminum in hemodialyzed patients and in rats injected with aluminum chloride: relationship to impaired bone mineralization. J Clin Pathol 32:832, 1979
34. Chan Y, Alfrey AC, Posen S, et al: The effect of aluminum on normal and uremic rats: Tissue distribution, vitamin D metabolites and quantitative bone histology. Calcif Tissue Int 35:344, 1983
35. Robertson JA, Felsenfeld AJ, Haygood CC, et al: Animal model of aluminum-induced osteomalacia: role of chronic renal failure. Kidney Int 23:327, 1983
36. Goodman WG, Gilligan J, Horst R: Short-term aluminum administration in the rat. J Clin Invest 73:171, 1984
37. Goodman WG, Henry DA, Horst R, et al: Parenteral aluminum administration in the dog: II. Induction of osteomalacia and effect on vitamin D metabolism. Kidney Int 25:370, 1984
38. Quarles LD, Dennis VW, Gitelman HJ, et al: Aluminum deposition at the osteoid–bone interface: an epiphenomenon of the osteomalacic state in vitamin D-deficient dogs. J Clin Invest 75:1441, 1985
39. Posner AA, Blumenthal NC, Boskey AL: Model of aluminum-induced osteomalacia: inhibition of apatite formation and growth. Kidney Int 29:S17, 1986

40. Meyer JL, Thomas WC, Jr: Aluminum and aluminum complexes. Effects on calcium phosphate precipitation. Kidney Int 29:S20, 1986
41. Cournot-Witmer J, Plachot JJ, Bourdeau A, et al: Effect of aluminum on bone and cell localization. Kidney Int 29:S37, 1986
42. Talwar HS, Reddi AH, Menczel J, et al: Influence of aluminum on mineralization during matrix-induced bone development. Kidney Int 29:1038, 1986
43. Andress DL, Ott SM, Maloney NA, Sherrard DJ: Effect of parathyroidectomy on aluminum accumulation in chronic renal failure. N Engl J Med 312:468, 1985
44. De Vernejoul MC, Marchais S, London G, et al: Increased bone aluminum deposition after subtotal parathyroidectomy in dialyzed patients. Kidney Int 27:785, 1985
45. Norris KC, Crooks PW, Nebeker HG, et al: Clinical and laboratory features of aluminum-related bone disease: differences between sporadic and "epidemic" forms of the syndrome. Am J Kidney Dis 6:342, 1985
46. Meema HE, Oreopoupos DG, Rapport A: Serum magnesium level and arterial calcification in end-stage renal disease. Kidney Int 32:388, 1987
47. Buccianti G, Bianchi ML, Valenti G: Progress of renal osteodystrophy during continuous ambulatory peritoneal dialysis. Clin Nephrol 22:279, 1984
48. Hruska KA, Teitelbaum SL, Kopelman R, et al: The predictability of the histologic features of uremic bone diseases by non-invasive techniques. Metab Bone Dis Relat Res 1:39, 1978
49. Andress D, Endress DB, Ott SM, Sherrard DJ: Parathyroid hormone in aluminum-bone disease: a comparison of parathyroid hormone assays. Kidney Int 29:587, 1986
50. Salusky IB, Coburn, JW, Brill J, et al: Bone disease in pediatric patients undergoing dialysis with CAPD or CCPI. Kidney Int 33:975, 1988
51. Ott SM, Andress DL, Nebeker H, et al: Changes in bone histology after treatment with desferrioxamine. Kidney Int 29:S108, 1986
52. Milliner DS, Ott SM, Nebeker HG, et al: Deferoxamine infusion test for diagnosis of aluminum-related osteomalacia. Ann Intern Med 101:775, 1984
53. Malluche HH, Smith AJ, Abreo K, Faugere M-C: The use of desferrioxamine in the management of aluminum accumulation in bone in patients with renal failure. N Engl J Med 311:140–144, 1984
54. Hodsman AB, Hood SA, Brown P, Cordy PE: Do serum aluminum levels reflect underlying skeletal aluminum accumulation and bone histology before or after chelation by deferoxamine? J Lab Clin Med 106:674, 1985
55. Meema HE, Rabinovich S, Meema S, et al: Improved radiological diagnosis of azotemic osteodystrophy. Radiology 102:1, 1972
56. Hodson EM, Howman Gilles RB, Evans RA, et al: The diagnosis of renal osteodystrophy: a comparison of technitium^{99} pyrophosphate bone scintigraphy with other techniques. Clin Nephrol 16:24, 1981
57. Karsenty G, Vigneron N, Jorgetti V, et al: Value of the ^{99}-mTc-methylene diphosphonate bone scan in renal osteodystrophy. Kidney Int 29:1058, 1986
58. Hodgson SF: Skeletal remodeling and renal osteodystrophy. Semin Nephrol VI:42, 1986
59. Sherrard DJ, Baylink DJ, Wergedal JE, Maloney N: Quantitative histological studies on the pathogenesis of uremic bone disease. J Clin Endocrinol 39:119, 1974
60. Sherrard DJ, Ott SM, Maloney NA, et al: Uremic osteodystrophy: classification, cause and treatment. p.254. In Frame B, Potts JT (eds): Proceedings of the Symposium on Clinical Disorders of Bone and Mineral Metabolism. Excerpta Medica, Amsterdam, 1984

61. Winney RJ, Cowie JF, Robson JS: Role of plasma aluminum in the detection and prevention of aluminum toxicity. Kidney Int 29:S91, 1986
62. Makoff DL, Gordon A, Franklin SS, et al: Chronic calcium carbonate therapy in uremia. Arch Intern Med 123:15, 1969
63. Fournier A, Moriniere P, Sebert JL, et al: Calcium carbonate, an aluminum-free agent for control of hyperphosphatemia, hypocalcemia, and hyperparathyroidism in uremia. Kidney Int 29:S114, 1986
64. Guillot AP, Hood VL, Runge CF, Gennari FJ: The use of magnesium-containing phosphate binders in patients with end-stage renal disease on maintenance hemodialysis. Nephron 30:114, 1982
65. O'Donovan R, Baldwin D, Hammer M, et al: Substitutions of aluminum salts by magnesium salts in control of dialysis hyperphosphatemia. Lancet 1:680, 1986
66. Schneider H, Kulke KD, Wever H, Streicher E: High effective aluminum-free phosphate binder. In vitro and in vivo studies. Proc EDTA 20:725, 1983
67. Witmer G, Margolis A, Fontaine O, et al: Effects of 25-hydroxycholecalciferol on bone lesions of children with terminal renal failure. Kidney Int 10:395, 1976
68. Recker R, Schoenfeld P, Letteri J, et al: The efficacy of calcifediol in renal osteodystrophy. Arch Intern Med 138:857, 1978
69. Sherrard DJ, Coburn JW, Brickman AS, et al: Skeletal response to treatment with 1,25-dihydroxyvitamin D in renal failure. Contrib Nephrol 18:92, 1980
70. Salusky IB, Fine RN, Kangarloo H, et al: "High-dose" calcitriol for control of renal osteodystrophy in children on CAPD. Kidney Int 32:89, 1987
71. Slatopolsky E, Weerts C, Thielan J, et al: Marked suppression of secondary hyperparathyroidism by intravenous administration of 1,25-dihydroxycholecalciferol in uremic patients. J Clin Invest 74:2136, 1984
72. Delmez JA, Dougan CS, Gearing BK, et al: The effect of intraperitoneal calcitriol on calcium and parathyroid hormone. Kidney Int 31:795, 1987
73. Milliner DS, Hercz G, Miller JH, et al: Clearance of aluminum by hemodialysis: effect of desferrioxamine. Kidney Int 29:S100, 1986
74. Hercz G, Salusky IB, Norris KC, et al: Aluminum removal by peritoneal dialysis: effect of intravenous versus intraperitoneal deferoxamine. Kidney Int 30:944, 1986
75. Windus DW, Stokes TJ, Julian BA, Fenves AZ: Fatal rhizopus infections in hemodialysis patients receiving deferoxamine. Ann Intern Med 107:678, 1987
76. Jeejeebhoy KN, Langer B, Tsallas T, et al: Total parenteral nutrition at home: studies in patients surviving 4 months to 5 years. Gastroenterology 71:943, 1976
77. Byrne WJ, Ament ME, Burke M, Fonkalsrud E: Home parenteral nutrition. Surg Gynecol Obstet 149:593, 1979
78. Targoff CM, Coburn JW, Ament ME, et al: Bone disease associated with total parenteral nutrition, a new syndrome. p.1171. In Norman AW, Schaeffer K, von Herrath D, et al (eds): Vitamin D: Basic Research and its Clinical Application. DeGruyter, Berlin, 1979
79. Shike M, Harrison JE, Sturtridge WT, et al: Metabolic bone disease in patients receiving long-term total parenteral nutrition. Ann Intern Med 92:343, 1980
80. Klein GL, Targoff CM, Ament ME, et al: Bone disease associated with total parenteral nutrition. Lancet 2(8203):1041, 1980
81. Klein GL, Horst RL, Norman AW, et al: Reduced levels of 1 alpha, 25-dihydroxyvitamin D during long-term total parenteral nutrition. Ann Intern Med 94:638, 1981
82. Shike M, Sturtridge WC, Tam CS, et al: A possible role of vitamin D in the genesis of parenteral nutrition induced metabolic bone disease. Ann Intern Med 95:560, 1981

83. Klein GL, Cannon RA, Diament M, et al: Infantile vitamin D-resistant rickets associated with total parenteral nutrition. Am J Dis Child 136:74, 1982
84. Klein GL, Alfrey AC, Miller NI, et al: Aluminum loading during total parenteral nutrition. Am J Clin Nutr 35:1425, 1982
85. Ott SM, Maloney NA, Klein GL, et al: Aluminum is associated with low bone formation in patients on chronic parenteral nutrition. Ann Intern Med 98:910, 1983
86. Vargas JH, Klein GL, Ott SM, et al: Metabolic bone disease associated with total parenteral nutrition: course after reducing aluminum content in parenteral solutions. Am J Clin Nutr (in press)
87. Morrissey J, Slatopolsky E: Effect of aluminum on parathyroid hormone secretion. Kidney Int (suppl.) 29:S41, 1985
88. Goodman WG, Henry DA, Horst R, et al: Parenteral aluminum administration in the dog: II. Induction of osteomalacia and effect on vitamin D metabolism. Kidney Int 25:370, 1984
89. Klein GL, Ament ME, Slatopolsky E, Coburn JW: Urinary mineral excretion during long-term total parenteral nutrition. p.89. In Coburn JW, Klein GL (eds): Metabolic Bone Disease in Total Parenteral Nutrition. Urban & Schwarzenberg, Baltimore, 1985
90. McCarron DA, Rankin LI, Bennett WM, et al: Urinary calcium excretion at extremes of sodium intake in normal man. Am J Nephrol 1:84, 1981
91. Lemann J, Lennon EG, Piering WR, et al: Evidence that glucose ingestion inhibits net renal tubular reabsorption of calcium and magnesium in man. J Lab Clin Med 75:578, 1970
92. Bengoa JM, Sitrin MD, Wood RJ, Rosenbert IH: Amino acid-induced hypercalciuria in patients on total parenteral nutrition. Am J Clin Nutr 38:264, 1983
93. Wood RJ, Bengoa JM, Sitrin MD, Rosenberg IH: Calciuretic effect of cyclic versus continuous total parenteral nutrition. Am J Clin Nutr 41:614, 1985
94. Coburn JW, Hartenbower DL, Massry SG: Modification of the calciuretic effect of extracellular volume expansion by phosphate infusion. Am J Physiol 220:44, 1971
95. de Verjejoul MC, Messing B, Modrowski D, et al: Multifactorial low remodeling bone disease during cyclic total parenteral nutrition. J Clin Endocrinol Metab 60:109, 1985
96. Shike M, Shils ME, Heller A, et al: Bone disease in prolonged parenteral nutrition:osteopenia without mineralization defect. Am J Clin Nutr 44:89, 1986
97. LIpkin EW, Ott SM, Klein GL: Heterogeneity of bone histology in parenteral nutrition patients. Am J Clin Nutr 46:673, 1987
98. Editorial: Cadmium-continuing enigma. Lancet 1:1421, 1983
99. Carlisle EM: Silicon: a requirement in bone formation independent of vitamin D. Calcif Tissue Int 33:27, 1981

9 Hereditary Disorders of Bone and Mineral Metabolism

Michael P. Whyte

Although all are rare, there is a great diversity of inherited disorders of bone and mineral metabolism. Some are endocrinopathies characterized by abnormalities in circulating levels of minerals, parathyroid hormone, and vitamin D metabolites; some result from enzyme deficiencies in osseous tissue or from disturbances in bone cells or matrix. In others, the pathogenesis is less well understood and the conditions are known primarily for their clinical and radiologic features. Cumulatively, the number of affected subjects is significant. This chapter provides a brief current review of some of the principal disorders.[1–5] Heritable forms of pseudohypoparathyroidism and vitamin D resistant rickets are discussed in Chapters 4 and 5, respectively.

OSTEOPETROSIS

Osteopetrosis (marble bone disease) occurs in two principal forms: an autosomal dominant (benign) type with few or no symptoms and an autosomal recessive (malignant) type that, unless treated, is usually fatal during infancy or early childhood.[5–7] Especially rare "intermediate" forms of osteopetrosis, inherited as autosomal recessive traits, manifest during childhood with some of the clinical problems of the malignant type, but do not appear to shorten life expectancy.[5–8] Recently, deficiency of the carbonic anhydrase II isoenzyme has been found in a fourth type. Correct diagnosis of the malignant versus the intermediate forms of osteopetrosis may require assessment of disease progression.

In malignant osteopetrosis, symptoms begin during infancy.[7] Nasal "stuffiness," an early observation, is attributable to malformation of paranasal and mastoid sinuses. Subsequently, there is failure to thrive and a variety of complications (Table 9-1) from increased bone density, including myelophtistic anemia that can be exacerbated by hypersplenism and hemolysis.

In the intermediate form(s), short stature, macrocephaly, cranial nerve deficits, ankylosed teeth with osteomyelitis of the jaw, recurrent fractures, and anemia may occur.[8]

In the benign form, most subjects are asymptomatic.[6] However, long bones are brittle and may fracture. Deafness, facial palsy, visual impairment, osteomyelitis of the jaw, psychomotor delay, carpal tunnel syndrome, and osteoarthritis have been reported.[6] A recent radiologic study suggests that there are at least two types.[9]

Standard biochemical indices of mineral homeostasis are generally unremarkable in the various forms. Serum acid phosphatase activity (derived from osteoclasts) is often increased. Serum calcitriol levels may be elevated in some patients with malignant osteopetrosis.

Radiographic studies are usually diagnostic (Fig. 9-1) for the osteopetroses.[1,2] Abnormal skeletal growth, modeling (shaping of individual bones), and remodeling produce a symmetrical increase in bone mass that is accompanied by additional characteristic features (Table 9-2). Osteosclerosis may occur as a developmental defect in benign osteopetrosis. Skeletal scintigraphy is useful to demonstrate fractures, osteomyelitis, and other abnormalities.

The pathogenesis of all true forms of human osteopetrosis involves defective bone resorption.[11] Osteoclast failure provides a diagnostic histologic finding (Fig. 9-2): remnants of calcified cartilage (unresorbed primary spongiosa) within bony trabeculae.[4] However, the clinical diversity of the osteopetroses suggests that numerous molecular defects that lead to impaired skeletal degradation will be found. Indeed, osteoclasts can be increased (malignant form especially), normal, or decreased in number and their nuclei may be especially numerous. Ruffled borders and clear zones (histologic features of active osteoclasts) may be absent. The pathogenesis of osteopetrosis could involve aberrations of the stem cell or its microenvironment that impair differentiation to fully active osteoclasts, or defects in the action of mature osteoclasts.

In malignant osteopetrosis, the marrow space is usually crowded with osteoclasts and fibrous tissue; this may contribute to the myelophtistic anemia

Table 9-1. Malignant Osteopetrosis: Signs and Symptoms

Nasal stuffiness	Delayed dentition	Leukoerythoblastic anemia
Large head	Short stature	Bruising
Frontal bossing	Genu valgum	Pneumonia
Hydrocephalus	Fracture	Hepatosplenomegaly
Nystagmus	Failure to thrive	Recurrent infection
Cranial nerve palsy		

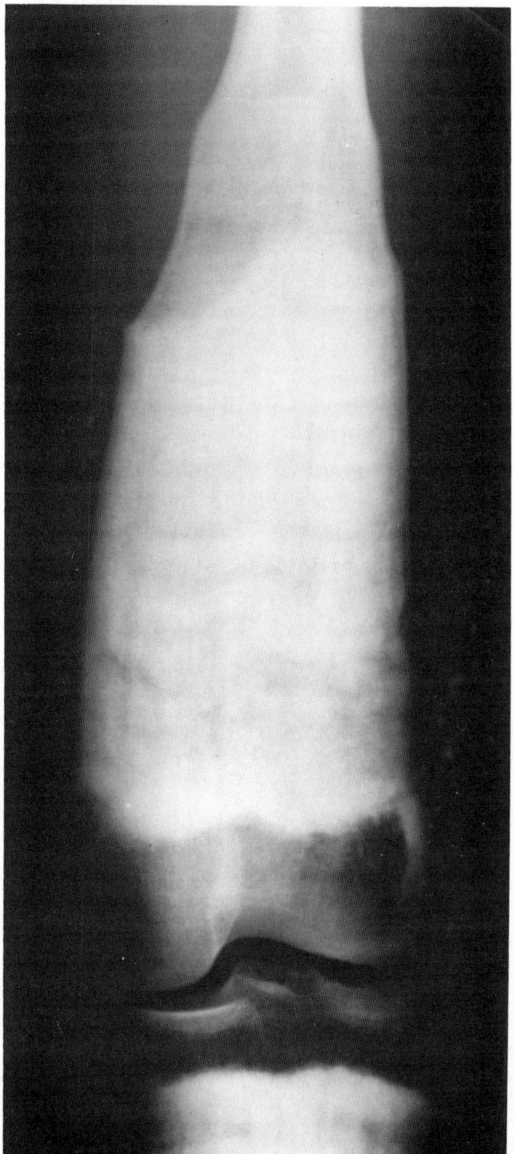

Fig. 9-1 Characteristic widening and dense transverse striations are present in the distal femoral and proximal tibial metaphyses of this 19-year-old woman with benign osteopetrosis.

Table 9-2. Malignant Osteopetrosis: Radiologic Features

Generalized symmetrical osteosclerosis
Cranial sclerosis with thick cranium
Underpneumatization of paranasal and mastoid sinuses
"Bone-in-bone" configuration in vertebrae
Transverse fractures of long bones
Widening of metaphyses and diaphyses
Alternating dense and lucent metaphyseal bands
Erosion of distal phalanges (rare)

(Fig. 9-2). Allogeneic bone marrow transplantation has been followed by reversal of neurologic, hematologic, radiologic, and histopathologic abnormalities in some cases of malignant osteopetrosis.[13,14] These studies indicated that functional osteoclasts, not osteoblasts, were of donor origin.[13] High-dose glucocorticoid therapy has been of benefit to several severe cases.[15] Similarly, brief trials of large doses of 1,25-dihydroxyvitamin D_3 (calcitriol) with a calcium-deficient diet have produced some evidence of increased bone resorption in a few cases of malignant osteopetrosis.[16] Improved hematopoietic function and decreased skeletal mass was also noted following this therapy in one adult with, apparently, an intermediate form.[17] Hyperbaric oxygenation is useful for osteo-

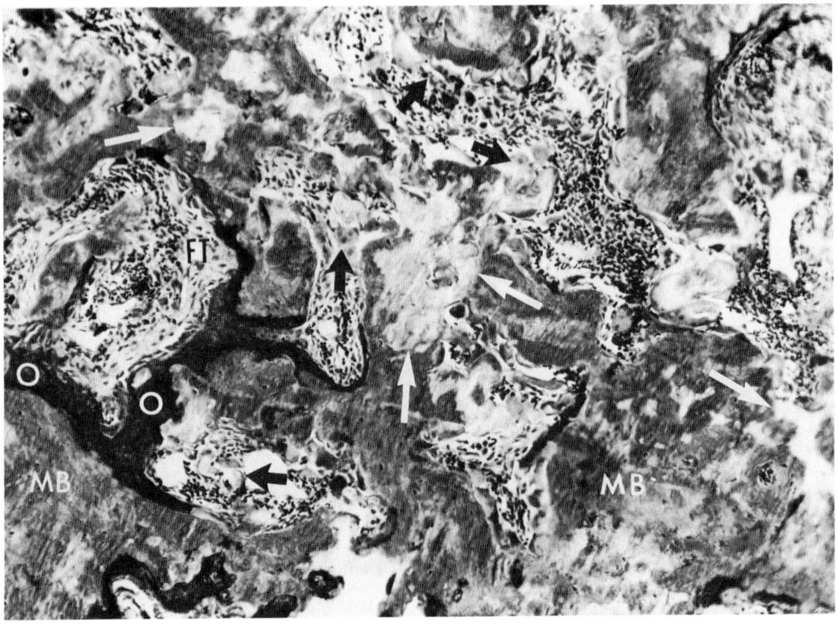

Fig. 9-2 Undecalcified iliac crest from an infant with malignant osteopetrosis shows many lightly stained areas of calcified cartilage (white arrows) within darkly stained, well-mineralized bone (MB). Abundant osteoid (O) covers the trabeculae in some areas. The marrow space is crowded with fibrous tissue (FT) and numerous osteoclasts (black arrows).

myelitis of the jaw. Surgical decompression of entrapped optic and facial nerves may be helpful.[18] Early prenatal diagnosis has been unsuccessful.[19]

CARBONIC ANHYDRASE II DEFICIENCY

Deficiency of the carbonic anhydrase II (CA-II) isoenzyme was identified in 1983 as the primary biochemical defect in the autosomal recessive syndrome of osteopetrosis, renal tubular acidosis (RTA), and cerebral calcification.[20] There is, however, clinical variability among affected families. Consanguinity is common. The disorder usually manifests in infancy or early childhood (Table 9-3), but appears to be compatible with long life.[21,22]

Anemia, if present, is usually mild; bone marrow is normal. Metabolic acidosis has been noted in neonates.[22] Distal RTA is well established; proximal RTA may also occur, but further studies of the renal acidification defect are needed.[23] The diagnosis is established by demonstrating profound deficiency of CA-II, but not CA-I, in erythrocyte lysates. CA-II levels are approximately half-normal in obligate (heterozygous) carriers.[20–22]

Radiologic features of CA-II deficiency are typical of osteopetrosis except that osteosclerosis may diminish spontaneously over years and cerebral calcification may appear at 2 to 5 years of age.[24] Histopathologic findings are characteristic of osteopetrosis.[24]

The molecular defect(s) in CA-II deficiency is unknown. Delineation of CA-II deficiency suggests an important physiologic role for this isoenzyme in the skeleton and kidney and perhaps in brain.

RTA in CA-II deficiency has been treated briefly with bicarbonate supplementation, but the long-term outcome has not been reported.[22] Conceiveably, treatment with bicarbonate could inhibit beneficial skeletal demineralization from the concomitant systemic acidosis.[24] Bone marrow transplantation is unlikely to correct the kidney defect.[23] Prenatal diagnosis has not been described.

PYCNODYSOSTOSIS

Pycnodysostosis, the disorder believed to have affected the painter Henri de Toulouse-Lautrec, is inherited as an autosomal recessive trait.[5] Parental consanguinity is common.[25] It is usually diagnosed during infancy or childhood from a great variety of skeletal abnormalities[25] (Table 9-4). Adult height is usually 4′3″ to 4′11″. Atypical patients have been reported.

Anemia is absent. Serum calcium and inorganic phosphate levels and alkaline phosphatase activity are generally normal.

Table 9-3. CA-II Deficiency: Signs and Symptoms

Developmental delay	Fracture	Apathy, muscle weakness, hypotonia and periodic hypokalemic paralysis from RTA
Failure to thrive	Mental subnormality (+/−)	
Short stature	Cranial nerve palsy	
Dental malocclusion		

Table 9-4. Pycnodysostosis: Signs and Symptoms

Disproportionate short stature	Proptosis	Hypoplastic nails
Relatively large cranium with fronto-occipital prominence	Open anterior fontanel and cranial sutures	Recurrent deforming fractures of legs
Small facies and chin	Genu valgum	Narrowed thorax (pectus excavatum)
Obtuse mandibular angle	Small square hands	Kyphoscoliosis
Ankylosis and malocclusion of teeth	Short clubbed fingers	Lumbar lordosis
High-arched palate	Acro-osteolysis or aplasia of terminal phalanges	Mental retardation (10%)

Radiologic features resemble those of osteopetrosis (generalized osteosclerosis and recurrent fractures), however, pycnodysostosis has the following additional findings: wormian bones, delayed closure of sutures and fontanels (prominently the anterior), obtuse jaw angle, thin clavicles with hypoplastic ends, partial absence of the hyoid bone, and aplasia or hypoplasia of the distal ribs and phalanges.[1,2,26] Unlike osteopetrosis, the bony contours are normal. Although long bones have sclerotic cortices and narrow medullary cavities, endobones (bone within bone) and radiodense metaphyseal striations are absent. Uniform osteosclerosis appears in childhood and increases with age. The calvarium and base of the skull are sclerotic; orbital ridges are dense. Facial bones, paranasal sinuses, and terminal phalanges are hypoplastic. Lumbosacral spondylolisthesis is not uncommon; lack of segmentation of the atlas and axis may occur.[1,2]

Histopathologic study reveals normal cortical bone structure, but osteoblastic and osteoclastic activity appear to be decreased.[27] Electron microscopy has suggested defective osteoclastic degradation of skeletal collagen, perhaps due to an abnormality in bone matrix or in the osteoclasts themselves.[27] Abnormal inclusions can also occur in chondrocytes.[28] Although calcium absorption from the gastrointestinal tract can be markedly increased, decreased bone resorption appears to account for the osteosclerosis.[29]

The genetic defect is unknown. Chromosomal abnormalities have been reported.[25]

There is no effective medical therapy for pycnodysostosis. Fractures usually heal at a satisfactory rate. Internal fixation of long bones is made difficult by their hardness. Patients are generally able to walk independently. Extraction of teeth is difficult; fracture or osteomyelitis of the mandible can occur.[25]

ENGELMANN'S DISEASE (PROGRESSIVE DIAPHYSEAL DYSPLASIA)

Progressive diaphyseal dysplasia is a developmental, autosomal dominant form of osteosclerosis with variable clinical and radiologic penetrance.[30] Some

Table 9-5. Engelmann's Disease: Signs and Symptoms

Leg pain	Palpable bony enlargement	Proptosis
Muscle wasting	Skeletal tenderness	Increased intracranial pressure
Gait disturbance	Enlarged head and prominent forehead	Delayed puberty
Decreased subcutaneous fat in limbs	Cranial nerve palsies	Hepatosplenomegaly

adult carriers have no radiographic abnormalities. In severe cases, osteosclerosis is generalized and involves nearly the entire skeleton. The disorder is characterized by gradual new bone formation along both the endosteal and periosteal surfaces of the cortices of tubular bones; patients have a variety of associated clinical problems (Table 9-5). All races are affected. Spontaneous clinical improvement with cessation of radiologic change has been described in adolescents.

Routine biochemical parameters of bone and mineral metabolism are usually unremarkable, although hypocalciuria and modest hypocalcemia may occur in severely affected individuals.[31] Serum alkaline phosphatase activity and the erythrocyte sedimentation rate can be increased. Mild anemia and leukopenia may be present.[31]

Radiologic studies characteristically show nearly symmetrical, spreading hyperostosis of long bone shafts.[1,2] Epiphyses are spared. Tibiae and femora are involved most frequently (Fig. 9-3). The age of onset, rate of progression, and degree of severity vary considerably. In the milder forms, which can present in adolescents or young adults, abnormalities are limited to long bones of the lower extremities. Although bone scanning and radiographic findings are usually concordant, the former may be unremarkable despite distinct radiographic changes and may reflect advanced (quiescent) disease. Bone scan abnormalities with only mild radiologic changes suggest early disease.[32]

Prednisone (small doses on alternate days) appears to be a very effective therapy. Relief of skeletal pain and histologic improvement of affected bone have been described.[33]

ENDOSTEAL HYPEROSTOSIS

Van Buchem Disease*

Endosteal hyperostosis has been reported in a severe autosomal recessive form (van Buchem disease) or in a relatively benign autosomal dominant form.[35,36] Both types are characterized by new bone formation on the endosteal (inner) surface of bone cortices (see also discussion of sclerosteosis).

* Note: A recent review of van Buchem disease in Holland and sclerosteosis in South Africa emphasizes the similarity of their clinical and radiographic features (which are more severe in sclerosteosis). Each disorder may, therefore, represent homozygosity for the same genetic defect where differences in expression are caused by modifying genes.[34]

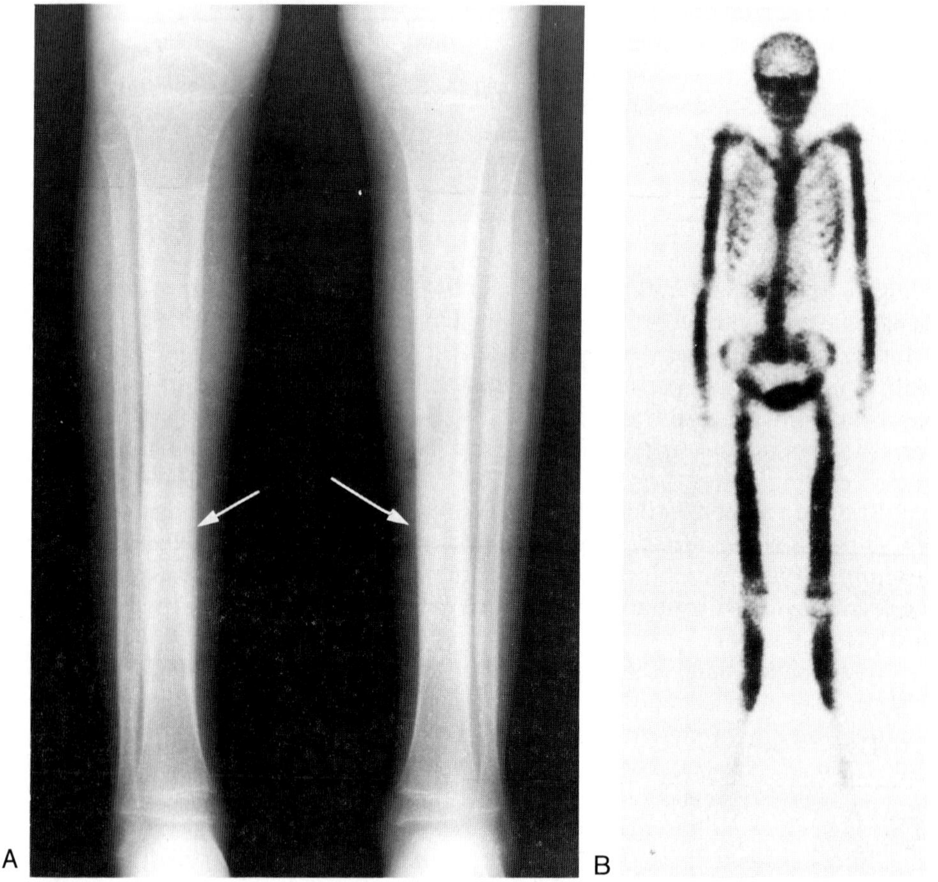

Fig. 9-3 **(A)** The tibiae and fibulae of this 4-year-old girl with Engelmann's disease are broad and show cortical thickening, especially in the distal tibiae (arrows). **(B)** Bone scan at age 16 shows characteristic symmetrical increased radionuclide uptake that is particularly striking in the shafts of the long bones.

In van Buchem disease, the jaw progressively and asymmetrically enlarges and the mandibular angle widens but without prognathism. Skull involvement during early childhood causes recurrent facial paralysis, deafness, and optic atrophy by narrowing cranial foramina. Clavicles and ribs are thickened. Long bones may be painful to pressure.[35]

Alkaline phosphatase activity in serum may be increased (bone isoenzyme), yet circulating levels of calcium and inorganic phosphate are normal.

Radiologic study shows properly shaped long bones that are dense from cortical widening from selective endosteal hyperostosis. Generalized osteosclerosis affects the base of the skull, facial bones, mandible, vertebrae, pelvis, and ribs.[1,2]

There is no effective medical treatment. Surgical decompression of narrowed foramina may be helpful in some cases with cranial nerve palsy.

Sclerosteosis*

Sclerosteosis, also an autosomal recessive disorder, is usually reported in subjects of Dutch ancestry (e.g., Afrikaner population of South Africa). During early childhood, there is overgrowth and sclerosis of the skeleton, especially the skull. Patients are tall and heavy[37]; the jaw has a very square appearance. Cranial nerve entrapment develops early. Raised intracranial pressure from a small cranial cavity and brain stem compression may occur. Syndactyly (due to cutaneous or bony fusion of the index and middle fingers) is a characteristic but variable finding. Patients are not prone to fractures. Intelligence is not affected. Life expectancy may be shortened.

Radiologic study, except for syndactyly, is normal in early childhood. Subsequently, there is progressive osteosclerosis and widening of the skull and mandible (including prognathism).[38] Ribs, pelvis, vertebral pedicles, and tubular bones are somewhat dense. Modeling defects occur in the long bones where the cortices are thickened.

Histologic studies of bone from an American kindred indicated that enhanced osteoblastic formation of skeletal tissue is a primary reason for the osteosclerosis.[39] There is no medical treatment. Syndactyly usually requires surgical correction. Surgery to correct prognathism is complicated by the dense mandibular bone.

HYPOPHOSPHATASIA

Hypophosphatasia is a form of rickets/osteomalacia that results from a generalized deficiency of activity of the tissue-nonspecific (liver/bone/kidney) alkaline phosphatase (ALP) isoenzyme; placental and intestinal ALP isoenzyme activity is normal.[40] Unlike in most forms of rickets or osteomalacia (see Chap. 5), serum calcium and inorganic phosphate levels are not subnormal. Furthermore, instead of manifesting increased serum ALP activity, the biochemical hallmark of hypophosphatasia is hypophosphatasemia. All races are affected. The age at presentation generally reflects the extremely variable clinical severity; that is, the earlier patients become symptomatic, the more severe the disease.[40] Five clinical forms are reported (Table 9-6). This inborn error of

Table 9-6. Hypophosphatasia: Signs and Symptoms in Various Clinical Forms

Perinatal	Infantile	Childhood	Adult	Odonto
Polyhydramnios	Failure to thrive	Premature loss of deciduous teeth	Premature loss of teeth	Premature loss of deciduous teeth
Stillbirth	Hypotonia	Short stature	Osteopenia	No radiologic abnormalities
Deformed limbs	Progressive rachitic deformities	Delayed walking	Recurrent metatarsal stress fractures	
Respiratory compromise, periodic apnea, and bradycardia	Flail chest	Rachitic deformities	Pseudofractures	
Fever	Pneumonia	Waddling gait	Chondrocalcinosis	
Intracranial hemorrhage	Wide fontanels		Pseudogout	
Irritability	Hypercalcemia/nephrocalcinosis			
Anemia	Craniosynostosis			
Seizures	Proptosis and hypertelorism			

* See footnote on p. 229.

metabolism illustrates that ALP is important for skeletal mineralization and dental development.

Perinatal hypophosphatasia is clinically apparent at birth and is always fatal. Subjects that are not stillborn live only a few days or weeks despite mechanical ventilation for flail chest secondary to severe rachitic disease. Infantile hypophosphatasia usually presents at a few months of age with failure to thrive and progressive rachitic deformity. Hypercalcemia/hypercalciuria with nephrocalcinosis then develops in some patients and seems to reflect dyssynergy between active gut absorption of calcium and decreased skeletal deposition of mineral. Raised intracranial pressure from functional synostosis of the skull (despite radiologically open fontanels) is common. About one-half of affected infants die; those who survive may have variable degrees of skeletal deformity. Childhood hypophosphatasia varies considerably in clinical severity. Premature loss of deciduous teeth (i.e., before age 5 years) is the most consistent clinical finding and reflects aplasia or hypoplasia of dental cementum that connects dentin to the peridontal ligament. Dental abnormalities may occur alone (odontohypophosphatasia) or with variable degrees of rickets detected radiologically. A waddling gait appears to indicate a concomitant myopathy (personal observation). The disease may remit clinically when growth plates fuse. Adult hypophosphatasia usually presents during middle age with pain from recurrent, slowly healing, metatarsal stress fractures or femoral pseudofractures.[41] Some individuals give histories to suggest that they had had rachitic disease during childhood as well. Occasional subjects, despite biochemical abnormalities consistent with hypophosphatasia, have life-long absence of clinical disease.

Laboratory diagnosis requires demonstration of hypophosphatasemia (age-dependent changes in serum ALP activity in control subjects must be taken into consideration). Quantitation of ALP isoenzyme levels in serum may be helpful in perplexing cases. Patients are often mildly hyperphosphatemic. Three phosphocompounds that appear to be natural substrates for ALP accumulate endogenously in all forms of hypophosphatasia: phosphoethanolamine (PEA), inorganic pyrophosphate (PPi), and pyridoxal phosphate (PLP).[42] Assay of urinary PEA levels is readily available and helps to support the diagnosis.

Radiologic studies, especially in the more severe forms, are characteristic if not diagnostic.[1–2,43] Perinatal hypophosphatasia results in extreme undermineralization of the skeleton that can be readily distinguished from osteogenesis imperfecta (see below) or severe skeletal dysplasias. Irregular extensions of growth plate cartilage into metaphyses (Fig. 9-4) is a radiologic finding that characterizes the rachitic disease of affected infants and children. Adults may have osteopenia, metatarsal stress fractures, femoral pseudofractures, and chondrocalcinosis.[41]

Histologic study of bone reveals rickets/osteomalacia but, without histochemical evaluation of ALP activity, is not diagnostic.[44] Demonstration of hypoplasia or aplasia of dental cementum is a reliable means of diagnosis.

Defective bone mineralization probably results from endogenous accumu-

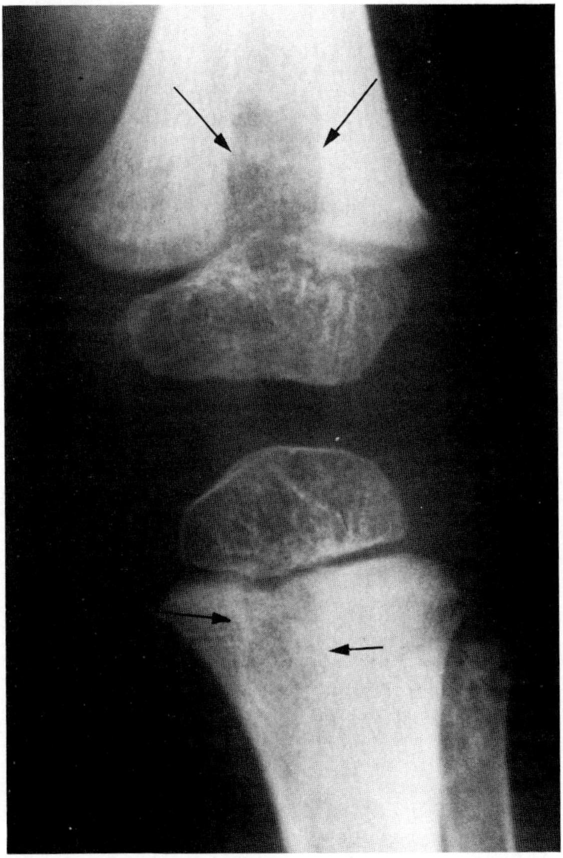

Fig. 9-4 Characteristic "tongues" of radiolucency (arrows) protrude into the metaphyses of a knee in this 2½-year-old boy with hypophosphatasia.

lation of PPi, which is an inhibitor of hydroxyapatite crystal formation.[40,45] Despite markedly elevated levels of plasma PLP (the cofactor form of vitamin B6), tissue levels of vitamin B6 appear to be normal in hypophosphatasia.[46] Accordingly, tissue nonspecific ALP seems to act as an ectoenzyme to control extracellular substrate levels. The pathogenesis of the myopathy is unknown.

The molecular defects for hypophosphatasia have not yet been elucidated, although a regulatory problem of tissue-nonspecific ALP gene expression appears to occur in some cases.[47] Family studies indicate that severely affected individuals have homozygous disease; mildly affected subjects appear to be heterozygotes.[40]

There is no effective medical treatment. Intramedullary rodding seems to be the best orthopedic approach to treatment of fractures and pseudofractures in long bones.[48] Prenatal identification of severe disease is accomplished best at about 16 weeks gestation by ultrasound study of the fetus and by assay (in an experienced laboratory) of ALP activity in cultivated amniotic fluid cells.[49]

MYOSITIS OSSIFICANS PROGRESSIVA

Myositis (fibrodysplasia) ossificans progressiva is an autosomal dominant disorder characterized by congenital skeletal anomalies together with recurrent painful episodes of heterotopic bone formation. It is transmitted with very variable expressivity.[5] More than 500 cases have been reported.[50] The disorder may be suspected at birth because of characteristic *Hallux valgus* with microdactyly.[1,2] Synostosis and hypoplasia of the phalanges and microdactyly of the thumb are also common congenital findings. Subsequent development of heterotopic bone formation in voluntary muscles and ligaments, however, establishes the diagnosis.[50,51] Cardiac and involuntary muscle is spared. Although the onset of ectopic bone formation is usually during the first decade of life, it is variable (in utero to early adulthood). Recurrent episodes of fever with tender and rubbery soft tissue swellings (sometimes after even minor trauma, sometimes spontaneously) are followed by ectopic calcification and then formation of osseous tissue. Initially, the sternocleidomastoid, shoulder girdle, and dorsal musculature of the trunk are involved. Subsequent ankylosis of the spine, rib cage, and shoulders may severely limit mobility and torticollis and scoliotic deformity can occur. Later, the proximal lower extremities may be affected. Distal limb musculature, however, does not calcify. Despite widespread ectopic bone formation, some patients live into the fifth decade; most, however, die sooner from respiratory complications due to restricted motion of the thorax.

In some cases only, routine laboratory studies show increased serum alkaline phosphatase activity.[52]

Radiologic studies[1–2] reveal the various congenital skeletal anomalies (absence or fusion of phalanges of the great toe and short first metacarpals and middle phalanges of the hands) and progressive ossification affecting fascia, tendons, aponeuroses, and other tissues (Fig. 9-5). Cervical vertebrae may be small and have thick pedicles and large spinous processes that undergo progressive fusion. Acetabular dysplasia is common. During periods of severe inflammation, portions of the skeleton can become osteopenic; otherwise, the bones are generally well mineralized.[1,2]

Histopathologic studies of early lesions show multifocal interconnecting nodules of fibroblasts within a connective tissue matrix. Subsequently, bone (or occasionally cartilage) occurs centrally. Fasciae, tendons, ligaments, and joint capsules may be involved. Cancellous bone that contains hematopoietic tissue appears in mature lesions.[50,51]

Paternal age appears to contribute importantly to the incidence of new dominant mutations. Indeed, most cases appear to be sporadic.[53] It is unclear, however, whether the disorder is due to a primary abnormality in skeletal muscle (myositis) or connective tissue (fibrodysplasia). Histologic and electromyographic abnormalities in muscle that precede connective tissue proliferation support the term *myositis* ossificans progressiva.

There is no satisfactory medical therapy. Treatment with the diphosphonate, disodium etidronate, has resulted in a variable response.[54] Warfarin therapy, to disrupt the γ-carboxylation of calcium-binding proteins in bone, has

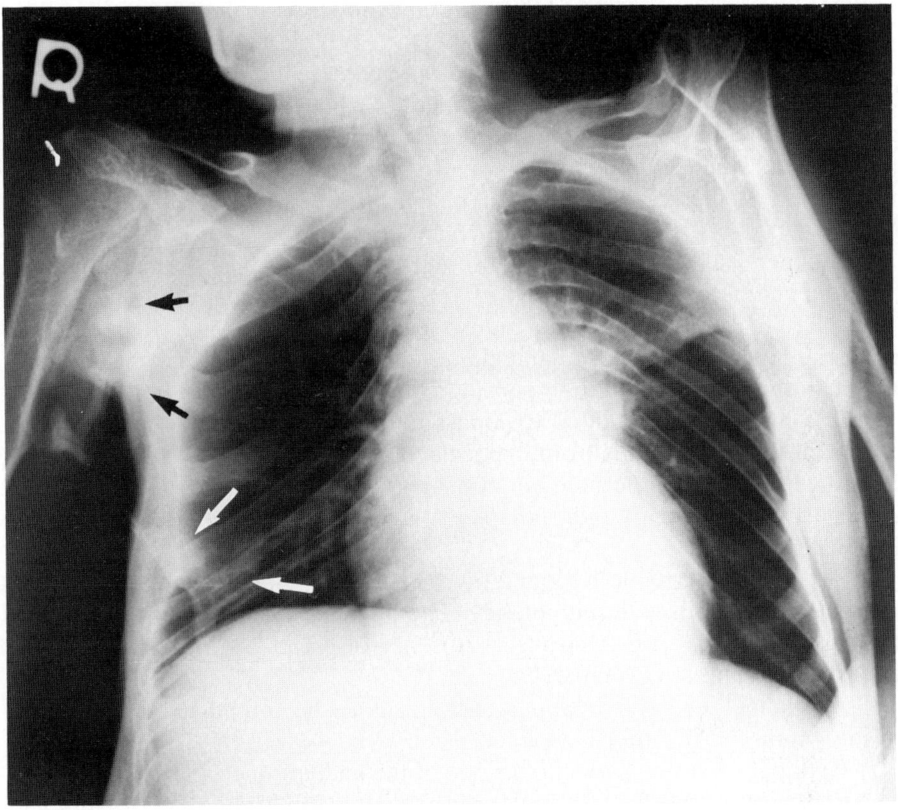

Fig. 9-5 Advanced heterotopic bone formation in the chest wall (white arrows) and especially the right shoulder (black arrowheads) has deformed the thorax of this 18-year-old boy with myositis ossificans progressiva.

been reported recently to decrease modestly urinary excretion of γ-carboxyglutamic acid but not to improve the ectopic calcification.[55] Trauma to muscle (including injections or surgical procedures) should be avoided, if possible, so as not to precipitate swellings. Surgery, however, may help to release joint contractures, increase the mandibular range of motion, or correct neurovascular entrapment. A brief course of high-dose etidronate disodium during the perioperative period may help to prevent trauma-induced calcification. Removal of calcified lesions may be followed by recurrence.

HYPOPARATHYROIDISM

Failure of the parathyroid glands to secrete parathyroid hormone, thus causing hypocalcemia (i.e., idiopathic hypoparathyroidism) generally occurs as a sporadic disorder. However, a variety of heritable forms have also been described.[5] In some of these conditions, the hypoparathyroidism is an isolated finding; in others, it occurs with additional endocrine or nonendocrine abnormalities (Table 9-7).

With mild hypocalcemia, subjects may experience paresthesias. If hypocalcemia is severe, clinical sequelae include carpopedal spasm, laryngospasm, and/or seizures. Long-standing and poorly treated disease may result in cataracts, dental enamel hypoplasia, paravertebral ligamentous ossification, mental retardation, dementia, basal ganglia calcification, and a variety of additional central nervous system problems.

Biochemical studies typically show hypocalcemia, hyperphosphatemia, and (depending on the sensitivity of the assay) low or inappropriately "normal" serum levels of immunoreactive parathyroid hormone. If parathyroid hormone levels are increased and glomerular filtration rate is normal, pseudohypoparathyroidism should be considered (see Chap. 4).

In kindreds with isolated hypoparathyroidism inherited as an autosomal dominant trait, symptoms from hypocalcemia may be mild and vary according to age.[56] Recently, in one such kindred, serum calcitriol levels were found to be normal (not subnormal) and perhaps explained these patients' only moderate hypocalcemia.[57]

Sex-linked recessive hypoparathyroidism (only males clinically affected) presents with seizures during infancy. The disorder has been described in just two large kindreds from Missouri.[58] Absence of parathyroid tissue appears to be a fundamental abnormality.[59]

Autosomal recessive hypoparathyroidism has been reported in a few families in whom the disorder is isolated.[60]

Hypoparathyroidism occurs as one of the endocrine problems in the autosomal recessive trait polyglandular autoimmune syndrome, type I, in which affected subjects may also have moniliasis, Addison's disease, chronic active hepatitis, pernicious anemia, alopecia, and primary hypogonadism.[61]

Kenny-Caffey syndrome is a form of dwarfism[62] associated with transient bouts of hypocalcemia from hypoparathyroidism, narrow medullary cavities of tubular bones, which gives the impression of osteosclerosis, and nanophthalmos. It is unclear if the dominant inheritance pattern is autosomal or sex-linked.[5] An abnormal parathyroid hormone has recently been reported in one case.[63]

Hypoparathyroidism, from defective secretion of or peripheral resistance to parathyroid hormone, can occur from hypomagnesemia. Primary hypomagnesemia may be inherited as an autosomal and sex-linked condition (see below).

Table 9-7. Idiopathic Hypoparathyroidism (Heritable Forms)

Isolated (AD, AR, SLR)	From primary hypomagnesemia (AR, AD, SLR)
Polyglandular autoimmune syndrome, type I (AR)	With lymphedema (recessive; AR? SLR?)
Kenny-Caffey syndrome (dominant; AD? SLD?)	With sensorineural deafness (AR?)

AR autosomal recessive; AD autosomal dominant; SLR sex-linked recessive; SLD sex-linked dominant.

Heritable syndromes of hypoparathyroidism with lymphedema[64] or sensorineural deafness[65] have been described.

DiGeorge's syndrome (congenital absence of the parathyroid and thymus glands: III and IV pharyngeal pouch syndrome) is considered a sporadic condition.

The variety of inherited forms of idiopathic hypoparathyroidism indicate that at least several molecular mechanisms will be uncovered. Thus far, linkage studies have failed to indicate a defect in the parathyroid hormone gene itself.[66,67] Hypoparathyroidism has been reported with a 10p deletion[68] and with ring chromosome 18.[69] Autoantibodies to parathyroid cells have been found recently in autoimmune hypoparathyroidism.[70]

Treatment usually consists of vitamin D or an active metabolite together with calcium supplementation and phosphate-binding antacid.[71] Allotransplantation of parathyroid glands has recently been used to treat intractable hypoparathyroidism.[72]

OSTEOGENESIS IMPERFECTA

Osteogenesis imperfecta (OI) (brittle bone disease) is a connective tissue disorder characterized by skeletal fragility and a variety of extraskeletal manifestations (Table 9-8) that appear to reflect a great many molecular defects that produce quantitative and/or qualitative abnormalities in the biosynthesis of Type I collagen.[73] Understandably, therefore, OI is characterized by very variable severity. Its major clinical findings are listed in Table 9-8. The widely used nosology formulated by Sillence[74] is based primarily on clinical presentation, radiologic findings, natural history, and apparent mode of inheritance. Detailed biochemical/molecular studies, however, are beginning to clarify the patterns of inheritance (see below).[73] Sillence type I OI is a well-characterized, autosomal dominant, clinically mild disorder characterized by recurrent fractures (especially during childhood), blue sclerae, deafness that manifests during early adulthood, and either absence or presence of dentinogenesis imperfecta (Type IA and IB, respectively). About one-third of cases are new mutations. Type II and III are severe forms that were previously believed to be autosomal recessive conditions. In type II disease (the perinatal (lethal) form), there is in utero onset with blue sclerae, "crumpled" bones, and severe generalized osteopenia. Type III is characterized by progressive deformity with severe growth failure, pale blue sclerae, and dentinogenesis imperfecta. Type IV patients have white sclerae, variable bone fragility, and deformity believed to be transmitted as an

Table 9-8. Osteogenesis Imperfecta: Signs and Symptoms

Osteopenia	High-pitched voice	Excessive sweating
Recurrent fractures	Short stature	Joint hypermobility
Blue sclerae	Triangle-shaped facies	Scoliosis
Early-onset deafness	Chest deformity	Herniae
Dentinogenesis imperfecta	Head appears large	Easy bruisability/thin skin

autosomal dominant trait.[74] However, the sizable number of subjects (families) that do not fit these categories well indicates that many molecular defects will be found.[73]

For all forms of OI, fractures tend to occur more frequently in the legs than arms, and may heal with exuberant callus formation. Intelligence is usually normal. Thoracic deformity predisposes to pneumonia.

Radiologic studies show variable degrees of generalized osteopenia and deformity from fractures[1,2] (Fig. 9-6A). Marked shortening of limbs from "telescoped" fractures, craniofacial disproportion with wide intertemporal diameter, and thoracic deformity occur in severe cases. Some patients have wormian bones in the skull (Fig. 9-6B). The pelvis may be triradiate. Thin cortices in the calvarium and especially in narrowed (gracile) long bones are a characteristic feature. So-called popcorn calcification, found predominantly at the knees and ankles, reflects a developmental abnormality in the epiphyses and metaphyses of major long bones from fragmentation of growth plates. Biconcave vertebrae or platyspondylia and basilar invagination of the skull occur in more severely osteopenic subjects.

Routine biochemical studies of mineral metabolism are usually unremarkable. Elevations in serum alkaline phosphatase activity and urine hydroxyproline occur in some patients. Subjects who are severely affected and growing poorly may be hypercalciuric.

Histologic studies of bone from patients with the severe forms of OI show thin collagen bundles on polarized-light microscopy. Bone remodeling is rapid and woven bone may be abundant. In more mild forms, bone is more lamellar. Some patients have excessive numbers of osteocytes within cortical bone.[4] Accordingly, activity of individual osteoblasts may be decreased although, overall, bone turnover is accelerated.

Sillence's classification suggested that severe types of OI were inherited as autosomal recessive traits.[74] More recent biochemical studies of type I collagen and its gene indicate that the most patients (even those in severely affected sibships) reflect heterozygous disease[73,75–78]; autosomal recessive forms appear to be less common than suggested previously. Occurrence of severe disease in siblings seems to be explained best by gonadal mutation rather than autosomal recessive inheritance.[74] About 5 to 7 percent of families with an infant with severe OI are at risk of having another affected child. Studies of collagen from cultivated skin cells are especially helpful in diagnosis.[73] OI is characterized by decreased production of type I collagen. The slow rate of formation of collagen often leads to excessive posttranslational modification of the protein helix. It is possible that some cases of OI are due to primary defects in the noncollagenous bone proteins.[73]

There is no effective medical therapy.[79] Orthopedic and physical/occupational therapy are the mainstays of treatment.[80] Leg bracing, when severely affected children begin to stand, is important. Scoliosis must be carefully evaluated for possible surgical intervention. Support groups such as the American Brittle Bone Society, Inc., and the Osteogenesis Imperfecta Foundation, Inc., are important sources of information and comfort for affected families. Progno-

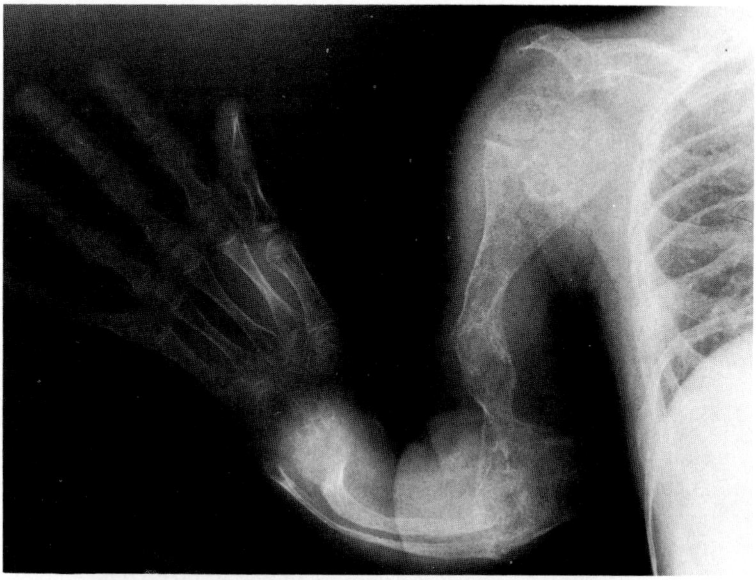

A

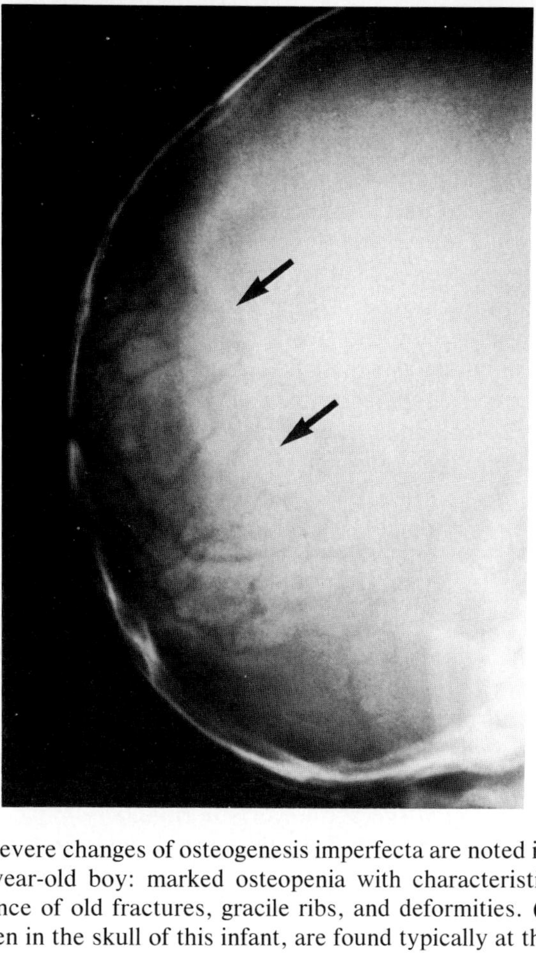

B

Fig. 9-6 **(A)** Severe changes of osteogenesis imperfecta are noted in the upper extremity of this 14-year-old boy: marked osteopenia with characteristic thinning of bony cortices, evidence of old fractures, gracile ribs, and deformities. **(B)** Wormian bones (arrows), as seen in the skull of this infant, are found typically at the lamdoidal suture.

sis is variable. Many patients experience fewer fractures once they reach adolescence. Diagnosis of some of the severe forms in utero has been possible by sonography (15 to 17 weeks' gestation),[81] and restriction fragment-length polymorphism studies appear to be promising for some affected kindreds.[82] Increased paternal age appears to be a risk factor for new dominant mutation.[83]

FAMILIAL BENIGN HYPERCALCEMIA (FAMILIAL HYPOCALCIURIC HYPERCALCEMIA)

Familial benign hypercalcemia (FBH), also called familial hypocalciuric hypercalcemia, can be mistaken for primary hyperparathyroidism. It is transmitted as an autosomal dominant trait with a high degree of penetrance.[5] Hypercalcemia is present from infancy.[84] Unlike in most patients with primary hyperparathyroidism, however, *urinary* calcium levels are not elevated, but normal or low[84–86]; that is, there is relative hypocalciuria. Despite moderate hypercalcemia, patients are generally well. Rarely, pancreatitis, chondrocalcinosis, or cholelithiasis is reported. However, some affected newborns have neonatal hyperparathyroidism with severe symptomatic hypercalcemia and osteopenia.[87]

As in primary hyperparathyroidism, serum inorganic phosphate concentration tends to be low or low–normal, but the serum magnesium level is not reduced but elevated. Despite the hypercalcemia, hypercalciuria does not occur and the fractional excretion of calcium helps to differentiate these patients from those with hypercalcemia of other causes. A simple diagnostic index is the ratio of renal calcium clearance to creatinine clearance. A value below 0.01 suggests FBH. Serum immunoreactive parathyroid hormone levels are usually normal. Hypercalcemia persists after partial parathyroidectomy; if all parathyroid tissue is removed, hypocalcemia follows. Circulating immunoreactive calcitonin levels are also generally normal.

Radiologic study of the skeleton is unremarkable. High-resolution parathyroid sonography appears to be a useful diagnostic tool since, in FBH, the parathyroid glands are not detectably enlarged as they are in primary hyperparathyroidism.[88]

Histologic studies, however, reveal that the parathyroid glands are about three times larger than normal in familial benign hypercalcemia, but significantly smaller than in primary parathyroid hyperplasia.[89] Parathyroid glands may be hyperplastic or normal.[89,90] We have recently observed a family in whom serum immunoreactive parathyroid hormone levels rise in affected individuals to elevated levels during the adult years (unpublished findings, 1988). A limited number of studies of bone tissue suggest that there may be accelerated bone remodeling[91] although skeletal mass is normal.[92]

FBH appears to reflect an abnormality in the "set-point" for the parathyroid glands together with a defect in the kidney tubules that leads to enhanced renal reclamation of filtered calcium. Urinary calcium excretion rates are about one-third those in primary hyperparathyroidism. Abnormalities in Ca^{++} transport in both of these tissues could be a common causative factor. Calcitriol levels have been reported to be low in FBH; they are increased in primary hyperparathyroidism.[93] Despite hypercalcemia, immunoreactive parathyroid hormone levels are not suppressed. Renal reclamation of filtered magnesium is also enhanced. Hypocalciuria will persist after total parathyroidectomy.[94] The basic defect may involve a blunted inhibitory response to hypercalcemia by the parathyroid glands leading to an abnormal "set-point" and to abnormal calcium and Mg^{++} reabsorption in the thick ascending section of Henle's loop.[95]

Definitive diagnosis requires demonstration of hypercalcemia in first-degree relatives. Affected family members should be identified and warned that their offspring are at risk of neonatal hypercalcemia. Serum calcium level should be assayed in newborns at risk.

HYPERPARATHYROIDISM

Primary hyperparathyroidism can occur as an isolated disorder that is transmitted as an autosomal dominant[96] or autosomal recessive[97] trait, or in association with hyperfunction of other endocrine glands; that is, type I and II multiple endocrine neoplasia.[98] In type I multiple endocrine neoplasia, powerful mitogenic activity for parathyroid tissue has recently been identified as a potential pathogenic factor.[98] In type II disease, medullary carcinoma of the thyroid with pheochromocytoma (Sipple's syndrome), a deletion of chromosome 20 has been found.[99]

HYPOMAGNESEMIA

Primary hypomagnesemia, apparently due to selective gastrointestinal malabsorption of Mg^{++}, has been reported in the offspring of first cousins.[100] The disorder, which appears to have been transmitted as an autosomal recessive trait, presents with neonatal convulsions from concomitant hypocalcemia. Hypomagnesemic tetany has also been reported to be inherited, apparently as an X-linked recessive trait.[101,102] In these cases also, convulsions with hypocalcemia occur in infancy. Calcinosis of heart, kidneys, and arteries can also develop. More recently, renal magnesium wasting with hypocalciuria has been described in two unrelated families in whom the inheritance pattern was consistent with autosomal dominant transmission.[103]

HYPERPHOSPHATEMIC TUMORAL CALCINOSIS

Hyperphosphatemic tumoral calcinosis is characterized by developmental ectopic calcification around major joints, especially the shoulder and hips. Angioid streaks of the retina may occur. Most affected subjects in North America have been black (Fig. 9-7). It is usually inherited as an autosomal recessive

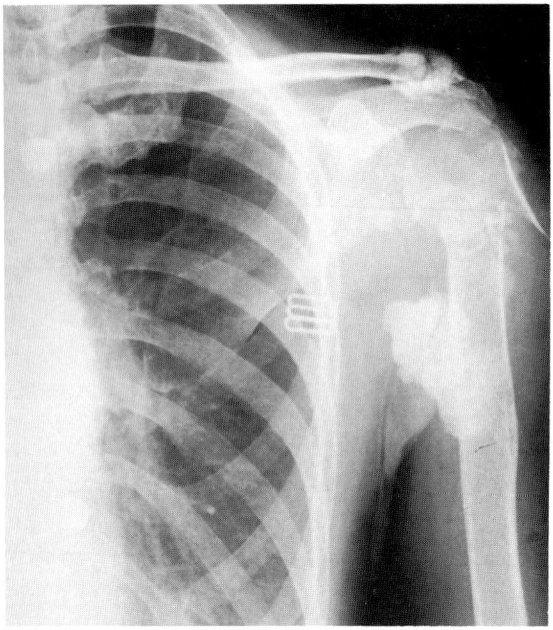

Fig. 9-7 Characteristic periarticular accumulation of calcium in a 58-year-old black woman with hyperphosphatemic tumoral calcinosis.

trait.[104] Recently, however, autosomal dominant transmission has been reported in a kindred where affected family members had teeth with well-developed enamel yet were hypoplastic and had bulbous roots, obliterated pulp cavities, and dentin abnormalities.[105] Serum calcitriol levels were elevated in only some of the subjects with calcinosis.[105]

Hyperphosphatemia is due to increased renal tubular reclamation of filtered phosphate. Enhanced calcitriol synthesis by the kidney appears to be a basic pathogenetic abnormality.[106] Phosphate deprivation has been reported to be helpful in some cases.[107]

OTHER

A great variety of additional hereditary disorders of bone and mineral metabolism have been characterized.[1–5]

Familial idiopathic hypercalciuria[108]—an autosomal dominant form of absorptive hypercalciuria—could be a mild form of hereditary hypophosphatemic rickets with hypercalciuria[109] (see Chap. 5).

Idiopathic hypercalcemia of infancy may, in some instances, be a distinct autosomal dominant disorder, or may be a form of William's syndrome or familial benign hypercalcemia (see above).[5]

Hypophosphatemic bone disease, an autosomal dominant disorder, is characterized by hypophosphatemia, a modest degree of short stature, bowing of the lower extremities, and radiographic changes that resemble a metaphyseal chondrodysplasia rather than rickets. For the same degree of hypophosphatemia, skeletal disease is less severe than in sex-linked hypophosphatemic rickets[110] (see Chap. 5).

Paget's disease of bone is not infrequently found to be familial. Both environmental and genetic factors probably account for this observation. Association with certain HLA types has been reported.[111] In some kindreds, there is a clear autosomal dominant form characterized by especially aggressive osteolytic disease, osteopenia, hypercalciuria, and deafness.[112]

The reader is referred elsewhere for information on the many other rare inherited disorders of bone and mineral metabolism that could not be described here.[1–5,113]

REFERENCES

1. Resnick D, Niwayama G: Diagnosis of Bone and Joint Disorders. 2nd Ed. WB Saunders, Philadelphia, 1988
2. Wynne-Davies R, Hall CM, Apley AG: Atlas of Skeletal Dysplasias. Churchill Livingstone, Edinburgh, 1985
3. Maroteaux P: Bone Diseases of Children. JB Lippincott, Philadelphia, 1979
4. Revell PA: Pathology of Bone. Springer-Verlag, Berlin, Heidelberg, 1986
5. McKusick VA: Mendelian Inheritance In Man. 7th Ed. Johns Hopkins University Press, Baltimore, 1986
6. Johnston CC, Jr., Lavy N, Lord T, et al: Osteopetrosis: a clinical, genetic, metabolic, and morphologic study of the dominantly inherited benign form. Medicine 47: 149, 1968
7. Loria-Cortes R, Quesada-Calvo E, Cordero-Chaverri E: Osteopetrosis in children: a report of 26 cases. J Pediat 91: 43, 1977
8. Kahler SG, Burns JA, Aylsworth AS: A mild autosomal recessive form of osteopetrosis. Am J Med Genet 17: 451, 1984
9. Andersen PE, Jr., Bollerslev J: Heterogeneity of autosomal dominant osteopetrosis. Radiology 164: 223, 1987
10. Park H-M, Lambertus J: Skeletal and reticuloendothelial imaging in osteopetrosis: case report. J Nucl Med 18: 1091, 1977
11. Marks SC, Jr.: Congenital osteopetrotic mutations as probes of origin, structure, and function of osteoclasts. Clin Orthop 189: 239, 1984
12. Shapiro R, Glimcher MJ, Holtrop ME, et al: Human osteopetrosis, J Bone Joint Surg [Am] 62: 384, 1980
13. Coccia PF, Krivit W, Cervenka J, et al: Successful bone-marrow transplantation for infantile malignant osteopetrosis. N Engl J Med 302: 701, 1980
14. Fischer A, Griscelli C, Friedrich W, et al: Bone-marrow transplantation for immunodeficiencies and osteopetrosis: European survey, 1968–1985. Lancet 2: 1080, 1986
15. Ozsoyla S: High dose intravenous methylprednisolone in treatment of recessive osteopetrosis (letter). Arch Dis Child 62: 215, 1987
16. Key LL, Jr., Anast CS: Calcitriol for congenital osteopetrosis (letter). N Engl J Med 311: 55, 1984

17. Delmas PD, Chapuy MC, Viala JJ, Meunier PJ: Improvement of adult congenital osteopetrosis with high doses of calcitriol (abstract 93). J Bone Mineral Res 2: (Suppl. 1), 1987
18. Lehman RAW, Reeves JD, Wilson WB, Wesenberg RL: Neurological complications of infantile osteopetrosis. Ann Neurol 2: 378, 1977
19. Golbus MS, Loerper MA, Hall BD: Failure to diagnose osteopetrosis in utero (letter). Lancet 2: 1246, 1976
20. Sly WS, Hewett-Emmett D, Whyte MP, et al: Carbonic anhydrase II deficiency identified as the primary defect in the autosomal recessive syndrome of osteopetrosis with renal tubular acidosis and cerebral calcification. Proc Natl Acad Sci USA 80: 2752, 1983
21. Sly WS, Whyte MP, Sundaram V, et al: Carbonic anhydrase II deficiency in 12 families with the autosomal recessive syndrome of osteopetrosis with renal tubular acidosis and cerebral calcification. N Engl J Med 313: 139, 1985
22. Ohlsson A, Cumming WA, Paul A, Sly WS: Carbonic anhydrase II deficiency syndrome: recessive osteopetrosis with renal tubular acidosis and cerebral calcification. Pediatrics 77: 371, 1986
23. Whyte MP, Hamm LL III, Sly WS: Transfusion of carbonic anhydrase-replete erythrocytes fails to correct the acidification defect in the syndrome of osteopetrosis, renal tubular acidosis, and cerebral calcification (carbonic anhydrase II deficiency) J Bone Mineral Res (in press)
24. Whyte MP, Murphy WA, Fallon MD, et al: Osteopetrosis, renal tubular acidosis, and basal ganglia calcification in three sisters. Am J Med 69: 64, 1980
25. Elmore SM: Pycnodysostosis: a review. J Bone Joint Surg [Am] 49: 153, 1967
26. Wolpowitz A, Matisson A: A comparative study of pycnodysostosis, cleidocranial dysostosis, osteopetrosis and acro-osteolysis. S Afr Med J 48: 1011, 1974
27. Everts V, Aronson DC, Beertsen W: Phagocytosis of bone collagen by osteoclasts in two cases of pycnodysostosis. Calcif Tissue Int 37: 25, 1985
28. Stanescu R, Stanescu V, Maroteaux P: Ultrastructural abnormalities in chondrocytes in pycnodysostosis. Nouv Med 437: 247, 1975
29. Cabrejas ML, Fromm GA, Roca JF: Pycnodysostosis. Some aspects concerning kinetics of calcium metabolism and bone pathology. Am J Med Sci 271/2: 215, 1976
30. Wilson FC, Hundley JD: Progressive diaphyseal dysplasia: review of the literature and report of seven cases in one family. J Bone Joint Surg [Am] 55: 461, 1973
31. Smith R, Walton RJ, Corner BD, Gordon IRS: Clinical and biochemical studies in Engelmann's disease (progressive diaphyseal dysplasia). Q J Med 46: 273, 1977
32. Kumar B, Murphy WA, Whyte MP: Progressive diaphyseal dysplasia (Engelmann's disease): scintigraphic-radiologic-clinical correlations. Radiology 140: 87, 1981
33. Naveh Y, Alon U, Kaftori JK, Berant M: Progressive diaphyseal dysplasia: evaluation of corticosteroid therapy. Pediatrics 75: 321, 1985
34. Beighton P, Barnard A, Hamersma H, van der Wouden A: The syndromic status of sclerosteosis and van Buchem disease. Clin Genet 25: 175, 1984
35. Van Buchem FSP, Prick JJG, Jaspar HHJ: Hyperostosis Corticalis Generalisata Familiaris (Van Buchem's Disease). Exerpta Medica, Amsterdam, Excerpta, 1976
36. Eastman JR, Bixler D: Generalized cortical hyperostosis (Van Buchem disease): nosologic considerations. Radiology 125: 297, 1977
37. Beighton P, Durr L, Hamersma H: The clinical features of sclerosteosis: a review of the manifestations in twenty-five affected individuals. Ann Intern Med 84: 393, 1976

38. Beighton P, Cremin BJ, Hamersma H: The radiology of sclerosteosis. Br J Radiol 49: 934, 1976
39. Stein SA, Witkop C, Hill S, et al: Sclerosteosis: neurogenetic and pathophysiologic analysis of an American kinship. Neurology 33: 267, 1983
40. Whyte MP: Hypophosphatasia. In Sciver CR, Beaudet AL, Sly WS, Valle D (eds): The Metabolic Basis of Inherited Disease. 6th Ed. McGraw-Hill, New York, 1981
41. Whyte MP, Teitelbaum SL, Murphy WA, et al: Adult hypophosphatasia: clinical laboratory, and genetic investigation of a large kindred with review of the literature. Medicine (Baltimore) 58: 329, 1979
42. Whyte MP, Mahuren JD, Vrabel LA, Coburn SP: Markedly increased circulating pyridoxal-5′-phosphate levels in hypophosphatasia: alkaline phosphatase acts in vitamin B6 metabolism. J Clin Invest 76: 752, 1985
43. Kozlowski K, Sutcliffe J, Barylak A, et al: Hypophosphatasia: review of 24 cases. Pediat Radiol 5: 103, 1976
44. Fallon MD, Teitelbaum SL, Weinstein RS, et al: Hypophosphatasia: clinicopathologic comparison of the infantile, childhood, and adult forms. Medicine 63: 12, 1984
45. Ornoy A, Adomian GE, Rimoin DL: Histologic and ultrastructural studies on the mineralization process in hypophosphatasia. Am J Med Genet 22: 743, 1985
46. Whyte MP, Mahuren JD, Fedde KN, et al: Perinatal hypophosphatasia: tissue levels of vitamin B6 are unremarkable despite markedly increased circulating concentrations of pyridoxal-5′-phosphatase (evidence for an ectoenzyme role for tissue nonspecific alkaline phosphatase). J Clin Invest 81:1234, 1988
47. Whyte MP, Magill HL, Fallon MD, Herrod HG: Infantile hypophosphatasia: normalization of circulating bone alkaline phosphatase activity followed by skeletal remineralization (evidence for an intact structural gene for tissue nonspecific alkaline phosphatase). J Pediatr 108: 82, 1986
48. Coe JD, Murphy WA, Whyte MP: Management of femoral fractures and pseudofractures in adult hypophosphatasia. J Bone Joint Surg [Am] 68: 981, 1986
49. Kousseff BG, Mulivor RA: Prenatal diagnosis of hypophosphatasia. Obstet Gynecol 57: 6 (Supplement) 9S, 1981
50. Connor JM, Evans DAP: Fibrodysplasia ossificans progressiva: the clinical features and natural history of 34 patients. J Bone Joint Surg [Br] 64: 76, 1982
51. Rogers JG, Geho WB: Fibrodysplasia ossificans progressiva: a survey of forty-two cases. J Bone Joint Surg [Am] 61: 909, 1979
52. Lutwak L: Myositis ossificans progressiva: mineral, metabolic, and radioactive calcium studies of the effects of hormones. Am J Med 37: 269, 1964
53. Rogers JG, Chase GA: Paternal age effect in fibrodysplasia ossificans progressiva. J Med Genet 16: 147, 1979
54. Smith R, Russell RGG, Woods CG: Myositis ossificans progressiva: clinical features of eight patients and their response to treatment. J Bone Joint Surg [Br] 58: 48, 1976
55. Moore SE, Jump AA, Smiley JD: Effect of Warfarin sodium therapy on excretion of 4-carboxy-L-glutamic acid in scleroderma, dermatomyositis, and myositis ossificans progressiva. Arthritis Rheum 29: 344, 1986
56. Martins L, Biscaia J, daMota HC: Asymptomatic autosomal dominant hypoparathyroidism in six family members of a symptomatic infant (letter). J Pediatr 106: 167, 1985
57. Nolten WE, Chesney RW, Dabbagh S, et al: Moderate hypocalcemia due to nor-

mal serum 1,25-dihydroxyvitamin D levels in an asymptomatic kindred with familial hypoparathyroidism. Am J Med 82: 1157, 1987
58. Whyte MP, Weldon VV: Idiopathic hypoparathyroidism presenting with seizures during infancy: X-linked recessive inheritance in a large Missouri kindred. J Pediat 99: 608, 1981
59. Whyte MP, Kim GS, Kasmonovich M: Absence of parathyroid tissue in sex-linked recessive hypoparathyroidism. J Pediatr 109: 915, 1986
60. Niklasson E: Family early hypoparathyroidism associated with hypomagnesaemia. Acta Pediatr Scand 59: 715, 1970
61. Ahonen P: Autoimmune polyendocrinopathy-candidiasis-ectodermal dystrophy (APECED): autosomal recessive inheritance. Clin Genet 27: 535, 1985
62. Lee WK, Vargas A, Barnes J, Root AW: The Kenny-Caffey syndrome: growth retardation and hypocalcemia in a young boy. Am J Med Genet 14: 773, 1983
63. Fanconi S, Fischer JR, Wieland P, et al: Kenny syndrome: evidence for idiopathic hypoparathyroidism in two patients and for abnormal parathyroid hormone in one. J Pediatr 109: 469, 1986
64. Dahlberg PJ, Borer WZ, Newcomer KL, Yutuc WR: Autosomal or X-linked recessive syndrome of congenital lymphedema, hypoparathyroidism, nephropathy, prolapsing mitral valve, and brachytelephalangy. Am J Genet 16: 99, 1983
65. Yumita S, Furukawa Y, Sohn HE, et al: Familial idiopathic hypoparathyroidism and progressive sensorineural deafness. Tohoku J Exp Med 148: 135, 1986
66. Ahn TG, Antonarakis SE, Kronenberg HM, et al: Familial isolated hypoparathyroidism: a molecular genetic analysis of 8 families with 23 affected persons. Medicine 65: 73, 1986
67. Schmidtke J, Kruse K, Pape B, Sippell G: Exclusion of close linkage beween the parathyroid hormone gene and a mutant gene locus causing idiopathic hypoparathyroidism. J Med Genet 23: 217, 1986
68. Greenberg F, Valdes C, Rosenblatt HM, et al: Hypoparathyroidism and T cell immune defect in a patient with 10p deletion syndrome. J Pediatr 109: 469, 1986
69. Olambiwonma NO, Ebbin AJ, Frasier SD: Primary hypoparathyroidism associated with ring chromosome 18. J Pediatr 80: 833, 1972
70. Brandi ML, Aurbach GD, Fattorossi A, et al: Antibodies cytotoxic to bovine parathyroid cells in autoimmune hypoparathyroidism. Proc Natl Acad Sci USA 83: 8366, 1986
71. Rakel RE: Conn's Current Therapy 1987. WB Saunders, Philadelphia, 1987
72. Zeng, Q: Allotransplantation of parathyroid glands to treat intractable hypoparathyroidism. Surgery 99:131, 1986
73. Hollister DW: Molecular basis for osteogenesis imperfecta. Curr Probl Dermatol 17: 76, 1987
74. Sillence D: Osteogenesis imperfecta: an expanding panorama of variants. Clin Orthop 159: 11, 1981
75. Bateman JF, Chan D, Walder ID, et al: Lethal perinatal osteogenesis imperfecta due to substitution of arginine for glycine at residue 391 of the alpha 1 (1) chain of type I collagen. J Biol Chem 262: 7021, 1987
76. Wenstrup RJ, Tsipouras P, Byers PH: Osteogenesis imperfecta type IV. Biochemical confirmation of genetic linkage to the pro alpha 2 (1) gene of type I collagen. J Clin Invest 78: 1449, 1986
77. Bonaventure J, Cohen-Solal L, Lasselin C, et al: Abnormal procollagen synthesis in fibroblasts from three patients of the same family with a severe form of osteogenesis imperfecta (type III). Biochim Biophys Acta 889: 23, 1986

78. Wallis G, Beighton P, Boyd C, Mathew CG: Mutations linked to the pro alpha 2 (1) collagen gene are responsible for several cases of osteogenesis imperfecta type I. J Med Genet 23: 411, 1986
79. Pederson U, Charles P, Hansen HH, Elbrond O: Lack of effects of human calcitonin in osteogenesis imperfecta. Acta Orthop Scand 56: 260, 1985
80. Ryoppy S, Alberty A, Kaitila I: Early semiclosed intramedullary stabilization in osteogenesis imperfecta. J Pediatr Orthop 7: 139, 1987
81. Merz E, Goldhofer W: Sonographic diagnosis of lethal osteogenesis imperfecta in the second trimester: case report and review. JCU 14: 380, 1986
82. Tsipouras P, Schwartz RC, Goldberg JD, et al: Prenatal prediction of osteogenesis imperfecta (OI type IV): exclusion of inheritance using a collagen gene probe. J Med Genet 24: 406, 1987
83. Carothers AD, McAllion SJ, Paterson CR: Risk of dominant mutation in older fathers: evidence from osteogenesis imperfecta. J Med Genet 23: 227, 1986
84. Law WM Jr., Heath H III: Familial benign hypercalcemia (hypocalciuric hypercalcemia): clinical and pathogenetic studies in 21 families. Ann Intern Med 102: 511-519, 1985
85. Marx SJ, Attie MF, Levine MA, et al: The hypocalcuiric or benign variant of familial hypercalcemia: clinical and biochemical features in fifteen kindreds. Medicine (Baltimore) 60: 397, 1981
86. Marx SJ, Spiegel AM, Levine MA, et al: Familial hypocalciuric hypercalcemia. The relation to primary parathyroid hyperplasia. N Engl J Med 307: 416, 1982
87. Marx SJ, Fraser D, Rapoport A: Familial hypocalciuric/hypercalcemia: mild expression of the gene in heterozygotes and severe expression in homozygotes. Am J Med 78: 15, 1985
88. Law WM, James EM, Charboneau JW, et al: High-resolution parathyroid ultrasonography in familial benign hypercalcemia (familial hypocalciuric hypercalcemia). Mayo Clin Prox 59: 153, 1984
89. Thorgeirsson U, Costa J, Marx SJ: The parathyroid glands in familial hypocalciuric hypercalcemia. Human Pathol 12: 229, 1981
90. Law WM, Carney JA, Heath H: Parathyroid glands in familial benign hypercalcemia (familial hypocalciuric hypercalcemia). Am J Med 76: 1021, 1984
91. Alexandre C, Chappard D, Riffat G: Bone histomorphometric analysis in familial hypocalciuric hypercalcemia. J Clin Pathol 36: 1319, 1983
92. Law WM, Jr., Wahner HW, Heath H III: Bone mineral density and skeletal fractures in familial benign hypercalcemia (hypocalciuric hypercalcemia). Mayo Clin Proc 59: 811, 1984
93. Law WM, Jr., Bollman S, Kumar R, Heath H III: Vitamin D metabolism in familial benign hypercalcemia (hypocalciuric hypercalcemia) differs from that in primary hyperparathyroidism. J Clin Endocrinol Metabol 58: 744, 1984
94. Attie MF, Gill JR, Stock JL, et al: Urinary calcium excretion in familial hypocalciuric hypercalcemia. Persistence of relative hypocalciuria after induction of hypoparathyroidism. J Clin Invest 72: 667, 1983
95. Wantanabe H, Sutton RAL: Renal calcium handling in familial hypocalciuric hypercalcemia. Kidney Int 24: 353, 1983
96. Christensson T: Familial hyperparathyroidism. Ann Intern Med 85: 614, 1976
97. Law WM, Jr., Hodgson SF, Heath H III: Autosomal recessive inheritance of familial hyperparathyroidism. N Engl J Med 309: 650, 1983
98. Brandi ML, Aurbach GD, Fitzpatrick LA, et al: Parathyroid mitogenic activity in

plasma from patients with familial multiple endocrine neoplasia type I. N Engl J Med 314: 1287, 1986

99. Babu VR, Jackson CE, Van Dyke DL: Chromosome 20 deletion in multiple endocrine neoplasia syndrome types 2A and 2B (abstract). Clin Res 30: 489A, 1982
100. Friedman M, Hatcher G, Watson L: Primary hypomagnesaemia with secondary hypocalcemia in an infant. Lancet 1: 703, 1967
101. Skyberg D, Stromme JH, Normann T, et al: Selective malabsorption of magnesium. An inborn error of metabolism. In Allan JD, et al (eds): Enzymopenic Anemias, Lysosomes, and Other Papers. Proceedings 6th Symposium of The Society for Study of Inborn Errors of Metabolism. E.A. Livingstone, Edinburgh and London, 1969
102. Teebi AS: Primary hypomagnesemia, an x-borne allele? Lancet I: 701, 1983
103. Geven WB, Monnens LA, Willems HL, et al: Renal magnesium wasting in two families with autosomal dominant inheritance. Kidney Int 31: 1140, 1987
104. Baldursson H, Evans EB, Dodge WF, Jackson WT: Tumoral calcinosis with hyperphosphatemia. A report of a family with incidence in four siblings. J Bone Joint Surg [Br] 51: 913, 1969
105. Lyles KW, Burkes EJ, Ellis GJ, et al: Genetic transmission of tumoral calcinosis: autosomal dominant with variable clinical expressivity. J Clin Endocrinol Metab 60: 1093, 1985
106. Steinherz R, Chesney RW, Eisenstein B, et al: Elevated serum calcitriol concentrations do not fall in response to hyperphosphatemia in familial tumoral calcinosis. Am J Dis Child 139: 816, 1985
107. Mozaffarian G, Lafferty FW, Pearson OH: Treatment of tumoral calcinosis with phosphorus deprivation. Ann Intern Med 77: 741, 1972
108. Mehes K, Szelid Z: Autosomal dominant inheritance of hypercalciuria. Eur J Pediatr 133: 239, 1980
109. Tieder M, Modai D, Samuel R, et al: Hereditary hypophosphatemic rickets with hypercalciuria. N Engl J Med 312: 611, 1985
110. Scriver CR, Reade T, Halal F, et al: Autosomal hypophosphatemic bone disease responds to 1,25-$(OH)_2D_3$. Arch Dis Child 56: 203, 1981
111. Fotino M, Haymovits A, Falk CT: Evidence for linkage between HLA and Paget's disease. Transplant Proc 9: 1867, 1977
112. Whyte MP, Fallon MD, Perry HM III, et al: Osteolytic Paget bone disease, osteopenia, and otosclerosis in four generations (in manuscript).
113. Beighton P: Inherited Disorders of the Skeleton. Churchill Livingstone, Edinburgh, 1978

Index

Page numbers followed by f denote figures; those followed by t denote tables.